Homeland Maternity

FEMINIST MEDIA STUDIES

Edited by Carol Stabile

A list of books in the series appears at the end of this book.

Homeland Maternity

US Security Culture and the New Reproductive Regime

NATALIE FIXMER-ORAIZ

UNIVERSITY OF ILLINOIS PRESS
Urbana, Chicago, and Springfield

1 2 3 4 5 C P 5 4 3 2 1
∞ This book is printed on acid-free paper.

Library of Congress Control Number: 2018057607

ISBN 9780252042355 (hardcover)
ISBN 9780252084140 (paperback)

Publication of this book was supported by funding from University of Iowa's Office of the Vice President for Research and Economic Development.

Contents

Preface

"Your body is a battleground." For the three years I worked as a community organizer for Planned Parenthood in the US South, the iconic art of Barbara Kruger—visually arresting in its split symmetry and color contrast across a woman's steady gaze—greeted me every morning as I opened my laptop. It felt real. I was in my early twenties, funneling my deepest rage and passion into statewide organizing for the 2004 March for Women's Lives against a steady stream of assaults on reproductive rights and dignity.

It is fair to say that this book began then. It has traveled with me, too—deepening alongside shifts in my career, spanning two pregnancies, the journey into parenthood, and vexed negotiations of reproductive technologies in the context of queer family formation. It is fueled by the endless urgency of queer, feminist, and antiracist struggle that eventually propelled my return to academic research and teaching, in search of answers that might help build a better world, beginning with our collective capacity to imagine and speak its possibility.

Much has changed for the worse. We face stunning hostility to sexual and reproductive self-determination, some of it painful in its familiarity and some the likes of which we haven't seen since the Comstock Era. In 2018, two of the three federal branches of US government are controlled by vocal opponents of reproductive, social, and economic justice. Mike Pence governed one of the most dangerous states in the nation for those pregnant and parenting before taking up residence in the Naval Observatory. And attacks on health care continue unabashed and unabated at the state level, with 431 anti-choice bills proposed in the first three months of 2017 alone.

Nevertheless, we persist. I am buoyed by the historic 2017 Women's March, in which an estimated 3.5 to 4.5 million people in the United States—roughly one in a hundred—took to the streets on the day following Donald Trump's inauguration, in solidarity with 250,000+ marchers worldwide. I am inspired by grassroots activists and organizations that insist on maternal dignity and reproductive justice in novel and affirming ways—for example, in the Mama's Bail Out Day campaign launched in 2017 by Southerners on New Ground, Color of Change, Black Lives Matter, and other allied organizations. I celebrate the growing number of bills proposed in state assemblies that aim to enhance reproductive health and dignity, even as the number of anti-choice bills continues to outpace them. And I admit a small, quiet solace in returning to the history of radical struggle for reproductive justice in my research, knowing that our work here and now travels farther and faster in its wake.

Much of this book was written before the Trump administration, and I imagine that the struggles detailed here will endure long after this particular nightmare ends. It is written in the spirit of resistance and resilience, that we might understand how our communicative habits shape—or distort—the possibilities of justice, and that we might find ways to bend those habits toward a vision of reproductive justice that includes us all.

Acknowledgments

I open with gratitude to the fierce advocates for reproductive justice then and now, including those I have had the privilege of working alongside: Janet Colm, Paige Johnson, Gwendolyn Neumeister, Mitchell Price, Misty Rebik, and Jamie Brooks Robertson especially. I am also grateful to my activist families and communities, including the Cuntry Kings, the Queer Yoga Collective, Likhaan, and Born After Roe, for building community, for creating art and beauty and things worth fighting for, and for struggling tirelessly on behalf of a better world.

To my stellar editor at the University of Illinois Press, Dawn Durante: enthusiastic thanks for the unparalleled clarity, expertise, and excitement you brought to this project. I am also deeply appreciative of Deborah Oliver's astute copyedits and the invaluable feedback provided by my anonymous reviewers that enhanced this project in countless ways.

Considerable financial and institutional support made this book possible. The University of Iowa provided me with pre-tenure leave, fellowship opportunities, and funding through the Digital Humanities Initiative and the Office of the Vice President for Research and Economic Development. The Organization for Research on Women and Communication funded research-related travel expenses, and the American Association of University Women generously supported my final year of dissertating, lending me the extraordinary freedom to write from abroad. I also remain deeply indebted to the University of North Carolina at Chapel Hill and its Department of Communication Studies for investing in me early on through the Caroline H. and Thomas S. Royster Fellowship.

Thanks to mentors and peers at Indiana University who nurtured my earliest intellectual curiosities, especially Bob Ivie, John Lucaites, Robert Terrill, and Sam McCormick. Faculty in the Department of Communication Studies at UNC–Chapel Hill have remained central to my professional and intellectual development, and I am particularly grateful to Bill Balthrop, Carole Blair, Ken Hillis, Jordynn Jack, Chris Lundberg, and Sarah Sharma. The unparalleled genius and generosity of two esteemed faculty members from this department continues to shape my life in immeasurable ways. To Robbie Cox, my PhD advisor, infinite thanks for your steady guidance, constructive criticism, intellectual and interpersonal generosity, and unwavering belief in me. To Julia Wood, my heartfelt gratitude for the infinite ways you have encouraged and made possible this journey—for your edgy and steadfast sisterhood, incisive feedback and sage advice, as well as the extraordinary time and care you have invested in my growth as a scholar and human being.

Brilliant peers make graduate studies possible and pleasurable, especially when you find yourself working alongside Katy Bodey, J. Nikol Jackson-Beckham, Elizabeth Nelson, Julia Scatliff O'Grady, David Supp-Montgomerie, Jenna Supp-Montgomerie, Freya Thimsen, Stace Treat, and Grover Wehman-Brown. A special shout-out to two senior peers from UNC-CH: Phaedra Pezzullo for offering her wisdom and wit at key turning points in my career, and Billie Murray, cherished friend, collaborator, and coconspirator.

I cannot imagine a better academic home than the one I have found at the University of Iowa. Utmost gratitude to my colleagues in the Departments of Communication Studies and Gender, Women's, and Sexuality Studies for pairing rigorous intellectual community with deep generosity and respect. Special thanks to my senior colleagues—especially Tim Havens, David Hingstman, Jiyeon Kang, Rachel McLaren, Kembrew McLeod, John Durham Peters, Darrel Wanzer-Serrano, Gigi Durham, Ellen Lewin, Leslie Schwalm, and Rachel Williams—for your mentoring, friendship, and making the mountain seem doable. The Friday writing party and CSA crew added levity and a healthy dose of irreverence to life on the tenure track—many thanks to E Cram, Andy High, Mary High, Jiyeon Kang, David Supp-Montgomerie, and Jenna Supp-Montgomerie for this. And to Leslie Baxter, Jeff Bennett, and Isaac West, thank you for your early guidance in navigating faculty life and for your enduring friendship and support.

The students at the University of Iowa are phenomenal. Thanks to those in my seminars and classrooms who spurred my thinking with their questions and insights, and especially to my doctoral advisees who also offered invaluable aid at different stages in this project. Heather Roy and Meg Tully provided thorough and timely research assistance, and Michelle Colpean was the most spectacular teaching assistant imaginable during a writing-intensive semester. Our department staff makes the daily grind of institutional life manageable; thanks to Jacquie Albrecht, Mike Hendrickson, Andrea Krekel, Kyle Marxen, Hope Miller, Sarah Moeller, Wanda Osborne, and Jenny Ritchie for their expertise.

Countless academic conversations, conferences, and opportunities have shaped the best in this book. I am grateful to the editors and anonymous reviewers who helped to refine my analysis and published portions of this manuscript in other outlets: Sara Hayden and Lynn O'Brien Hallstein, Joan Faber McAlister, and Kent Ono. To my writing comrades—Peter Campbell, Vincent Pham, and Alyssa Samek—thank you for engaging every corner of this project with boundless insight and care, sometimes at a moment's notice. The theoretical framework for the book was profoundly enriched in a POROI (Project on the Rhetoric of Inquiry) workshop, especially with feedback from Jeff Bennett, Frank Durham, Naomi Greyser, and Deborah Whaley. Shelly Gulati has provided a reliable sounding board from the earliest years of junior faculty life. And I am fortunate to find myself in a field of brilliance, with growing networks of folks who inspire—in addition to those already named, Bonnie Dow, Karma Chávez, and Sara McKinnon deserve a special shout-out.

An early version of chapter 2 appears in "(In)Conceivable: Risky Reproduction and the Rhetorical Labors of 'Octomom,'" *Communication and Critical/Cultural Studies* 11, no. 3 (2014): 231–49, and brief excerpts from the introduction and first chapter are informed by my short forum essay, "Contemplating Homeland Maternity," *Women's Studies in Communication* 38, no. 2 (2015): 129–34. A previous version of the analysis presented in chapter 3 is available in "No Exception Post-Prevention: 'Differential' Biopolitics on the Morning After," in *Contemplating Maternity in the Era of Choice: Explorations into the Discourses of Reproduction*, edited by Sara Hayden and Lynn O'Brien Hallstein (Blue Ridge Summit, PA: Lexington Books), 27–48.

My family never falters in their belief in me, even when I do. I cherish the steadfast presence of my parents, Tim and Carson—from their big, embracing love to their willingness to help juggle the not-so-small minutiae of daily life, including impromptu childcare, house projects, family meals, and so much more. My mom especially excels at showing up when I need her the most—and as my first editor (a thankless job indeed when providing feedback to an adolescent), she shaped my earliest writing impulses. My siblings, Lindsay and Dylan, are passionate, principled, and downright hilarious—and they are two of the best built-in friends one could ask for. Over thirteen years ago, I lucked into the open arms of an extraordinary family-in-law—much love and gratitude to Michele, Teri, Rich, Charlie, John, Val, Vangie, Chuck, Jason, Gilda, Jeff, and Lesli. And I am no less fortunate in community kin. I am so thankful for the longstanding camaraderie of Jamie Brooks Robertson, Emily Hamer Hunt, and Luke Stepleton. Sarina Martini, Kimberly Hendricks, and Monica Basile offered exceptional compassion and expertise in my transition to motherhood; Gwendolyn Neumeister, Erin Helm, Maddie Hinrichs, and Marty Milder are the extraordinary humans who provided love and care for my children in many of the hours I devoted to this book, and I am profoundly grateful for their ongoing presence in our lives. And from Bingham to Becker and beyond, I feel outrageously lucky to reside in the orbit of David Supp-Montgomerie and Jenna Supp-Montgomerie. To Jenna in particular, my heartfelt gratitude for a string of pivotal conversations over coffee, your unbridled support and awesome solidarity. If family is a metaphor and model for collective life, then all of you are living proof that a better world—a *much* better world—is possible indeed.

I close with profound gratitude to my partner, Vanessa, and with a dedication to the two extraordinary young people who have most recently made their way into our world. To Emmons and Celso, this is for you. And to Vanessa, thank you for being a steady compass, for bearing countless caffeinated nights, for talking rhetoric and reproductive justice with more sincerity, enthusiasm, and regularity than one could ever reasonably ask of another human being. Thank you for nourishing my spirit with your creative genius, impulse for adventure, mad culinary skills, and enduring love. Thank you for dreaming and believing and sharing the journey. The gift of you makes all things possible.

Homeland Maternity

Introduction

Homeland Maternity, the New Reproductive Regime

In 2014, Tamara Loertscher was charged by the State of Wisconsin with posing a "substantial risk" to her fourteen-week fetus.[1] Unemployed and unable to afford her thyroid medication, the twenty-nine-year-old former nursing aide eventually sought care for hypothyroidism and depression when she suspected she was pregnant. Providing a full account of her medical history to her doctor, Loertscher disclosed that she had self-medicated for her condition with methamphetamine and marijuana prior to discovering her pregnancy. She expressed her strong desire to have a healthy pregnancy and baby, and was voluntarily admitted to the hospital's unit for behavioral health. During her brief stay, a social worker reported Loertscher to county officials for illicit drug use in violation of the state's Unborn Child Protection Act.[2] Subsequently held at the hospital against her will and denied legal counsel, Loertscher arrived at an initial hearing to discover that the state had appointed an attorney to represent her fetus. The court ordered Loertscher to be placed in an inpatient drug treatment facility indefinitely. When she refused to comply, Loertscher was incarcerated in a county jail for eighteen days. In state custody she was denied prenatal care, threatened with a Taser, and placed in solitary confinement for thirty-six hours for refusing a pregnancy test.[3] Her eventual release was predicated on, among other things, regular drug tests at Loertscher's expense—all of which were negative. The state of Wisconsin considers her a child abuser, which bars employment in her field of nursing and prevents her from volunteering someday in her child's school.[4]

Several weeks prior to giving birth to a healthy baby in early 2015, Loertscher filed a lawsuit against the State of Wisconsin, initiating a legal battle that is winding through the federal courts as this book goes to press.[5]

Wisconsin is not anomalous but rather at the forefront of a disturbing trend. Loertscher joins Rinat Dray, Marlise Muñoz, Purvi Patel, and countless other women across the country recently deprived of fundamental human rights in the name of fetal health and protection. As the concept of "risk" is used to position women against fetuses, women have been arrested and detained for refusing a Caesarean, attempting a home birth, falling down a flight of stairs, disclosing addiction, and attempting suicide.[6] State actions against pregnant women—including incarceration, involuntary commitment, and forced medical interventions—are on the rise in the United States and are disproportionately imposed on low-income women, immigrant women, and women of color.[7] While a district court decided in Loertscher's favor, the state appealed the decision and in July 2017 the US Supreme Court weighed in briefly to stay an injunction—in short, permitting the State of Wisconsin to continue to prosecute pregnant women like Loertscher under its Unborn Child Protection Act.[8] Loertscher's story points to a frightening pattern of state intervention that compels women to eliminate all manner of prenatal risk, inflicting severe punishment—and, ironically, new risks—when they falter in the impossible task of ensuring a perfect uterine environment for their pregnancies.

At the same time that pregnant women are increasingly criminalized, the requirements of motherhood are intensified. In 2016, former Homeland Security advisor and mother of three Juliette Kayyem issued a clarion call to US mothers in *Security Mom: An Unclassified Guide to Protecting Our Homeland and Your Home*. Urging mothers to embrace the passé moniker with a new twist, Kayyem asserts that a "'security mom' can and should mean a woman who plans and prepares as she raises her children in a world where anything can happen." Her inspiration came by way of an e-mail from a cousin who, in soliciting advice on precautionary parenting in a post-9/11 world, "clarified what [Kayyem] had always suspected—there is something missing from our nation's security efforts." The glaring omission, for Kayyem, was the fundamental connection between the homeland and the home: "The safety of our nation is dependent on skills that we [mothers] already practice to keep ourselves and our children safer at home, in our communities. And those of us who work in homeland security failed to disclose this one basic fact: You are a security expert, too."[9] Blending memoir and self-help, Kayyem urges a rethinking of homeland security, in which the security of the state was articulated to quotidian maternal sensibilities. Her book is described as "smart, manageable guidelines for keeping your family safe in an unpredictable world. From stocking up on coloring books to stashing duplicate copies of valuable papers out of state, Juliette's wisdom does more than just prepare us to survive in an age of mayhem—it empowers us to thrive."[10] In *Security Mom*, mothering is of explicit value to domestic affairs—central, in fact, to the security of the nation itself.

The criminalization of Loertscher and Kayyem's call to rethink motherhood and security are not unrelated. Consider the following parallels. First, in each instance, pregnant and parenting women are made relentlessly responsible for circumstances beyond their control. Loertscher is part of a startling trend in which the state punishes women for failure to eliminate prenatal risk; Kayyem's manifesto renders maternal vigilance central to the safety of children—and entire communities—in a world fraught with insecurities. Second, motherhood subsumes the claim to personhood as any concept of individual human rights is made ancillary to those of the fetus or child. Despite Loertscher's clear and urgent need for health care services, the State of Wisconsin positioned her as a threat to her unborn child and supplied criminal interrogation, arrest, and detention instead. According to Kayyem, being a security mom is an all-consuming endeavor, exacting exceptional diligence, labor, and wholesale devotion to family. Finally, in each instance pregnancy and motherhood are intimately entwined with the nation, its recent investments and dominant logics. Both stories turn on discursive features (e.g., "risk" and "security") of homeland security culture—a term that I use to signal both an early twenty-first-century state formation as well as a felt exigence in a post-9/11 United States that has filtered into routine ways of relating to one another and to the world. Loertscher's story signals the intense, if also unevenly distributed, policing of pregnancy by the state under the banner of fetal risk; Kayyem's book recasts motherhood—and presumably wealthy, white, heteronuclear motherhood—explicitly in the service of national goals and desires. Thus, each of these stories is differently, but also profoundly, shaped by what I refer to as *homeland maternity*. I designate this term in order to theorize a significant force within US reproductive regimes of the early twenty-first century—namely, the relationship between motherhood and nation within homeland security culture.

In naming homeland maternity, I argue that motherhood and nation are deeply enmeshed and mutually constitutive. Each of the chapters that follow centers a site of analysis wherein discursive alignments of motherhood and nation are present and persistent—a site where homeland security culture shapes reproductive politics just as motherhood and reproduction are imagined to bolster the project of building and securing the nation. Homeland maternity, thus, joins two bodies of literature: feminist studies of maternal and reproductive politics and critical scholarship on homeland security culture. Regarding the former, homeland maternity extends existing feminist scholarship on the politics of motherhood and reproduction. Grounding recent public struggles within a broader cultural terrain, the concept of homeland maternity clarifies connections between national security and the strict regulation of sexuality, reproduction, and family formation in the early twenty-first century. Homeland maternity specifies how *national security is tethered to securing the domestic and reproductive body*. The recent history of reproductive politics is deeply inflected by the dominant discourses of homeland security culture—from public debates over the availability of birth control and the uptick in crisis pregnancy centers to the privileging of fetal personhood and subsequent deprivations of pregnant individuals' rights and liberties. Critically tending to these discourses—to related rhetorics of security, risk, emergency, and crisis—*Homeland Maternity: US Security Culture and the New Reproductive Regime* traces how homeland security culture shapes the tumultuous terrain of contemporary reproductive politics, with an eye toward the possibilities of reproductive justice.

This book also specifies a new arena of attention for scholarship dedicated to mapping the form and function of homeland security culture across a range of public policies, practices, and politics.[11] Historically speaking, the project of securing the nation has long exceeded explicit political efforts and investments, such as foreign diplomacy, immigration policy, and the use of military force. The project of security enlists domesticity as requisite to the future of the nation, which has often meant governing reproduction through the differential surveillance and control of women's bodies and behaviors.[12] Thus, the cultural alignment of motherhood and nation is evident at several key historical moments in the United States from the colonial era to postwar containment culture and into the present.[13] Homeland maternity stands as the most recent iteration of this persistent trend, reviving familiar tropes and normativities as it accommodates postfeminist ideologies, deepening neoliberalism, and the surveillance state.

Naming homeland maternity provides a critical point of departure for intervening in the conditions that fuel contemporary forms of reproductive injustice. Homeland maternity draws attention to motherhood and reproduction as thoroughly implicated in homeland security culture and, reciprocally, clarifies how the logic of homeland security culture shapes contemporary US reproductive politics. Homeland maternity provides a vocabulary through which we might better understand how, why, and under what circumstances pregnancy is figured as patriotic—whether in fertility campaigns aimed at young professional women or in the high-profile celebration of US military wives serving as commercial surrogates for infertile couples at home and abroad.[14] Homeland maternity includes, for example, the quiet colonization of comprehensive reproductive health clinics by crisis pregnancy centers, the revival of traditional beliefs about gender and motherhood that "take feminism into account,"[15] and the elevated status of the fetus that renders pregnant women vulnerable to forced interventions, arrests, and detention. It signals a context in which the concept of fetal personhood regularly eclipses claims to reproductive or maternal rights, in which pregnancy itself is increasingly medicalized and managed by experts, a culture in which risk in any form—but particularly that related to the future of the nation and its citizenry—is to be avoided at all costs. In short, this book is an attempt to account for the recent history of US reproductive politics—stubbornly inflected by, but also active in shaping, collective life in post-9/11 homeland security culture.

I begin with a history, detailing motherhood and nation as deeply enmeshed and mutually constitutive, in order to understand homeland maternity more thoroughly in light of its antecedents. Then, drawing the past into the present, I turn to theorizing homeland security culture itself as a primary context for more recent reproductive and maternal politics. My concluding remarks center critical frameworks and offer an outline of chapters.

Histories of Motherhood and Nation

Alignments between motherhood and nation are not new. Reproduction has long been a site for negotiating cultural anxieties, most often at the expense of women. As historian Rickie Solinger reminds us, "Official discussions about reproductive politics have rarely been women-centered. More often than not, debate and discussion about reproductive politics—*where the power to manage women's reproductive capacity should reside*—have been part of discussions about *how to solve certain large social problems facing the country*" (original emphasis).[16] A wealth of feminist scholarship has documented the relationship between pregnancy and power in US history; some of this scholarship highlights the centrality of reproductive politics to nation, particularly in moments of national crisis and heightened patriotism. Tracing a genealogy of relationships between motherhood and nation allows me to ground homeland maternity within relevant histories of gender, race, coloniality, national identity, and belonging. Stories like those of Loertscher and Kayyem thus become legible—less anomalous than synecdochic, symptoms of long-standing patterns of cultural practice and belief.

Reproduction, Motherhood, and Racializing the Nation

The strict regulation of reproduction proved central to early state formation and colonialism, codifying white supremacy at the founding of the new US republic. Early laws legitimized white, propertied forms of intimacy—for example, banning interracial marriage between white women and black men as early as the seventeenth century and prohibiting slaves from marrying altogether. For wealthy white women, motherhood was imagined as the primary vehicle for patriotism, citizenship, and civic virtue. In her germinal study of republican motherhood, historian Linda K. Kerber explores the historical persistence of motherhood as the primary justification for women's political participation, noting its roots in the late eighteenth century: "In the years of the early Republic a consensus developed around the idea that a mother, committed to the service of her family and to the state, might serve a political purpose . . . through the raising of a patriotic child."[17] Drawing on popular ideologies, including the "cult of true womanhood,"[18] the white, upper-class family was figured as central to nurturing the nation, and white women of means were urged to birth sons who would inherit the fledgling republic. In other words, rather than participate directly in democracy, wealthy white women of the Revolutionary era were to perform citizenship through domesticity. Although the rearing of wealthy white children typically exploited the labor of enslaved black women as primary-care providers, white women were nonetheless constituted as the bearers of moral guidance and virtue, rendered responsible for cultivating their sons' investments in civic participation and state leadership. This understanding of republican motherhood lends nuance and specificity to one dimension of a multifaceted historical phenomenon—that is, the negotiation and management of women's reproductive and childrearing capacities as a national resource.

Republican motherhood stands in stark contrast to the maternal histories of indigenous women, black women, and poor white women in conditions of servitude in the United States.[19] Systemic reproductive abuses of women are similarly embedded within the project of nation building, inextricably tied to broader systems of racial domination and the colonization of the Americas. In the context of US slavery, for example, while republican motherhood was marshaled to establish white wealth across generations, enslaved women were denied legal recognition as mothers, their children born into bondage and designated by law as a slaveholder's property. Early colonial laws established the legal status of a child, either bonded or free, as contingent on the status of the mother. Thus, biracial children born to enslaved women became the property of the slaveholder; biracial children born to white women contributed to a growing population of free people of color, thus fueling the establishment of antimiscegenation laws and strict enforcement of white women's fidelity within marriage.[20] Relatedly, propertied white men's rape of black and indigenous women was essential to perpetuating slavery and reinforcing white supremacy, as historian Rickie Solinger notes: "the reproductive capacity of enslaved and native women was the resource whites relied on to produce an enslaved labor force, to produce and transmit property and wealth across generations, to consolidate white control over land in North America, and to produce a class of human beings who, in their ineligibility for citizenship, underwrote the exclusivity and value of white citizenship."[21] Denying legal recognition of motherhood or kinship codified slaves as property without claim to family, ancestry, or national belonging.[22] Women resisted by refusing compliance—fighting off rape, committing to partners of their choosing, creating extended networks of kin, shielding enslaved children from white slaveholders' brutalities, providing forbidden forms of care under the cloak of night, and attempting self-induced abortions. Even so, this violent occupation of women's bodies and reproduction under slavery was a key component in racializing the nation.[23]

The use of reproductive and sexual violence as weapons of racial domination characterizes a broad pattern of reproductive injustice in the United States. Documenting myriad brutalities inflicted on indigenous populations, Andrea Smith demonstrates how the colonization of the Americas relied on violent assertions of white patriarchal control. Early narratives detailing the gruesome rape and dismemberment of Native women are woven throughout European settlers' records of war against indigenous peoples, attesting to the centrality of sexual violence to colonization and genocide.[24] In another example, beginning in the mid-nineteenth century, Native boarding schools were established in communities across the United States in order to, in the words of Carlisle Indian School founder Richard Pratt, "kill the Indian and save the man."[25] Boarding schools destroyed Native communities and cultures. Over a hundred thousand indigenous children were removed from their families—they were forced to speak English, trained for menial labor based on strict gender binaries, and subject to horrific physical and sexual abuse by pro-assimilationist missionaries.[26] These and other more recent examples, from sterilization abuse to medical experimentation, demonstrate how attacks on Native women's bodies and efforts to exert control over Native reproduction and family formation persist as powerful weapons of white supremacy, patriarchy, and genocide.[27]

Immigration is another key site for policing the borders and bodies of national belonging. From the Alien and Sedition Acts of the late eighteenth century through the Trump administration's attempts to ban travel and migration from

Muslim-majority nations, culturally legible claims to US entry and citizenship have long been shaped by the perceived threat of the political, ethnic, and religious Other; these fears have been negotiated in part through the strict regulation of immigrant women's bodies and behaviors.[28] Historically, US immigration policies have privileged "selective" immigration and family reunification, targeting for exclusion those imagined as threatening to white, hetero-patriarchal norms. For example, early selective immigration laws barred most immigration from Asian nations but specifically targeted Asian women, curtailing the possibility of family formation for Asian men who were subject to antimiscegenation laws, and providing a precedent for early twentieth-century policies that excluded all Asian immigration with the exception of Filipinos, who were then under US rule.[29] In concert with nativist panics regarding "race suicide" and declining white birth rates in the late nineteenth century, pregnant immigrant women faced increasing barriers to entry and family reunification laws were unevenly applied to preclude immigrants of color from citizenship while working to codify European families as "white" and to affirm "white families . . . [as] desirable and consonant with the interests in the nation."[30]

Restrictive immigration policies and practices were intensified in the early twentieth century, fueled by isolationist cultural sentiment and increasing support for eugenics and scientific racism. Post–World War I restrictions included literacy tests and quotas; as a result, over 85 percent of immigration was effectively designated for Northern and Western Europeans.[31] For immigrant women allowed entry or conditional entry to the United States, sexuality was tightly regulated in accordance with heteronormative domesticity. Lesbians were refused at the border; immigration authorities rigorously inspected the homes where single women were to reside, conducted marriages for engaged women on the dock prior to entry, and frequently deported poor immigrant women on the grounds of pregnancy.[32] In short, the strict exclusion of pregnant women, lesbians, and immigrant women of color, in combination with antimiscegenation laws, inhibited family formation outside of dominant, white heteronuclear norms. In this way, immigration policies and practices reveal clear historical investments in regulating sexuality, reproduction, and family formation as central to the project of nation building.

As these histories demonstrate, the concept of nation has, since its inception, relied on regulating maternal and reproductive labor. It is a pattern traceable into and throughout the twentieth century. For example, while the early birth control movement argued on behalf of voluntary motherhood and originated within radical activisms of the Progressive Era, these alliances were quickly dissolved as birth control campaigns found mainstream support and expression in eugenics.[33] In this collaboration, Angela Davis explains, the birth control movement was "robbed of its progressive potential, advocating for people of color not the individual right to *birth control*, but rather the racist strategy of *population control*" (original emphasis).[34] State-funded family planning programs as early as the 1930s targeted low-wealth communities and communities of color, who otherwise struggled for access to quality health care and public services. These government programs made birth control readily available and actively promoted its use.[35] Similarly, in the postwar era, "overpopulation" roused significant panic and debate. While situated squarely in the midst of the US "baby boom," public concern did not center on the domestic demographic experiencing the sharpest increase in birth rates—white middle-class women.[36] Instead, public anxieties focused on the birth rates of women of color and low-wealth women, both in the United States and the Global South. These anxieties coincided with a loosening of US immigration restrictions designed to curry international favor during the Cold War, as well as hard-won expansions of welfare provisions that enabled low-wage workers to leave exploitative conditions and afforded greater access to state services.[37] No longer a cheap source of labor, low-wealth communities, immigrant communities, and communities of color were soon considered "surplus" and targeted for state population control policies, including federally funded sterilization.[38]

The history of sterilization in the mid- to late-twentieth century clarifies the differential politics of motherhood and reproduction in no uncertain terms. At its height in the 1970s, sterilization was the fastest growing birth control method in the country. But while white women of means had difficulty locating a doctor willing to perform this procedure and were often required to obtain their husbands' consent, other women were particularly vulnerable to sterilization abuse—specifically, black, Puerto Rican, and indigenous women, as well as women on welfare, who were threatened with refusal of services if they did not consent.[39] A 1973 lawsuit revealed the extent of sterilization abuse in the US South, where an estimated 100,000 to 150,000 low-wealth women, almost half of them African American, were sterilized annually under federal programs. Sterilization abuse frequently occurred as women sought routine medical attention and were subsequently sterilized by the attending physician without warning or consent, a practice so widespread that it was commonly referred to as a "Mississippi appendectomy."[40] Sterilization abuse was not limited to marginalized communities in the US South, however. By 1968, over one third of women of reproductive age in Puerto Rico were sterilized through an aggressive campaign waged by private agencies and the US and Puerto Rican governments; another federally funded campaign in the 1970s sterilized over a quarter of Native American women, and in some cases eliminated entire tribes.[41] In short, the reproductive abuse of women and communities of color has long been central in maintaining white supremacy in global and domestic settings.

The postwar experiences and expectations of middle-class white women were markedly different. Far from being subjected to forced sterilization or targeted by state family planning services, white women's domesticity and motherhood were valorized and encouraged across a variety of contexts. Tracing the sentiments of republican motherhood into post–World War II containment culture, Elaine Tyler May documents the revival in the cult of domesticity that infused white suburban motherhood with national purpose, noting its celebration of early marriage, contained heterosexuality, and traditional gender roles as uniquely American and anticommunist. Thus, private life was not a retreat from public affairs but rather codified as an embodied commitment to it: "Procreation in the cold war era took on almost mythic proportions," May writes. "Through children, men and women . . . demonstrated their loyalty to national goals by having as many children as they could."[42] While men were implicated in the national impulse toward the nuclear family, the postwar reproductive consensus was particularly salient for white women, as motherhood and domesticity were elevated once more and idealized in a postwar suburban form. In an era of nuclear threat and cultural containment, maternity was figured, yet again, as pivotal to securing the home front.

The habits and requirements of containment culture signal patterns that are explored for their contemporary resonance throughout this book. Take, for example, the national panic induced by sex outside of straightness and marriage, from the McCarthy-era lavender scare and the forced surrender of "illegitimate" white children to suburban white couples, to the recent history of heated public debates over same-sex marriage, sex education, and the stigmatization of teen sexuality and pregnancy in popular culture. In another parallel, post–World War II containment culture transformed white Hollywood sex symbols into domestic goddesses and contented mothers. A similar pattern emerges in contemporary celebrity maternity, perhaps most clearly evidenced in Angelina Jolie's reinvention from bisexual-badgirl-bombshell to ideal citizen and global mother.[43] And, as if to anticipate Kayyem's call, the so-called opt-out revolution of the early twenty-first century profiled the exodus of professional white women from prestigious jobs and careers for a domestic agenda, a trend that recalls the midcentury suburbia of Betty Friedan's feminine mystique.[44] Postwar containment culture is thus a powerful precedent for homeland maternity in its resurrection of traditional gender roles, emphasis on gender normativity and white women's domesticity, as well as its reification of the white suburban nuclear family as a strategy of security and mode of governance. Each of these examples underscores how homeland maternity functions as an historically specific yet patterned articulation between motherhood and nation.

Contemporary Motherhood and Homeland Security Culture

The discursive alignment of motherhood and nation is yet to be explicitly named and theorized as a coherent system of regulation in twenty-first century contexts. In so doing, homeland maternity extends three critical insights advanced by scholars of contemporary maternal and reproductive politics. First, recent scholarship on motherhood theorizes its all-encompassing and uncompromising character, but is less attentive to how these expectations of motherhood underwrite the nation and national belonging. Referred to as "intensive mothering," the "mommy mystique," or what Susan Douglas and Meredith Michaels term "the new momism," contemporary motherhood recasts traditional gender politics in new relational terrain, that which is "not about subservience to men ... [but rather] about subservience to children."[45] Domesticated, intensive mothering is an ideology predicated on individual perfection and personal responsibility for the health and well-being of children. Reanimating nostalgic notions of wealthy white "virtuous" motherhood—and significantly, I argue, in service of national imaginaries—these responsibilities are assigned to women, guided by experts, and relentless in locating children at the center of women's lives.

Intensive mothering borrows on mainstream feminism in its interpellation of women, as Lynn O'Brien Hallstein argues: "rather than *compete* with feminism, the new momism began to *integrate* feminist ideas and the rhetoric of choice explicitly" (original emphasis).[46] Motherhood itself, for example, is articulated through the logic of "choice," increasingly stripped of its political import and strictly relocated to the realm of the personal. Thus, as women "opt in" to motherhood, they are made solely responsible for managing the choice to parent, fueling the conditions for what Judith Warner refers to as the "perfect madness" of contemporary motherhood: "The mess of the Mommy Mystique—the belief that we can and should control every aspect of our children's lives, that our lives are the sum total of our personal choices, that our limitations stem from choosing poorly and that our problems are chiefly private, rather than public, in nature—is *not* an individual problem. . . . It is a social malady . . . a way of privatizing problems that are social in scope and rendering them, in the absence of real solutions, amenable to one's private powers of control."[47] Notably, the mommy mystique recalls Betty Friedan's classic second-wave feminist text, highlighting parallels between motherhood in contemporary and containment culture with one significant exception—ideologies of contemporary motherhood are decidedly postfeminist. They adopt the language of mainstream feminism (i.e., "choice" and "empowerment") in the service of an agenda that depoliticizes women's lives and struggles. Deeply rooted in the new economic order, postfeminism signals a world in which feminism has been "taken into account,"[48] a world in which feminism is done, over, and no longer necessary. It appropriates the language of feminism as it undermines feminism's radical impulse toward structural transformation—in personalizing and individualizing, postfeminism reduces the political to the personal once more. Not only is this a world in which individual solutions reign supreme, but it is also one in which structural conditions such as lack of childcare or livable wages are positioned as personal problems, the result of poor decision making or individual character flaws. In short, postfeminism makes women exclusively responsible for ongoing structural inequities, and does so, insidiously, under the banner of feminism itself.[49] Postfeminist mothering has been rightly critiqued for its tidy coherence with late capitalism,[50] but it has been less interrogated for reviving mythic maternities consonant with nationalist nostalgia for "the way we never were,"[51] a task that this book takes up.

Second, scholars have traced the role of risk in shaping the experiences and expectations of contemporary motherhood. For example, Julie A. Wilson and Emily Chivers Yochim explore how working- and middle-class mothers support their families in an era of privatized risk through "mamapreneurial" endeavors, striving to manage economic instability through digital and home-based labor.[52] Risk also filters into the everyday demands of care for children. Integrating risk into the ideology of intensive mothering, Joan Wolf defines "total motherhood" as that which: "reveals the vexations of a risk culture: the fixation on planning and the ongoing drive to control the future through the proper selection and application of scientific knowledge; the individualization and privatization of responsibility for lifestyles, particularly in matters of health; overlapping reverence and disdain both for science and technology and for all things natural; the inescapable moral dimension of risk analysis; and the reflexive construction of self-identity."[53] Total motherhood relies on personal responsibility and self-sufficiency in the care, nurturance, protection, and cultivated successes of children; it expects that mothers anticipate and mitigate all potential harm by developing a range of professional expertise, from child nutrition and psychology to consumer products safety. As Loertscher's case against the State of Wisconsin demonstrates, total motherhood is a moral code that begins at least by conception, but perhaps even earlier, in what Miranda Waggoner refers to as the "zero trimester."[54] Recent scholarly attention to risk in the context of mothering provides a point of departure for considering how reproductive and maternal politics are not only inflected by risk but reshaped by the homeland security state and its attendant cultural logics. In *Homeland Maternity*, I argue for an expansion of this line of inquiry by situating risk alongside other discursive constructs central to homeland security culture—namely security, emergency, and crisis.

Third, homeland maternity broadens the scope and implications of critical motherhood studies by attending to various maternal identities and reproductive struggles. Intensive mothering feeds acute and exacting demands, but it also functions powerfully to codify the trope of the "bad" mother as its constitutive outside. Put another way, ideologies of intensive mothering sculpt a different world for those pregnant and parenting outside of wealth, whiteness, US citizenship, or heteronuclear family formation. With a few notable exceptions, as Raka Shome astutely observes, wealthy "white heterosexual . . . mothers engage in mothering through an *affirming* relation with the nation-state. In contrast, mothers of color—especially working-class or poor mothers of color—have historically, and even today in most Anglo-dominant nations, engaged in mothering *against* the dominant norms of the nation-state" (original emphasis).[55] Intensive mothering propels this dynamic—as "good" motherhood is recast as all-encompassing and self-sufficient, the steady erosion of the welfare state is justified in turn. The effects are vicious and cyclical—the moralizing insistence on personal responsibility compounds the stigma attached to those who fall short of feeding, clothing, educating, and nurturing their children according to impossible ideals. Moreover, the ideology of intensive mothering renders the criminalization of "other" mothers possible. This is a world in which alarming trends take hold—one in which marginalized mothers are detained for crimes they are not convicted of and incarcerated for defending themselves against abusive partners.[56] One in which mothers are demonized for seeking state assistance and under constant threat of foster care removal even though minimum-wage employment offers neither rest nor mobility for the working poor. One in which pregnant women—like Loertscher—are incarcerated for disclosing to health care providers their addiction.[57] Thus, the ideology of intensive mothering is a dependent formation that relies on the pathology and criminality assigned to "other" mothers—to those who dare to parent while poor or undocumented or ill or addicted. These binary constructions of motherhood—good and bad, celebrated and criminalized, necessitating promotion or punishment—are accorded greater weight and velocity in moments of collective crisis as the figure of the child (or even that of the fetus) stands in for the future of the nation.

In theorizing homeland maternity, I argue for the immediacy of nation in understanding trends that celebrate and censure mothers and that shape US reproductive politics in the early twenty-first century. Motherhood is a key site in the production and maintenance of homeland security culture—it is a site that tends to fracture along lines of race, class, sexuality, age, marital, and immigration status. Indeed, homeland security culture possesses a resonance that adheres not only to security checks at airports and the defense of borders, but is similarly vested in reproduction and domesticity. Extending a long history of securing the nation through reproductive control, and particularly in moments of crisis, homeland maternity as a conceptual framework enables the interrogation of the conditions under which women are able (or unable) to assert control over their reproductive, maternal, and relational lives. And as a heuristic, homeland maternity also suggests the possibilities of invention, intervention, and redress. Its full theorizing necessitates, however, a robust understanding of homeland security culture itself.

Interrogating Homeland Security Culture

"Homeland security" simultaneously hails and exceeds the formal architecture of the state. It is typically understood vis-à-vis the former, as a referent to seismic shifts that include a restructuring of intelligence operations, preemptive foreign policy, and the proliferation of citizen surveillance and policing in the name of an opaque and endless so-called War on Terror. I use the phrase "homeland security state" to refer to these and other transformations in official modes of government. But homeland security is not limited to the state. It is centrally concerned with the nation as an imagined community.[58] In other words, homeland security functions ideologically, as a set of affective resonances attached to national identity and belonging that authorizes the state in its current form. Investigating it necessitates tending critically to both the power of sovereign governing apparatuses and the politics of everyday life. Thus, I use the phrase "homeland security culture" to refer broadly to the state in concert with the felt quality of life in post-9/11 US culture—including the rise in neoconservativism, postfeminist gender politics, as well as heightened nationalism, nativism, and US exceptionalism.

Theorizing homeland security culture is less a claim about the "effects" of 9/11 than it is an attempt to account for how the events of 9/11 provided a catalyst for reanimating familiar notions of security, nation, and citizenship.[59] "Homeland security" draws on Cold War conceptualizations of national security, substituting terrorism for communism as the single most imminent threat to US safety and global dominance.[60] Post-9/11 Cold War continuities include a governing apparatus reliant on agencies originally designed to combat communism (including the Central Intelligence Agency and the National Security Agency), as well as reinscriptions of citizenship and national identity that hinge on neo-conservative nostalgia, indiscriminate patriotism, and a silencing of dissent.[61] In short, the residue of postwar containment culture inflects the architecture of the state as well as everyday life in the early twenty-first century, even as homeland security culture is distinct in its shift toward preemption.

Preemption functions powerfully as paradigm in homeland security culture. Privileging "the power of imagination over the power of fact—suspicions over evidence," preemption relies on radical speculation to visualize the contours of all possible worlds.[62] It is neither primarily invested in accuracy (prediction) nor in probability (risk), exceeding the bounds of precision and estimation with its emphasis on capacious imagination. Scholars have traced how the logic of preemption undergirds the homeland security state at a variety of sites. For example, preemption swiftly displaced deterrence as the reigning doctrine of post-9/11 military and intelligence operations—from state justifications for the invasion of Iraq to the findings of the 9/11 Commission, which faulted intelligence agencies for a "failure of imagination" and lauded "agencies that had 'speculated' about . . . suicide hijackings."[63] Coining the term *premediation*, media scholar Richard Grusin argues that preemption sculpts a post-9/11 US media regime tasked with readying for all possible futures: "[its] fundamental purpose is to preclude that no matter what tomorrow might bring, it will always already have been premediated."[64] Thus, premediation names the requisite media logics that render anticipatory state action inevitable. In the homeland security state, radical speculation supplants scientific assessments of probability and possibility—forging a world in which present action hinges on riotous imagination, and in anticipation of our worst nightmares.

The logic of preemption is often couched as risk, however, even as preemption exceeds risk in centering imagination as the locus of anti-terror policy in domestic and international arenas.[65] Put another way, risk is frequently the rhetorical vehicle for authorizing preemption in homeland security culture. It is a powerful one. Risk functions discursively to cordon off undesirable outcomes, naming some practices excessive or unconscionable, and others optional; it defines normativitives, polices boundaries, and shapes pedestrian practices, attitudes, and beliefs. Risk has received extensive scholarly attention—it is theorized as a centerpiece of contemporary life, a form of "manufactured uncertainty" distinguished from danger or disaster by its unique temporality and assumption of human agency.[66] Marked not by realness but by the potential to "becom[e] real,"[67] risk is orientated toward unknowable futures; it positions humans as response-able agents and warrants decisive action in the present.

As Ulrich Beck writes, risk "is existent *and* non-existent, present *and* absent, doubtful *and* suspect. In the end it can be assumed to be ubiquitous and thus grounds a politics of prevention . . . assuming that the threat which does not (yet) exist really exists" (original emphasis).[68] As risk is imagined as the primary condition that sculpts our world, then preemption offers its requisite mode of management—constituting the primary logic through which we calculate and avoid, manage and deter, predict and prevent in a world replete with rapid transformation.

The 9/11 terrorist attacks on New York and Washington, D.C., mark a moment of intensification in the politics of risk and a point of departure for preemption as paradigm. As the vulnerability of the United States was made visible on a global stage, risk was rendered a defining feature of twenty-first-century US life and marshaled to bolster a politics of prevention no matter the cost. The centrality of risk to homeland security culture signals a world of proliferating possibilities and related uncertainties, distinct insofar as they are of our own making and thus subject to preemptive management through emerging modes of expertise and governance. In short, preemption is deeply reliant on the logic and rhetoric of risk, even as it exceeds the repertoire of risk to authorize any number of ruthless actions under the banner of homeland security. Notably, the insistence on preemption includes attempts to govern those pregnant and parenting through the culture of intensive mothering (evidenced by Kayyem) or through state violence against pregnant people (as in the case of Loertscher). Understanding the full significance and implications of these stories, however, requires first an elaboration of homeland security as a state apparatus and cultural politics.

Homeland Security and the State

The preemptive paradigm fuels the rapid expansion of two defining features of the homeland security state: surveillance and policing.[69] As feminist and critical race scholars have detailed, state surveillance and policing are not new. They constitute the very foundation of the settler state—violently circumscribing the lives of those most vulnerable, including black and brown communities, women, racialized immigrants, and poor people.[70] The 9/11 attacks catalyzed the intensification of surveillance and policing, however, through unprecedented technological capacity and state investment. The exponential growth of the security industry—topping $350 billion in 2012 in the United States alone—undergirds the rapid development of surveillance technologies, the outsourcing of security to private citizens and industries, and mounting violations of constitutional rights and privacy in the United States.[71] Moving from margin to center in the homeland security state, surveillance and policing are distinguished by their ubiquity, extensive infrastructure, and the urgency of the War on Terror. In this context, chronic forms of state violence against marginalized communities are compounded while white, middle-class citizens are rendered increasingly (if also differently) vulnerable to the homeland security state. Significantly, surveillance and policing are two sides of the same coin—one cultivates self-discipline and lateral observation; the other ensures strict sovereign enforcement when neoliberal governmentality fails to induce compliance.

Post-9/11 surveillance pivots on deepening neoliberal governmentality, concentrating power through its dispersion. This is evidenced, for example, by extensive citizen surveillance programs that range from the National Security Agency's warrantless wiretapping to the Department of Homeland Security's 2010 "If You See Something, Say Something" campaign to promote local reporting of "suspicious" activity to local authorities.[72] Foucauldian theories of governmentality account for such apparatuses, which are distanced from formal political institutions but aim to exert authority, govern through freedom, and "conduct conduct" nevertheless.[73] Power operates insidiously through a "loose assemblage of agents, calculations, techniques, images and commodities" that enlists individual actors and governs through related rationalities of individual choice and responsibility.[74] As Nikolas Rose and Peter Miller note, "personal autonomy is not the antithesis of political power, but a key term in its exercise, the more so because most individuals are not merely the subjects of power but play a part in its operations."[75] Governmentality turns our attention from centralized, sovereign structures to more dispersed locales, as myriad forms of authority are enlisted alongside a disciplined citizenry to manage responsibilities once considered public, from health and welfare to the security of the nation. Extensive citizen surveillance is thus recursive: trafficking in fear, docility, and allegiance to the state, surveillance itself is rendered mundane and inevitable.

Moreover, the homeland security state relentlessly positions risk and security as personal responsibilities. These responsibilities are contingent on an autonomous, enterprising, and disciplined citizen-subject to mitigate and manage the complexities of an uncertain world. Thus, in a key inversion of the welfare state, citizens absorb the work of domestic security in everyday life, as James Hay and Mark Andrejevic note: "In the era of Homeland Security, constant re-training and self-education in techniques for securing the self, the home, and the homeland become yet another set of required skills for the multitasking citizen-subject. An ethic of self-care is invoked in contrast to disparaged forms of dependency on the state and its institutions."[76] Linking national belonging to the integration of security and defense into everyday life, recent scholarship demonstrates how homeland security has become quotidian, from airport checkpoints and campaigns to secure the home, to interactive websites such as Ready.gov that encourage citizens to engage the war on terror through information gathering and preparedness.[77] This logic shifts responsibility from the public to the private sphere, casting the political as personal and mobilizing privacy "not just as a sphere for submission to expert guidance, but as the locus of responsibility and action."[78] From genetic counselors to financial risk advisors and home security experts, proliferating modes of expertise dedicated to the reduction of risk compel an "empowered" citizenry to seek guidance in securing everyday life, leaving James Hay to assert "Homeland Security as the new Social Security."[79]

The function of governmentality is usefully understood alongside transformations in contemporary biopolitics, particularly when considering reproduction and motherhood in the homeland security state.[80] Biopower has indeed shifted alongside capitalism; it is less reliant on exerting sovereign control over the health of the population than it is on what Nikolas Rose terms "ethopolitical" modes of governance.[81] In lieu of centering on disease or pathology, ethopolitics are concerned with the enhancement and optimization of life on a molecular level and at its earliest stages. Enlisting reprogenetic technologies,[82] ethopolitics focus on our increasing capacity to determine, shape, and intervene in human life at virtually any and all of its stages, from fetal gene therapies to biotechnical enhancement and optimization.[83] A constellation of forces—including the preemptive paradigm and postfeminist "choice" politics—collide to craft an ethopolitical imperative that demands informed, responsible decision making in consultation with new forms of expertise that include bioethicists, fertility counselors, and genetic engineers.[84] In a trend eerily reminiscent of republican motherhood, patients are saddled with the expectation to "exercise biological prudence, for their own sake, that of their families, that of their own lineage, and that of their nation as a whole."[85] This brave new world responsibilizes the self as it details the role of experts in governing "life itself" through freedom, blurring the boundaries between choice and determination, coercion and consent.

Pregnant and parenting individuals are particularly subject to interpellation within this biopolitical terrain. Take, for example, the intense medicalization of pregnancy. As prenatal life is increasingly imagined as a site of optimization, as innovations in reproductive and genetic technologies broaden the potential to determine the shape and the cadence of life on all scales, pregnancy gets tangled in a web of constraints masquerading as reproductive self-determination, often at the expense of social justice and even human diversity.[86] Reprogenetics—a term that highlights the steady integration of genetic testing and counseling into standard prenatal care—has rightly drawn sharp feminist critique for its eugenic tendencies, for its ushering in of what Dorothy Roberts refers to as a "new reproductive dystopia" wherein women are compelled to manage genetic risk as a condition of responsible citizenship as the state sheds support for children and families writ large and for children with disabilities specifically.[87] Moreover, the language of mainstream feminism is appropriated to forward this agenda, recasting concepts such as "autonomy" and "choice" so as to render extensive medical counsel and intervention inevitable.[88] Far from expanding reproductive freedom, as Silja Samerski astutely observes, "the professional imputation of this new autonomy makes women powerless while holding them responsible."[89] Samerski's astute remarks are written in the context of her study of genetic counseling but are applicable to myriad modes of governmentality that shape maternal health and politics in the context of homeland security.[90]

This shift toward surveillance and governmentality, however, does not signal an abandonment of sovereign rule—far from it. Overt state action, including violence, remains central to the homeland security state when other forms of authority fail—when governing through freedom does not or cannot serve the interests of the state. This is clearly evidenced in the examples I offer at the opening of this book, but of course pregnant and parenting women are not the sole targets of policing and state violence. The rise of the homeland security state has wrought an alarming uptick in draconian forms of policing and a normalization of the "state of emergency" that suspends the rule of law in favor of the exception.[91] Frightening trends in post-9/11 policing exemplify this point. From Wall Street to Ferguson to Standing Rock, law enforcement officials have donned riot gear, acquired military-grade weaponry, and driven armored vehicles into assemblies of unarmed protesters. Reports have detailed numerous instances of brutal state violence against protestors (as well as journalists and legal observers): baseless arrests, unmerciful beatings, denial of medical care, sexual assault, and the use of chemical agents, stun grenades, pepper balls, rubber bullets, sound cannons, flex cuffs, and other so-called less lethal weapons to terrorize protestors.[92] In addition to inflicting immediate and serious harm, these weapons can result in permanent—even fatal—injuries such as neuropathy, hearing loss, and brain damage.

Poor communities, immigrant communities, and communities of color have long faced state and state-sanctioned brutalities in a system designed to protect whiteness, citizenship, and wealth. What distinguishes policing in the context of homeland security, however, is its rapid escalation, militarization, and mainstreaming. A federal program, initiated through the post–Cold War National Defense Authorization Act, authorized the transfer of military weapons and gear to civilian law enforcement to bolster efforts in the War on Drugs.[93] The implications are difficult to understate. This program funneled high-tech military equipment—including firearms, aircraft, and tactical vehicles—into local police departments, often into the hands of officers ill-equipped to use them. A new subset of the security industry flourished, targeting domestic law enforcement as an untapped but lucrative client for services and technologies. Industry conventions like Urban Shield, funded in part by the US Department of Homeland Security, continue to draw local law enforcement to showcase the latest in surveillance technologies and weaponry. Federal "antiterror grants" totaled over $34 billion in the decade following 9/11, ensuring a steady stream of funding for the amassing of weaponry and riot gear by state and local police.[94] The federal weapons program eventually garnered greater public scrutiny in the wake of Black Lives Matter, but even measured attempts by the Obama administration to curtail the scope of weapons transfer drew sharp criticism.[95]

The consequences of militarized policing have been devastating. Various reports detail egregious human rights abuses as well as the steady erosion of public trust.[96] Permanent injuries to Occupiers, Black Lives Matter activists, and #NoDAPL water protectors have been traced to weaponry from two major security contractors, as well as to Cold War–era arsenals.[97] The crude display of military might—state officials in full riot gear, tanks rolling into residential communities, midnight raids on peaceful encampments, chemical agents shot point-blank into the faces of nonviolent protestors—renders policing itself hypervisible, a turn fueled by the circulation of images of state violence through social networking platforms. In this strident exhibition of domestic arms, the nation is figured as a war zone. Political dissent is read against the grain of patriotism, and protestors are shamed and silenced by a politics of civility.[98] As everyday citizens, residents, and communities are recast as enemy combatants in the eyes of the homeland security state, policing as state occupation and suppression becomes the modus operandi. Each of these trends is deeply disconcerting when considered in isolation. In concert, the homeland security state is clarified as that which imagines its largest threat to be democracy itself.

The logic of preemption undergirds and sustains these trends. Moreover, just as preemption authorizes exceptional state violence against organized communities within the United States, so too does it promulgate a host of abusive practices in immigration and foreign policy. Examples include preventive detention, preemptive war, extraordinary rendition and torture, and, most recently, the unconscionable separation of undocumented children from their parents at the United States–Mexico border as an alleged strategy of deterrence, a story sparking national outrage as this book goes to press. My purpose here is not to detail these trends in their entirety, but rather to note them as evidence of the power and ubiquity of preemption—a doctrine that fuels the proliferation of surveillance and policing in both domestic and international arenas, and dwells at the heart of the homeland security state.

Homeland maternity thus privileges the reliance on neoliberal governmentality as a defining characteristic of the homeland security state, while noting the sovereign architecture necessary to ensure its normalizing grasp. The incarceration of Tamara Loertscher offers an example of violent state intervention under the banner of risk; in another, we might consider the unprecedented professional disciplining of Dr. Michael Kamrava, stripped of his medical license in 2011 by the Medical Board of California due largely to his role in Nadya Suleman's conception of octuplets (see chapter 3). My focus on governmentality does not exempt the sovereign state, its traditional functions and modes of enacting authority. But Kamrava and Loertscher mark an extreme—formal interventions deemed necessary when women, at odds or in concert with experts or authority figures, refuse to govern themselves. At the heart of this project is a desire to trace the more subtle discursive logics that render such state action possible, reasonable, or even pedestrian. This task not only requires attention to homeland security as it pivots on preemptive state action, but it also directs our concern to culture and the politics of everyday life in the new millennium.

Everyday Life in Homeland Security Culture

Homeland security culture both signals and exceeds the state, referencing a post-9/11 sociopolitical order that censures dissent, circumscribes civil liberties, relies on exclusion, and pairs draconian policing at home with flagrant lawlessness abroad.[99] Homeland security culture refers to a vision of nation and national belonging that celebrates nativism, nationalism, indiscriminate patriotism, and an adherence to resurging conservativism and normative "family values."[100] It is a defining characteristic of early twenty-first-century US public culture—evident in the architecture of the state and other cultural institutions, integrated into popular film and television, woven into the fabric of everyday life, and a powerful force shaping the recent history of reproductive and maternal politics in the United States.[101]

The rhetorical shift from Cold War–era "national security" to post-9/11 "homeland security" is significant. The appropriation of the term "homeland" itself broke with more familiar patriotic patois—prior to 9/11, no US president had referred to the nation as "homeland," even in moments of national crisis.[102] As Amy Kaplan notes, the "homeland" is tied to mythic beliefs in "native origins . . . ancient ancestry, and notions of racial and ethnic homogeneity."[103]

Imagining the nation as a homeland under siege in the early twenty-first century possesses a powerful double function. It fuels an anxious sense of porous boundaries and borders alongside racialized notions of belonging. References to the "homeland" have long signaled "diasporic nostalgia and desires," and, as Nicholas De Genova writes, "discursively re-figures US citizens as ineffably alienated from their own 'native' entitlement to the comfort of unproblematic belonging."[104] The vernacular privileging of "homeland" incites US nationalism and nostalgia apace with a felt sense of "radical insecurity,"[105] shoring up neoconservative ideological commitments and political priorities—including those related to domesticity—in the wake of the 9/11 terrorist attacks.

The homeland is thus an abrupt departure from familiar idioms of nation. And yet, homeland security culture possesses a powerful precedent in Cold War–era containment culture.[106] Much like communism in the Cold War era, terrorism could come from anyone anywhere at any time. Affectively marked by this heightened sense of endless insecurity,[107] homeland security culture is, as Jennifer Gillan explains, "both a makeover of, and a return to, 1950s style Containment Culture that divides the world into two camps, fetishizes national security, and establishes uncritical support [to the nation] as a value unto itself, and makes 'personal behavior part of a global strategy.'"[108] In the absence of any clear sense making or explanatory apparatus for the terrorist attacks, "it was the cold war that echoed most loudly across the post-9/11 landscape."[109] Familiar terminologies were deployed in characterizing the attacks—live reports on the World Trade Center drew an immediate parallel to the bombing of Pearl Harbor, the site "became 'ground zero'—a term long associated with nuclear targets,"[110] and, in an ill-fated attempt to merge the World War II Axis powers and Reagan's Evil Empire through metaphor, President George W. Bush called for public support against an "axis of evil." The Cold War metaphor reverberated far beyond the immediacy of the attacks, shaping homeland security culture through a revival of containment culture practices and attitudes—for example, in touting consumption as patriotic, reanimating traditional gender roles, idealizing traditional family values, silencing political dissent, threatening free speech and civil liberties, and targeting people of African, South Asian, Southeast Asian, and Southwest Asian descent in antiterrorist efforts.[111]

Significantly for the purposes of this project, homeland security culture is shaped by postfeminism even as its gender politics often include overt antifeminism.[112] As Susan Faludi deftly demonstrates in her study of the cultural response to 9/11, the terrorist attacks were collectively imagined as an emasculinization of the nation; its antidote swiftly asserted through a renaissance of virile manhood.[113] Indeed, emulating a persistent pattern of containment culture resuscitation and its attendant forms of gender discipline, the rise of homeland security culture fueled a neofifties gender melodrama that reinvigorated masculinist heroism and its feminine counterpart, domesticity and dependence. Media focused on "security moms" stockpiling food and obsessing over their children's safety, while single professional women were reportedly lonely and aiming to opt out of careers and into marriage.[114] Independent women were publicly chastised while pregnant widows and the "'manly men' at ground zero" were lauded extensively as brave and selfless patriots; taken together, these patterns form a consistent whole: "What mattered was restoring the illusion of a mythic America where women needed men's protection and men succeeded in providing it. What mattered was vanquishing the myth's dark twin, the humiliating 'terror-dream' that 9/11 had forced to the surface of national consciousness."[115] Save the grieving mothers and widows of 9/11 afforded copious publicity, women were expected to disappear from leadership and public life within the immediate post-9/11 US landscape.

These gender politics, as Faludi notes, did not bode well for feminism. Feminist journalists such as Susan Sontag and Katha Pollitt bore the brunt of public censure and allegations of treason—far beyond that of their male peers—for daring to suggest reflexivity in the wake of the attacks.[116] Contemporary feminist concerns were dismissed as superfluous at best, but more frequently demonized for leading the nation astray and heightening national insecurity; the allegations were twofold: "women's liberation had 'feminized' our men and, in so doing, left the nation vulnerable to attack."[117] Conservative women were immediately put to work in service of this agenda, from Karen Hughes and Ann Coulter to self-proclaimed "dissident feminist" Camille Paglia, each equating feminism with terrorism—for example, in framing reproductive rights as incompatible with the post-9/11 revaluation of life, reprimanding so-called career women for their lack of domestic aspiration, and maligning feminist challenges to patriarchal norms while asserting a revival in traditional masculinity as the antidote to national insecurity. The widows of 9/11 were culturally lauded as long as they remained chaste and in grief; those radicalized by the terrorist attacks, those widows who demanded answers and demonstrated some success in getting them, were reviled. And the very notion of security was retooled toward antifeminist ends—"hijacked," as Carol Stabile and Carrie Rentschler note, "as an alibi for a series of economic policies, political decisions, and military actions that have had the effect of making many women throughout the world infinitely less secure."[118] In short, the only "feminism" allowed to flourish in the wake of 9/11 was decidedly postfeminist—not only a feminism stripped of its radical politics, but one retooled in the interests of patriarchy, capitalism, and US imperialism.

Clarifying this resuscitation of containment culture gender regimes, which are made pliable and more insidious through the reigning logic of postfeminism, is pivotal to understanding homeland security culture writ large, and homeland maternity specifically. From Pat Robertson's blaming of gays, lesbians, and abortion rights supporters for 9/11 to the use of the terrorist attacks to mobilize donations for pro-life causes, the threat of women in control of their own sexuality, reproduction, and motherhood was discursively aligned with terrorist threats to the nation. While these sentiments may seem extreme, I argue that they function as a kind of canary in the coal mine—signaling relationships between motherhood and nation, between reproduction and homeland security, that play out meaningfully in a variety of more subtle, but no less dangerous, contexts. The reigning logic of homeland security culture—reliant on rhetorics of security, risk, emergency, and crisis—possesses a powerful velocity and salience that not only shapes public justifications for citizen surveillance, torture, and the fortification of national borders, but that also constrains sexual and reproductive agency. *Homeland Maternity* explores to what extent, and under what conditions, motherhood and reproduction are aligned with the interests of homeland security; it illuminates how motherhood and nation are inextricably interwoven, perhaps differently, but no less now than ever before.

Locating Homeland Maternity: On Method and an Outline of Chapters

My analysis is guided by an ethic of reproductive justice and by my training as a feminist rhetorical critic. Reproductive justice has been widely embraced as a necessary corrective to the inadequacies of reproductive choice.[119] As a mobilizing concept and rhetorical claim, "choice" has been rightly and thoroughly critiqued for centering women of means and privilege, for its inability to secure reproductive freedom and dignity for all women.[120] As opposed to rights or justice, choice is imagined as superfluous, elite, and rendered subject to the judgment of others. It is often subsumed by individualism and facilitates the privatization of matters that are fundamentally political in scope—for example, mothers on welfare are regularly accused of poor decision making, and this emphasis on "bad choices" deflects attention from the structural dimensions of poverty such as persistent gendered inequities and economic injustice. Put simply, reproduction and motherhood—and indeed, feminism itself—have been reduced to choice at their own peril. The crude equation of feminism with individual choice—*any* choice—robs feminist politics of their ongoing salience, force, and transformative potential through critique. What began decades ago as an earnest and resonant claim to self-determination—jurisdiction over one's body, fertility, sexuality—has been depoliticized through myopic obsessions with personal preference, mobilized in service of the new economic order, and subsequently articulated in defense of a range of practices that may or may not serve a vision of social justice or feminist politics. In short, "choice" has diminished the political to the personal once more.

As an organizing tool and critical paradigm, reproductive justice is rooted in the struggles of women of color, both in the United States and in the Global South. The term itself was coined by twelve African American women in 1994 on the heels of the International Conference on Population and Development in Cairo.[121] Inspired by their collaborations with feminists of color from around the globe, these twelve women discussed their frustrations with the pro-choice framework and sought a means to articulate reproductive rights as part of a broader human rights and social justice agenda.[122] As Loretta J. Ross explains, reproductive justice offers "a theory, strategy and practice for organizing against . . . multiple, interlocking reproductive violences . . . by placing Indigenous women and women of color at the center of [its] lens."[123] Thus, reproductive justice advocates center their work on the belief that every human "has the right to have a child, not have a child, and parent the children"[124] they have, illuminating one of the primary distinctions between reproductive justice and pro-choice advocacy. Pro-choice movements have historically focused almost exclusively on the right to decide *not* to bear children—a reflection of the ways in which whiteness, heteronormativity, and class privilege inform mainstream feminist advocacy and the experience of compulsory motherhood. The histories of women marginalized by and within heteronuclear white supremacist culture are decidedly dissimilar to compulsory motherhood, and in fact reveal the opposite—sustained, institutionalized efforts to curtail or prohibit fertility and motherhood. Reproductive justice takes this as its starting point, and interrogates contemporary issues with a cultivated sensitivity to these histories and experiences.

Reproductive justice is a framework increasingly conversant with the struggles of trans and nonbinary communities. The desire to birth and/or parent children in dignity is not one limited to cisgender women, and the language I use in this book attempts to grapple with the complex realities that shape diverse experiences with pregnancy and parenting. In some cases, the policing of pregnancy is explicitly about the policing of *all* cisgender women of reproductive age—regardless of their ability or desire to carry, birth, or parent children. In this way, there is a specificity to the cisgender misogyny embedded in homeland maternity—and a reason to name it as such. Accordingly, when in reference to narratives, historical practices, or other instances particular to cisgender women, my language reflects these conditions and points more specifically to considerations of cis sexism and misogyny in the politics of pregnancy and reproduction. Still, the policing and surveillance of reproduction ensnares people from across the gender spectrum, at times providing much common ground in the struggle for reproductive justice among those who identify as trans, nonbinary, or cisgender. Thus, I also use broader, more inclusive language in particular moments throughout this book to reflect how trans and nonbinary individuals are similarly subject to these, and other unique, hostilities. Following the lead of Loretta Ross and Rickie Solinger, I aspire imperfectly toward language both inclusive and specific, oscillating between "women" and "mothers" and "pregnant and/or parenting individuals" according to context.[125] This nexus of reproductive and gender justice is rich with possibility, calling for ongoing scholarship and critical attention.

As a rhetorical critic, I gather and read a range of artifacts that bear meaningfully on figurations of motherhood and reproduction in homeland security culture. My archive includes newspaper articles, public campaigns, advertisements, popular film and television, legal documents, and advocacy efforts by professional associations and nongovernmental organizations. In so doing, I build on a vibrant tradition of rhetorical scholarship that that embraces criticism "in the artistic mode."[126] It is a tradition that understands illumination as its first impulse, a tradition that invests in the critical process as fundamentally creative, generative, and world making.[127] While the sites of inquiry in the chapters that follow may seem divergent at first glance, I aim to articulate connections among fragments of culture in order to map continuities and consistencies; to locate, in Raymond Williams's terminology, "a felt sense of the quality of life at a particular place and time."[128] The selected case studies are spatially and temporally bracketed in distinct ways; rather than assume discrete beginnings and ends, however, the aim of this project is to trace striking consistencies across time and space as powerful, interanimating cultural formations.[129] Without laying claim to causality or intentionality, in *Homeland Maternity* I assemble and interrogate a rich archive of public discourse, with a cultivated sensitivity to how particular rhetorical acts and utterances are made salient in broader cultural contexts.

Each instance of homeland maternity explored in the following chapters focuses on a controversy or cultural phenomenon in recent US history (1) centered on reproduction and motherhood, (2) wherein the rationalities of homeland security culture shaped public thinking through rhetorics of security, risk, emergency, and crisis, (3) in ways that served a vision of nation, and (4) garnered significant attention—dominating news headlines for months (even years), reverberating through media, popular culture, state assemblies, and/or Congress, and generating a wealth of public interest and debate. That is to say, each chapter centers on a site where the discursive alignment of motherhood and nation is present and persistent, where the logic of homeland security culture shapes reproductive politics and, significantly, where motherhood and reproduction are figured as central to homeland security within dominant discourse. Although I focus some attention on instances where clear and egregious violations of human rights have occurred, the longer case studies foreground moments of homeland maternity that are more subtle, illustrating the quotidian contexts that undergird alignments between motherhood and nation and fuel the conditions necessary to police motherhood and reproduction in the ways that we currently—and increasingly—do. In other words, I attend to those discourses that normalize, even render necessary, more extreme forms of surveillance and policing of those pregnant and parenting in everyday US contexts. These sites are not meant to be exhaustive, but function rather as representative anecdotes that illustrate well the defining features of homeland maternity and its implications.

As history would suggest, homeland maternity enlists wealthy, white domesticity in the project of security. In chapter 1, "Securing Motherhood on the Home Front," I examine the post-9/11 surge in pronatalism that aligned white, professional women's fertility with national security. Two cultural sites are of particular interest in this case study. First, I interrogate the "opt-out revolution" of the early twenty-first century that profiled an exodus of professional women from elite careers in favor of full-time domesticity, a trend reminiscent of postwar white suburbia but refigured in the context of postfeminist culture. Second, I study the proliferation of fertility campaigns that targeted young professional women in the latter part of the decade, offering lifestyle directives and encouraging the use of assisted reproductive technologies to secure the possibility of pregnancy later in life. I argue that these pronatalist campaigns are usefully understood in concert, clarifying the discursive valorization of domesticity and motherhood for women of means as a critical dimension of homeland security culture.

But not all mothers are equally celebrated. Homeland maternity directs attention to how the fertility of particular women is relentlessly promoted, even as others are punished for reproductivity that is read against the grain of the nation. The second chapter, "Risky Reproduction and the Politics of Octomom," explores the case of Nadya Suleman (more widely known as Octomom) and the cultural politics of "risk" in reproduction. I examine public discourses surrounding the birth of the Suleman octuplets, tracing related rhetorics of pathology and risk that marked Suleman as a threat to be contained while masking dominant logics of race, class, and family formation through the ethos of medical expertise. In this chapter I explore how the rhetoric of risk governs women differentially, policing the borders of maternity and asserting the primacy of medical authority in maintaining these borders. Furthermore, as risk is rhetorically evoked to position women against their pregnancies, I argue that this fundamentally shifts the gaze of the clinic—decentering women, elevating the fetus, and fueling the discursive conditions necessary for the deprivation of pregnant women's rights and liberties. Thus, Suleman's story is situated alongside frightening trends toward state criminalization and punishment of pregnant women across the country, as evidenced recently in the state of Wisconsin's cruel treatment of Tamara Loertscher.

Attempts to govern motherhood and fertility according to dominant ideologies are also intimately entangled with the politics of purity and youth sexuality. The third chapter, "Post-Prevention? Conceptualizing Emergency Contraception," analyzes public debates surrounding the availability of emergency contraception (EC) over the counter. From 2001 to 2006, as FDA officials wrestled with the parameters of EC availability, the perceived significance and implications of a novel form of pregnancy prevention—specifically, a means of preventing pregnancy *after* unprotected sex—fueled cultural panics regarding sexual purity and young people's sexual and reproductive decision making. I argue that EC was discursively managed through rhetorics of "emergency" that drew on the ethos of science, emphasized normative family planning and sexual restraint, and disciplined women differentially according to longstanding (classed, racialized) hierarchies of maternal worth. In so doing, I note how advocacy for EC accessibility relied on antiabortion cultural sentiment and the intrinsic value of sexual "purity." Eventually placed behind the counter and subject to pharmacist refusal clauses and recipient age requirements, I explore how the reclassification of EC unevenly relocates and intensifies surveillance of women's sexual and reproductive lives within homeland security culture.

In the final chapter, I investigate how rhetorics of crisis in the context of homeland maternity have reshaped contemporary reproductive politics. In "Crisis Pregnancy and the Colonization of the Clinic," I critically account for the significance of crisis teen pregnancy narratives in homeland security culture (e.g., *Juno, 16 and Pregnant, Glee,* and *Teen Mom*) alongside the colonization of comprehensive women's health clinics by the evangelical crisis pregnancy center movement. First, I consider how crisis teen pregnancy narratives resuscitate containment culture normativities with a postfeminist twist. In dominant entertainment media, the containment culture disappearance of pregnant white teenagers is adapted to contemporary contexts as crisis pregnancy narratives offer teens neoliberal risk tutorials—tools for self-governance that emphasize postfeminist empowerment through prematernal and maternal prudence and responsibility. Rhetorics of "crisis" pregnancy resonate beyond television and film, however. I thus attend also to the rhetorics of crisis mobilized by federally funded evangelical crisis pregnancy centers, clarifying how they are implicated in the public defunding and closure of abortion clinics across the country. This is, to be sure, clear and sobering evidence of the steady uptick in the policing and coercion of women's reproductive lives in recent US security culture.

Taking recent immigration policies related to pregnancy and motherhood as a point of departure, the conclusion considers the implications of homeland maternity and examines potential modes of resistance to it, including strategies of co-optation, subversion, and other modes of rhetorical invention and reinvention. This final chapter is written in the spirit of exploration and provocation. It highlights and develops emerging channels of challenge and transformation, edging us toward the promise of reproductive justice beginning with the very words we speak.

Motherhood in the context of homeland security culture is a site of intense contestation—at once a powerful form of currency and a target of unprecedented assault. As reproductive bodies are imagined to threaten national security, either through supposed excess or deficiency, a culture of homeland maternity intensifies the requirements of pregnancy and parenting as it works to discipline those who refuse to adhere. Securing the nation has long entailed the surveillance and control of reproduction and motherhood. What follows is an investigation of this pattern in its most recent instantiation, committed to the belief that we can—and must—make other worlds possible.

CHAPTER 1

Securing Motherhood on the Home Front

It's often a child who helps us "touch the face of God" . . . Nothing drove this point home more powerfully than the terrible events of September 11, 2001. The awful carnage of that morning convinced many of us that our lives were filled with a great deal of noise and clamor. . . . In a post–September 11 world we may be able to better appreciate how much we need our children.

—Sylvia Ann Hewlett, *Creating a Life*

In spring of 2002, economist Sylvia Ann Hewlett was met with much critical acclaim for her book, *Creating a Life: Professional Women and the Quest for Children*. Her study chronicled deep but unspoken maternal longing among the professional elite: "There is a secret out there, a painful, well-kept secret: At mid-life, between a third and half of all high-achieving women in America do not have children. . . . By and large, these high-achieving women have not chosen to be childless. The vast majority yearn for children."[1] Publicly lauded for sounding the infertility alarm bell, Hewlett achieved what Susan Faludi referred to as "the media trifecta: *Oprah*, *60 Minutes*, and the cover of *Time*."[2] *Creating a Life* sparked an onslaught of attention to age-related infertility; it also generated significant feminist criticism for its tendency to scold women for allowing their careers to, in the words of one of Hewlett's interviewees, "obliterate [their] 30s."[3] Hewlett argued nonetheless that these women's stories, their largely failed "attempt[s] to snatch a child from the jaws of menopause," were valuable as cultural heuristics, but also because they implored "the next generation to pay attention. By doing so, twenty-something women might be able to avoid the cruel choices that dogged the footsteps of their older sisters."[4] The "creeping nonchoice," that is, of childlessness by professionally successful women. High-achieving women's fertility and childbearing, according to Hewlett, are not just personal but political matters, with dire implications for the nation should they be curtailed: "the more concrete and tangible rewards [of children] go to the nation. Competent, well-developed children become productive workers who boost the GNP and pay their taxes. They also become responsible citizens who vote and otherwise contribute to society. . . . Having it all, it turns out, is a good idea—for individual women and for the nation."[5] This linking of national interests to elite women's childbearing is perhaps remarkable in its candor, but it is also historically familiar as well as consonant with post-9/11 nostalgia and the white, middle-class return to home and hearth.

Widespread circulation of anxieties over elite women's childbearing—or lack thereof—is a key dimension of homeland maternity. Infertility panics and attendant pronatalist campaigns often align wealthy and/or white motherhood with the interests of the nation in pedestrian contexts, shoring up the logic necessary to surveil and police motherhood in myriad ways both subtle and overt. Indeed, while Hewlett's cautionary tale of age-related infertility reverberated across the homeland security landscape—even in spite of its exaggerated claims and conclusions[6]—her sound critique of the structural forces impeding family and work integration for US women was largely ignored.[7] Instead, age-related infertility panic was catalyzed and repeated across a range of settings—including pharmaceutical advertisements, celebrity memoirs, a burgeoning blogging community, and public awareness campaigns sponsored by assisted reproductive technology (ART) industry organizations and women's magazines. Take, for example, a campaign sponsored by the American Society for Reproductive Medicine, launched just before 9/11. Billboards displayed prominently in public transit systems in Chicago, New York, and Seattle displayed an upside-down baby bottle in hourglass form, warning women that "advancing age decreases your ability to have children," as narratives of domestic nostalgia—featuring single urban professionals' renewed interests in marriage and premature speculations about a post-9/11 baby boom—made headlines in the months immediately following the attacks.[8] Dominant media featured stories on declining fertility rates, and preemptive DIY-style fertility guides appeared regularly in women's magazines, educating readers on how to optimize the "pre-pregnant"[9] body through diet and exercise, and warning women not to wait until it was "too late." Blockbuster superhero films resuscitated narratives of feminine vulnerability and signaled, as Carol Stabile notes, "a desire for [masculine] secular saviors," as postfeminist chick flicks tempering women's professional aspirations via romance and domesticity were, in Diane Negra's words, "energized after 9/11 because they were so conversant with other social discourses that advocated traditionalism as the 'right' response to a changed national climate."[10] And, in the wake of the 2007 recession, the American Fertility Association launched a series titled "Manicures and Martinis" in Manhattan, aimed at educating professional women in their twenties and thirties on the "reality of the biological clock" and fertility preservation,[11] lest financial hardship necessitate work outside of the home. In short, Hewlett's message achieved a high degree of resonance not as an aberration, but rather for its consistency with other cultural phenomena that reified motherhood for white women of means in homeland security culture.

Historical precedent is instructive in understanding the currency of infertility panics in recent years. Rooted in antifeminist backlash and white supremacist ideologies, cultural myths have long maintained infertility as a disease of affluent white women who dare to delay childbearing in pursuit of other goals. In the late nineteenth century, in the midst of first-wave feminism, the US medical establishment viewed infertility as an affliction brought on by young women's supposedly audacious behavior—including educational or career aspirations, contraceptive use, or active sex lives with their husbands.[12] Feminist scholars have traced the infertility myth as a prominent theme in pronatalist 1980s narratives that worked to discipline feminist gains of the mid-twentieth century, and women themselves, in its articulation of infertility to a specific demographic: the educated, thirtysomething, professional white woman.[13] In other words, not unlike rape culture scripts, when it comes to infertility, women have asked for it. In their refusal to adhere to gendered norms that posit motherhood as the ultimate expression of white, well-to-do femininity—in pursuing education, careers, or pleasurable sex in lieu of traditional family life—women have secured their own demise. Despite considerable evidence that women's reproductive health has only been enhanced as a result of greater gender equality and opportunities, despite that infertility rates have remained relatively stable for over a century, the myth of feminism as the root of infertility persists.[14]

Cultural discourses constitutive of infertility epidemics are also wed to the logic of white supremacist culture. Dominant infertility narratives position middle-class, white women's reproduction at the center of national panic, despite consistent evidence of the disproportionate impact of infertility on low-wealth communities and communities of color due in large part to health care access disparities.[15] Several conservative public figures have gained widespread repute in forecasting a public crisis due to the unmet maternal obligations of educated white and/or Western women and the reproductive excesses of "undesirable" populations; popular titles include *The Birth Dearth*, *The Bell Curve*, and *What to*

Expect When No One's Expecting.[16] In short, the logic of eugenics is decisively present, not just in the collective imagining of an infertility epidemic, but also in the business of assisted reproduction. A multibillion-dollar industry has emerged alongside the contemporary infertility "epidemic" that reflects and perpetuates inequities; women who use infertility services are disproportionately privileged with regard to education, income, race, marital status, and age because primary barriers to assisted reproductive technologies are economic, geographical, and cultural.[17] Infertility is culturally figured as a problem for women with social and cultural capital, simultaneously reifying white motherhood, underscoring the tragedy of white infertility, and articulating infertility services to white women and families. The fertility panics that marked homeland security culture proved no exception to this history.

I examine early twenty-first-century infertility anxieties and the powerful surge in pronatalism in this chapter to illuminate how homeland maternity hinges on longstanding alignments between elite women's childbearing and the security of the nation. My argument advances that of other feminist scholars who have theorized a return to nostalgic domesticity that reigned supreme in post-9/11 US culture, from the emergence of "hegemonic familialism" and a return to a "nesting nation," to a revival of traditional gender roles and the amplification of intensive mothering.[18] With an explicit focus on how motherhood is not only celebrated and intensified but also deeply enmeshed in the logic of nation and homeland security, I explore two specific cultural moments central to understanding the revival of republican motherhood as *homeland maternity*, each unfolding in the wake of a catastrophic event—the terrorist attacks on September 11, 2001, and the global recession that began in 2007. I first examine the so-called opt-out revolution of the early twenty-first century that alleged an exodus of professional white women from prestigious jobs and careers for a more domestic agenda. Second, I consider the proliferation of fertility campaigns that targeted upwardly mobile young professional women, encouraging fertility vigilance and the consumption of assisted reproductive technologies to secure the possibility of pregnancy later in life. These pronatalist campaigns are usefully understood in concert, clarifying the valorization of elite women's domesticity and motherhood as a critical dimension of security efforts on the home front.

Opting Out on the Home Front

In addition to shining a spotlight on infertility and the biological clock, Hewlett's *Creating a Life* reignited debates concerned with "having it all," cultural shorthand for gendered expectations that women juggle second- and third-shift labor while employed full-time outside of the home. But even as Hewlett herself raised difficult questions regarding "the brutal demands of ambitious careers" and "the asymmetries of male-female relationships"[19] that disproportionately burden women's attempts to meld work with family, a more palatable explanation of gendered disparities took hold in dominant cultural imaginaries. In the words of Patricia Sellers in *Fortune* magazine, "Apparently it's not that women can't get high-level jobs. Rather, they're choosing not to."[20] This sentiment was consonant with a range of neo-traditionalist discourses arresting the US home front in the wake of the 9/11 attacks, from the resurging popularity of masculinist superheroes at the box office to the silencing of political dissent and broad support for preemptive aggression in foreign policy.[21] Dominant media figured domesticity as the new feminism—pitting working mothers against stay-at-home mothers and fueling the so-called mommy wars[22] in lieu of a rigorous examination of the structural impediments to juggling family and employment. Flattening structural critiques in favor of individualism and exhibiting the postfeminist penchant for personal choice, the extolled solution to the ticking biological clock and the relentless demands of paid labor was for elite women to simply "opt out."

In October 2003, "The Opt-Out Revolution" appeared as the cover story for the *New York Times Magazine*. Journalist Lisa Belkin claimed that accomplished professional women were "opting out" in droves, exiting high-stakes, powerful careers to embrace full-time domesticity.[23] These were the women who, according to Belkin, were supposed to lead in public life—those able to reap the benefits of second-wave feminism wholesale, earning advanced degrees from prestigious universities and ascending in their professions. Instead, the greatest beneficiaries of mainstream feminism were rejecting the workplace. In answer to the question, "why don't women run the world?," Belkin quipped, "maybe it's because they don't want to," and eventually concluded that, in stay-at-home motherhood, perhaps they already do. The opt-out narrative quickly captured widespread attention—Belkin's feature was the most e-mailed *New York Times* article of the year,[24] and "opting out" quickly gained traction as a social trend story. Grounding its authority in repetition as opposed to fact,[25] the opt-out revolution triggered a series of high-profile news reports on a younger generation of privileged women trading careerism and the corporate ladder for an embrace of full-time motherhood and domesticity. Within months, the opt-out narrative was featured on *60 Minutes* and the *Today Show*, appeared on the covers of *Time*, *Fortune*, and *Fast Company*, and was widely discussed in other news outlets and the burgeoning blogosphere.[26] Asserting an exodus from paid labor into full-time domesticity—particularly among white, middle-to-upper-class women—is a recurrent theme in journalism; the opt-out narrative has been resuscitated and rehashed at various intervals since at least the postwar era.[27] In 2003, however, Belkin's exposé struck at the heart of concerns over motherhood, work, and citizenship in the homeland security culture.

Feminist scholars were quick to interrogate the opt-out narrative, challenging its fundamental assumptions and politics. First, and perhaps obviously, opting out celebrates a narrow demographic of elite motherhood—specifically, white, highly educated, married, straight mothers.[28] Opt-out narratives feature mothers who attended Ivy League institutions and launched prestigious careers in finance, marketing, education, and government. Additionally, opt-out narratives offer little by way of data. Empirical research refuted the fundamental claims of the opt-out narrative as myth.[29] Longitudinal economic data reveal that the workforce participation of women with children has risen considerably since 1984; while the rate of increase has slowed in the last two decades, the overall trend continues upward.[30] When professional women do step off the fast track in their careers, it is far less often evidence of an enthusiastic embrace of motherhood and domesticity than it is a reluctant surrender to structural barriers that impede the integration of work and families.[31] Thus, research suggests that "opting out" in the professional elite is less a matter of choice than it is a lack of choice, including inflexible hours and work culture, few meaningful part-time options or telecommuting possibilities, and a dearth of female mentors in management.[32]

Still, despite these structural inequities, highly educated mothers are more likely to remain in the workforce than their working-class counterparts.[33] As Pamela Stone and Lisa Ackerly Hernandez note, college-educated mothers have the highest labor force participation rates of all mothers, and the "typical" stay-at-home mother "is not college-educated and white, but rather Hispanic, less educated, and likely a recent immigrant." This is due in large part to comforts afforded the professional class, which include higher pay, greater control over working conditions, and access to benefits. Low-wage workers, in contrast, have "no control over the conditions of work, no vacation or sick days, and little bargaining power, [they] lose or quit jobs and cycle in and out of the labor force to meet their family needs."[34] Thus, despite more acute conditions of need, working-class mothers are often overlooked in public discussions of work and motherhood. The opt-out narrative that emerged in the years following 9/11 and prevailed until the Great Recession—extolling the virtues of wealthy white stay-at-home motherhood—stood in stark contrast to dominant discourses surrounding working- and poverty-class mothers who are frequently berated for their mothering, shamed for any reliance on public assistance, and punished for anything less than full-time employment.[35] The opt-out narrative ignored the systemic challenges that working mothers face and exacerbated race and class divisions in omitting discussion of structural solutions. Aligning whiteness and wealth with "good" mothering, the opt-out narrative elevated motherhood as the most significant contribution that wealthy white women might make to collective life, while simultaneously circulating alongside disciplining discourses aimed at poverty- and working-class mothers.

Feminist scholars have also interrogated the opt-out narrative for its reliance on postfeminist, neoliberal rhetorics of choice.[36] The rhetoric of choice elides the structural conditions that differentially constrain women, relentlessly relocating conversations about the challenges facing working parents, and mothers in particular, to a matter of individual women's desires.[37] Belkin's article draws on "choice" repeatedly, for example: "It's not just that the workplace has failed women. It is also that women are rejecting the workplace."[38] The framing of women's individual motivations for "rejecting the workplace" took various forms within the opt-out narrative. These included, for example, a biological pull toward motherhood, a definition of success distinct from that of male peers, or even gendered gaps in intelligence and ambition: "'Sometimes I worry that [women are] really just a little bit lazier,' Sears says. But in my heart of hearts, I think it's really because we're smarter. Maybe evolution has endowed us with the ability to turn back our rheostat faster, to not always charge ahead after one all-consuming thing.'"[39] Whether biological or cultural in its proffered rationale, however, women *as mothers* were figured as fundamentally different than men. The focus on their individual desires and decision making borrowed on gender essentialism, obscured systemic barriers to mothers' workforce participation, and deflected serious considerations of power. Rich or poor, over- or under-resourced, the rhetoric of choice directed working mothers to resolve the structural conditions that hinder the integration of work and family through personal decision making. Thus, as Mary Vavrus notes, the rhetoric of choice was mobilized to assert "feminist credential[s] while simultaneously rationalizing and excusing workplace practices that discriminate against women and mothers." Held personally responsible for remediating institutional concerns such as a lack of childcare or equal pay, women were blamed for their inability to "think outside the box" should they fail to identify solutions.[40]

The opt-out narrative, then, has sustained warranted critical attention on multiple fronts, including for its elitist focus, lack of empirical support, and postfeminist politics that hold individual women responsible for systemic injustice. I revisit the opt-out narrative in order to interrogate a significant dimension of its form and function previously overlooked—specifically, its embeddedness within homeland security culture and related norms and values. Taking existing feminist analyses as a point of departure, I argue that the so-called opt-out revolution provides a clear example of homeland maternity, relentlessly relocating motherhood at the center of privileged women's lives and articulating maternal citizenship to broader cultural notions of security. In its celebration of wealthy, white motherhood, the opt-out revolution revived a version of republican motherhood responsive to dominant twenty-first-century ideologies—a version of republican motherhood that borrowed on gender essentialism while taking feminism into account.[41] In what follows, I trace the significance of the opt-out narrative to homeland maternity through its insistent focus on women of means, their mothering as their most significant contribution to public life, and, in a postfeminist twist, the articulation of opting out as the apex of women's empowerment. These claims bolster the significance of mothering to securing the homeland, emphasizing opting out as a means of managing a vulnerable world within the nuclear family unit.

Opting Out: Enacting Postfeminist Motherhood as Citizenship

The narrow elitism of the opt-out narrative positions elite women as exemplary mothers, worthy of public attention and accolades, resuscitating a twenty-first-century version of republican motherhood that aligned wealthy, white motherhood with the ideals of nation and citizenship. It is not simply that opt-out mothers were celebrated for their homemaking, but even more specifically for their maternal ambition—for their individual assertions that full-time motherhood was the most important use of their time and labor. As one stay-at-home mother told the *New York Times Magazine*: "I think some of us are swinging to a place where we enjoy, and can admit we enjoy, the stereotypical role of female/mother/caregiver. . . . I think we were born with those feelings." Fulfillment through mothering was naturalized and applauded through references to biology and differences between the sexes, as expressed by Duke University graduate, former attorney, and opt-out mom Vicky McElhaney Benedict: "'This is what I was meant to do. . . . I hate to say that because it sounds like I could have skipped college. But I mean this is what I was meant to do at this time. I know that's very un-p.c., but I like life's rhythms when I'm nurturing a child.'"[42] Another full-time mother, a former analyst with the Congressional Budget Office, affirmed this sense of maternal gratification in her interview with *60 Minutes*: "I think there's a lot of focus on what I'm sacrificing by staying home. And what's hard to articulate is how much I get back . . . I do it really—a lot of it is for me. I enjoy seeing and being with my children."[43] Underscoring traditional gender norms and family values conservativism, opt-out "revolutionaries" were culturally lauded for their embrace of *maternal citizenship*—not for their accomplishments in finance, government, or education, but rather, in their thorough dedication to raising children and embrace of the ideology of intensive mothering.

The logic of intensive mothering was reinforced throughout the opt-out narrative, even in the rare instance in which structural constraints on mothers' choices were explicitly discussed. A brief, counterpoint article embedded within the extended coverage of opting out in *Time*, titled "Why Women Have to Work," details the financial concerns that barred many women from staying at home. In emphasizing affordability (or lack thereof), however, its conclusions cohere with the aspirational telos of the opt-out narrative: "Why are today's mothers working so hard, putting in long hours at home and at the office? For the money."[44] The choice to continue working is referred to here as "no choice at all." In short, whether staying in the workforce or stopping out along the way, opt-out narratives asserted a new generation of US mothers as united in the belief that stay-at-home motherhood was ideal, if not always available to families. The return to traditionalism was frequently positioned in generational terms: "Gen Xers 'didn't want to have to make the kind of trade-offs the previous generation made. They're rejecting the stresses and sacrifices. . . . Both women and men rated personal and family goals higher than career goals.'"[45] Perhaps not surprisingly, however, only mothers were profiled in the opt-out exodus from the workplace, often figured as a kind of gendered generational realism: "What seems new is that while many of their mothers expected to have hard-charging careers, then scaled back their professional plans only after having children, the women of this generation expect their careers to take second place to child rearing."[46] In other words, despite feminist strides of the twentieth century that made it possible for some women to ascend in elite professions, women's fundamental desires had not changed. Rather, in a new generation of aspiring mothers, attitudes regarding work and family readjusted to align with women's "natural" interests in child-rearing and domesticity.

This emphasis on a generational divide functioned to frame opting-out as the most recent evolution in women's empowerment, a theme underscored in two distinct ways. First, opt-out narratives insisted that this was not a return to postwar containment culture, as in the *60 Minutes* report that posed the question: "Do any of [these mothers] wake up and say, 'I'm June Cleaver. I'm living in the '50s?,'" quickly refuting this sentiment with the words of opt-out mothers themselves: "'I don't think we are. I think that's wrong . . . I worked for 20 years after college. And so my experience in leaving to have children is different.'"[47] This point was readily and repeatedly emphasized: "These women say they don't feel they have anything to prove. They have been successful, and if they want to take some time out to be with their kids, why shouldn't they?"[48] Belkin's interviewees concurred: "'I am not a housewife. Is there still any such thing? I am doing what is right for me at the moment, not necessarily what is right for me forever'"; and "'Don't make me look like some 1950s Stepford wife. . . . I use my legal skills every day.'"[49] In other words, generational distinctions are marked within opt-out narratives so as to render any analogies to the 1950s erroneous, as Belkin clarifies: "Talk to any professional woman who made this choice, and this is what she will say. She is not her mother or her grandmother. She has made a temporary decision for just a few years, not a permanent decision for the rest of her life. She has not lost her skills, just put them on hold."[50] Similarly, in *Time*: "most of these women are choosing not so much to drop out as to stop out, often with every intention of returning . . . contrary to some popular reports, [this] is not a June Cleaver–ish embrace of old-fashioned motherhood but a new, nonlinear approach to building a career and an insistence on restoring some kind of sanity."[51] Rest assured, then, that this was not your postwar suburbia—generational differences included education, professional opportunity, and choice. Opting-out is distinct, in short, because women were actively locating motherhood at the center of their lives. Their maternal dedication resounded across post-9/11 US culture, garnering remarkable public attention and praise.

Second, and relatedly, the opt-out narrative advanced a failed account of mainstream feminism, repositioning opting out as the new women's empowerment. Relying heavily on choice rhetoric, opt-out narratives often puzzled over women's "rejection of the workplace," and used it as an index for the fundamentally misguided nature of twentieth-century feminist goals: "Look around these days, and you'll find women in positions of real power: a woman at the helm of the National Security Council, two Supreme Court justices, and female board members of every Fortune 100 company. It's just as it was supposed to be 40 years after women got in the front door. But look for the women of the next generation—the ones everyone assumed would follow in droves behind them, and you're likely to find many of them walking right back out and staying at home."[52] In lieu of using the opt-out revolution to underscore the urgency of feminist struggles for better working conditions, many of these narratives positioned opting out as the fullest expression of feminism itself. As *60 Minutes* interviewee Lisa Frelinghuysen explained: "I think the women's rights movement was very much about giving women choices and respecting the many choices that women make."[53] Or, in the words of opt-out mom Jeannie Tarkenton: "Women today, if we think about feminism at all, we see it as a battle fought for 'the choice.' For us, the freedom to choose work if we want to work is the feminist strain in our lives."[54] Thus, figuring traditional domestic arrangements as lifestyle preferences that were feminist simply by virtue of being "chosen," no matter how constrained or privileged those choices may be, these narratives faulted feminist ideology with generating unrealistic expectations and casted opting out as the contemporary exemplar of the freedom to choose.

Motherhood as Citizenship and Security in a Post-9/11 Nation

Opt-out narratives also advanced the notion of motherhood as a vehicle for citizenship and security for women of means. For example, opting out was frequently figured as the best means of safeguarding children in a context affectively marked by proliferating uncertainty and insecurity. Opt-out narratives positioned children's well-being and protection as uniquely maternal, both in their manifestation and in their inferred solution. In the words of Lisa Frelinghuysen: "I was afraid that if I was working, there would be no parent there with the children. And I wanted to experience getting to know my children, being there in a consistent way."[55] Children were figured as vulnerable in the absence of dedicated maternal care: "seeking clout in a male world does not correlate with child well-being. Today, striving for status usually means leaving your children with an au pair who's just there for a year, or in inadequate day care."[56] Thus, gender essentialism and maternal devotion were rendered requisite to children's safety and security. Moreover, ensuring that safety was figured as the core of feminine ambition: "So it's not that women aren't competitive [in the workforce]; it's just that they don't want to compete along the lines that are not compatible with their other [maternal] goals."[57] Similarly, in the 2004 *Time* cover story, "The Case for Staying Home," reporter Claudia Wallis generalized this sentiment to those of working mothers as a whole: "most women who step out of their careers find expected delights on the home front, not to mention the enormous relief of no longer worrying about shortchanging their kids. . . . Others appreciate a slow pace and being there when a child asks a tough question."[58] Thus, in opting out, women were "relieved" from concerns for their child's well-being and development, reinforcing the centrality of maternal care for children as well as various ills avoided through a woman's assertion of her primary caregiving role. Notably, the use of the term *home front* conjured the gravitas of domicile within US domestic affairs, articulating the importance of mothering in protecting and securing the interests of nation *within* its borders vis-à-vis the protection of the white, middle-class nuclear family itself.

The security interests of the nation were, on occasion, explicitly referenced within the opt-out narrative. For example, national concerns were woven into the fabric of opt-out mothering. As one opt-out mom noted in her interview with *60 Minutes*: "I think there's some people with preconceived notions that because I'm at home with my children all day, I must be preparing husband-delight casserole in a cocktail dress. The mothers['] groups get together and talk about Iraq policy."[59] Just as these remarks highlighted a clear break from retro visions of stay-at-home mothering, so too did they articulate opt-out motherhood as *uniquely* concerned with safety and security, signaled by attention to domesticity alongside concern over foreign policy. Indeed, this opt-out mom suggested that unlike their stressed and harried employed peers, opt-out mothers were able to dedicate significant time to matters of national concern. Moreover, this *60 Minutes* report aired in October 2003, when public controversy within the United States was steadily mounting in response to the military invasion and subsequent occupation of Iraq;[60] comments such as these aligned the labor of opt-out mothers with the most pressing political matters of the nation.

Another example of this alignment between (opt-out) motherhood and national interests was expressed in a series of anecdotes related to women in the public sector. In the opt-out exposé, Belkin noted some exemplary cases of female professionals who "have chosen to leave their high-powered jobs, most voluntarily, for lives that are less intense and more fulfilling. It's why President Bush's adviser Karen Hughes left the White house, saying her family was homesick and wanted to go back to Austin."[61] Mobilizing a twenty-first-century version of republican motherhood, maternal sacrifice was rendered in the service of the nation and its future citizenry. Belkin continued, shifting the focus from family and children in general to daughters specifically, underscoring the uniquely maternal responsibility for reproducing normative US families and gender relations: "And it's why Wendy Chamberlin, who was ambassador to Pakistan, resigned, because security concerns meant she never saw her two young daughters."[62] Both Hughes and Chamberlin were widely lauded for their decisions,[63] a phenomenon difficult to imagine possessing a paternal or masculine equivalent. Readers were invited to infer that women long dedicated to public service placed family first. This was, importantly, not only a priority that superseded professional employment writ large, but functioned as a venerated substitute for public service to the nation. It is a rationale rendered commonsensical through longstanding alignments of motherhood and nation—alignments that conflate elite white motherhood and citizenship and that allow white, wealthy families to function synecdochically for nation. As the United States was deeply entrenched in two wars overseas and the divisive cultural politics of so-called family values, elite motherhood was extolled as a substitute for high-ranking positions in foreign policy and security; opting out was cast as a means of managing the home front during times of heightened insecurity and vulnerability. Echoing broader cultural investments in homeland maternity, opt-out narratives functioned as a site for the figuration of elite motherhood as a central mode of post-9/11 citizenship. Its dictates reflected the ideologies of intensive mothering or the "new momism," but they were also notably and intimately written through the rhetoric of nation and security.

These mythic norms and narratives surrounding opt-out motherhood began to shift, however, in response to new economic realities. In 2007, as the global economy faltered, new narratives began to emerge around work and motherhood. Stay-at-home dads made headlines as women headed back to work—figured as the opt-out generation who wanted back in, applauded for a willingness to help their families weather the economic storm.[64] As one former breadwinner in the professional elite commented to the *New York Times* with respect to his recent unemployment: "frankly, having a wife who works or can readily join the work force is a good risk-management strategy."[65] But even as elite women's education and earning power eclipsed opting out as a "risk-management strategy," obligatory maternal responsibility persisted nonetheless. Motherhood proved no less culturally significant, but rather demanded different forms of management in the context of economic hardship. As opting out gave way to "leaning in," fertility preservation became a critical site of public concern, once again promoting elite women's childbearing and parenting in response to national insecurities.

Freezing for the Future

The pronatalist zeitgeist that followed in the wake of 9/11 shifted in response to new economic realities. From 2007 to 2009, as the United States suffered the worst economic recession since the 1930s, opting out and the mommy wars receded in dominant imaginaries as new maternal narratives emerged. During the economic crisis, campaigns aimed at young cosmopolitan women promoted fertility preservation through lifestyle enhancement and biomedical consumption. In the years of economic recovery that followed, fertility preservation discourses accelerated as changing trends in family and employment catalyzed additional public concerns. First, gendered segregation in employment fueled disparities in job loss during (and after) the recession.[66] Men were more vulnerable to unemployment—the economy shed 5.4 million jobs held by men compared to 2.1 million jobs held by women. While the recovery favored men, it was not enough to compensate for initial job loss—five years after the recession had officially ended, more than one in six men ages twenty-five to fifty-four were out of work, and 40 percent of those not working had been searching for employment for six months or more.[67] Second, job losses coincided with an uptick in multigenerational housing, declining rates in marriage and birth, and soaring numbers of breadwinner moms and stay-at-home dads.[68] As each of these trends commanded press, anxious speculation about family formation and the future of the nation captured the limelight. Headlines warned of a baby bust as mothers took primary responsibility for the economic security of their families and an increasing number of millennials were allegedly embracing, in the words of a 2013 *Time* cover, "The Childfree Life" (subtitled "When Having It All Means Not Having Children)."[69]

In the midst of revitalized conversations regarding work and family, newly infused with pronounced concern for the US economy and birth rate, Facebook executive Sheryl Sandberg published *Lean In: Women, Work, and the Will to Lead*.[70] The book remained on the *New York Times* bestseller list for months as mainstream media anointed Sandberg "the new voice of revolutionary feminism."[71] Prominent feminist thinkers however, including bell hooks and Susan Faludi, critiqued Sandberg's "faux feminism" for its trickle-down philosophy, ignorance of race and class, and misguided insistence on personal responsibility in response to structural disparities.[72] *Lean In* proved wildly successful nonetheless—a fact that can be attributed not only to its ambitious marketing campaign and star-studded celebrity network but also for its timing. Sandberg's book struck at the heart of public anxieties related to professional women's parenting in the wake of the Great Recession. Put simply, leaning in was the cultural corrective to opting out. Leaning in captured mainstream attention not only for its perky, postfeminist employment ethic, but also for its insistence on "having it all"—advocating an exuberant embrace of both work and motherhood. Corporate and opportunistic, this version of "feminism" simultaneously promoted women's reproductivity while shoring up postrecession labor demands.

I note economic data and the heated public discussions sparked by *Lean In* to better contextualize the form and function of postrecession fertility preservation discourses. Despite the facts that most fertility problems are unrelated to age, infertility impacts males and females equally, and the average decline in female fertility prior to age forty is slower and less consequential than headlines indicate,[73] dominant public discourse suggested otherwise. Popular women's magazines were particularly vocal about infertility, and the panic was palpable. Headlines blared: "Protect Your Fertility: What You Can Do Now to Safeguard Your Chances of Motherhood Later"[74] and cautioned against waiting "too long" and "playing Russian roulette with your chance to be a mom."[75] In unsettling references to the body as an appliance or depreciating asset (e.g., "baby-making machinery"),[76] readers were drawn into the preemptive paradigm and urged to plan for conception one, five, or even ten years in advance. Magazines offered "preconception checklist[s]" and promoted a range of preventive "lifestyle tweaks" in order to safeguard fertility, "from when to have sex to what not to eat."[77] Consistent themes punctuated these "pre-baby correction course[s]":[78] achieving a "healthy" body mass index (BMI), consuming a whole-foods diet, regular exercise and vaccinations, stress management, relaxation, and abstinence from caffeine, nicotine, alcohol, and other substances. The advice echoed a trend toward what Miranda Waggoner terms "anticipatory motherhood," wherein women's health care is eclipsed by prenatal care, regardless of maternal status or intent.[79] As managing fertility was likened to combat (e.g., "Women once waited until their biological clocks had almost popped a spring before bringing out the big guns"), "smart young women" were figured as powerful agents in determining the course of their reproductive lives by leaving nothing "to chance."[80] Thus, the promise of a fertile future hinged on savvy, postfeminist consumption—investing in knowledge acquisition and acting in accordance with its dictates. Much like other postfeminist health narratives, the DIY fertility guides in popular women's magazines figured women as both "vulnerable" and "empowered,"[81] assumed the primacy of domesticity in women's lives, and asserted their responsibility to secure the possibility of motherhood for the future.

As women were goaded to take charge of their fertility amid postrecession realities, a breakthrough in reproductive medicine captivated mainstream publics, emerging right alongside the clarion call to lean in. Oocyte preservation, or egg freezing, was widely celebrated for silencing the biological clock, leveling the professional playing field, and rendering menopause passé. Pioneering women in journalism and academia such as Diane Sawyer and Marcia Inhorn endorsed egg freezing to their protégées[82] as private fertility clinics, third-party brokers, and professional associations targeted young female professionals through posh educational soirees.[83] Cryopreservation was featured in the 2012 PBS documentary *My Future Baby* and two popular books blending journalism and memoir: Rachel Lehman-Haupt's 2009 *In Her Own Sweet Time* and Sarah Elizabeth Richards's 2013 *Motherhood, Rescheduled*. Egg freezing provided sensational headlines from *Bloomberg Businessweek* to *Bust* magazine, and its public profile was heightened through celebrity: in 2012 Kim Kardashian decided to freeze her eggs in her early thirties, bringing viewers with her on *Keeping Up with the Kardashians*.

The sudden interest was not necessarily due to the novelty of egg freezing, for it was not a new reproductive technology. Early attempts at egg freezing were designated experimental due to low rates of fertilization and pregnancy success, and selectively made available to women of childbearing age who were facing severe medical prognoses. However, the development of a new technique—vitrification, or flash freezing—enabled its mainstreaming. Based on new and promising success rates, the American Society for Reproductive Medicine lifted its experimental label on oocyte preservation in 2012, a decision endorsed by the American College of Obstetricians and Gynecologists,[84] and one that fueled public interest and the availability of services.[85] With age figured throughout dominant discourses as the ultimate nonnegotiable, the promise of freezing the biological clock via oocyte preservation arrived just in the nick of time.

My analysis in the remainder of this chapter centers on the treatment of egg freezing in dominant publications aimed at women of reproductive age, including feature articles in mainstream news outlets, popular women's magazines, and the 2012 monograph *Motherhood, Rescheduled* penned by award-winning freelance writer Sarah Elizabeth Richards. Egg freezing commanded the spotlight in the midst of frenzied public attention to securing the possibility of motherhood—particularly for women whose childbearing has long been imagined as a vehicle for nation building. As opting out proved increasingly untenable even for women of extraordinary means, dominant discourses regarding motherhood and fertility insisted on a different kind of security. Rather than position opt-out motherhood as a form of homeland security, the logic of security was marshaled to preserve elite women's fertility and motherhood through cryopreservation.

The logic of security was predicated on preemption and functioned on two distinct levels, one individual and another collective. First, egg freezing discourses aimed at women of reproductive age focused on the personal, affective dimensions of infertility. These discourses traded on the logic of preemption—exacerbating fertility panics and promising to assuage them simultaneously through the personal security made available through cryopreservation. Second, these discourses converged with those aimed at a broader population to underscore the cultural gains of egg freezing, celebrating its development as an expression of twenty-first-century feminism and promoting a form of personal security that squared comfortably with the demands of the nation.

Preempting Infertility and the Personal Quest for Security

Popular women's magazines devoted significant attention to egg freezing, often fueling fertility panics even as they demonstrated some sensitivity to the difficult emotional terrain of infertility. The lead to a 2013 series of articles "all about your eggs" in *Cosmopolitan* read: "You're panicked at the idea of having kids now and panicked at the idea of not having them later. . . . When it comes to fertility, has freaking out become the new normal?"[86] A cover story in *Bust* magazine titled "Chill Out" offered little affirmation of childfree women or critique of dominant fertility panics—despite a headline that might suggest otherwise—but rather championed egg freezing technologies. The writer erroneously declared: "Most of us know that by the time we hit 30, our fertility is on the decline. But what many don't realize is that the slide is a fast one."[87] In media coverage of egg freezing, women were confronted with alarming and inaccurate statistics, reminded that fertility "peaks" in their twenties and "plunges" in their thirties.[88] An essay in *Cosmopolitan* titled "Should You Freeze Your Eggs?" warned: "Female fertility declines slightly around age 28 and then plunges after 35. Not only do eggs decrease in number, but they are also more likely to be damaged, which can prevent fertilization."[89] Lest clarity be lacking, the article continued: "So why should egg freezing be on your radar? Although the procedure was originally aimed at women nearing 40, the fact is, 20- and early 30-somethings are the best candidates." The prose is situated alongside a full-page photo of small, brown bird eggs resting on ice, as an indecorous caption declared: "Just like these, your eggs have an expiration date."[90] Fertility panic was thus simultaneously acknowledged and exacerbated. Despite scientific evidence that challenges popular myths regarding age-related infertility, the savvy, independent woman was bombarded with inaccurate information about her ticking biological clock and her responsibility to *do something* about it, specifically in the form of biotechnology consumption.

As fertility panics were exacerbated and assuaged, women were urged to take charge—to act preemptively so as to preserve their fertility and, relatedly, their future. Egg freezing was positioned as insurance, a powerful means of building a personal safety net, a sense of security: "When a woman freezes her eggs, two things happen: She comes to terms with the fact that her fertility is fading, and she invests significant time, energy and money in protecting that asset."[91] Mobilizing the metaphor of investment and risk management, egg freezing was constituted as, in one writer's words, "a baby insurance policy."[92] As biological insurance, egg freezing was imagined as an investment in one's future reproductivity and motherhood: "Freezing now is insurance (sort of) for later. According to the latest census, 18 percent of women don't have a child by age 44, and for those with a master's degree or higher, it spikes to 24 percent—not always by choice."[93] Echoing Hewlett's thesis, egg freezing discourses noted a "fertility penalty" for high-achieving women and described oocyte preservation as a process that allowed women to take control of their reproductive and maternal destinies. This sentiment is expressed in a first-person narrative in *Glamour*: "As I punched the 7 key, it hit me: I was two years past the magic age of 35, when fertility starts to plummet—and I still didn't have kids. . . . I might not have enough time to 'think about it some more' before I became infertile. I restarted the elliptical and resolved to *do* something, and six months later, I walked out of the recovery room at a fertility clinic where doctors had extracted 13 eggs from me, eight of which were deemed good enough to freeze."[94] This writer noted that she wasn't freezing because of a medical diagnosis; rather, as a "social freezer" she was "building a career and a fabulous life, and since some of the 300,000 eggs you have at puberty disappear every day, you want to save a few good ones *just in case*" (original emphasis).[95] Egg freezing, then, is figured as risk management, as an investment that affords some measure of protection from infertility and the promise of maternal security in later life. The rhetoric of indemnity was bolstered by industry professionals, evidenced, for example, in the naming of third-party broker EggBanxx and articulated by Dr. Jamie Grifo of the prestigious New York University Fertility Center: "Right now, it's kind of an insurance policy to be your own egg donor, but with limited success. And that's the way we present it, so that women can make an informed decision and decide if it's worth the time and energy and money."[96] While the metaphor of investment occasionally included vague references to the wealth that egg freezing necessitates, its primary function was to fold egg freezing into articulations of postfeminist responsibility for managing one's life, on a literal—biological and molecular—level.

The biological security purchased through egg freezing as a form of "insurance" was reinforced through repeated emphasis on the psychological dimensions of egg freezing: "With every egg I stashed away, I moved further away from the persona of the sad girl whose baby-making window was closing and back to the hopeful girl who always had *someday*" (original emphasis).[97] Egg freezing discourses emphasized resulting calm, confidence, and relief from the pressures of the biological clock. *Vogue* interviewed "willowy 35-year-old media company executive" Leah, who confessed: "Freezing my eggs is my little secret. . . . I want to feel there's a backup plan. I don't want to waste the next few years in a state of panic, or feel terrible every time I hear that one of my married friends is pregnant."[98] Indeed, egg freezing was regularly situated as a solution to cultural pressures regarding aging and infertility, as marketing executive and Eggsurance blogger Brigitte Adams explained: "I think what it did emotionally for me, and what it does for a lot of women, is it gives you this sense of calmness. . . . It's a hell of a lot better than sitting back and waiting for my life to fly by."[99] This sense of personal control through preemption is affirmed and promoted by experts, as Sarah Elizabeth Richards recounts after attending a seminar on egg freezing: "Dr. Georgia Witkin, the clinic's house psychologist, told us what the chunk of cash really bought us: a sense of control over our lives. 'It's just in case,' she explained. 'It's not that women plan to use them. They just want to know they've done everything they could.'"[100]

This emphasis on personal control and security was emphatically normative, refuting common characterizations of egg freezing as frivolity or materialism. The psychological benefits of egg freezing were not centered on *relieving* cultural pressures surrounding heteronuclear family formation and childbearing, but rather as *better facilitating* this possibility, obliging women to "get serious" about their romantic and personal lives: "Why doesn't a woman who freezes her eggs ever get credit for proactively seeking a solution to her so-called problem of waiting to have a baby? Why isn't she celebrated for enduring hormone shots and emptying her bank account in order to have a better chance of finding a partner and father for her children, avoiding birth defects, and becoming financially secure so she can hold up her end of marriage or support a family?" Here we have a clear figuration of egg freezing as consonant with traditional US family formation, a means for women to manage—on an individual level—new economic realities alongside the mythic American dream. Indeed, the writer continues, offering an explicit tie to values of nation: "This 'take charge' attitude is one of our most fundamental American values. Seen this way, egg freezing isn't an act of desperation or indulgence. Rather, it's an act of love for her future family."[101] Tapping into a rich cultural archive, egg freezing was figured at the center of a constellation of sacrosanct US values—family, love, and hope—alongside the requirements of citizenship that include self-reliant individualism and exerting control over one's future, both for oneself and the nation.

This alignment of egg freezing with "American values" was not an anomaly. The sentiment was reinforced through rigorous assertions of traditional white femininity, as egg freezing was articulated as an important aid for women whose lives and fertility "veered off course."[102] Long-term romance and heteronuclear family formation were imagined as outcomes of oocyte preservation: "once you put eggs on ice, it can impact your dating life in dramatic ways. Rena, 37, a media consultant in Washington, D.C., put away 31 eggs from multiple rounds of freezing three years ago. She says she now feels more calm and confident."[103] Thus, egg freezing functioned as a vehicle for a familiar and resonant femininity. Not only did women "relax," but they were drawn to motherhood with considerable resolve: "Paul [my boyfriend] had awakened my longing to have children, but the act of freezing made me commit to it."[104] Other women's reflections on post-freezing priorities underscored renewed romantic ambition: "She was done wasting time waiting for love and was simply managing her [romantic] pipeline as she would a project for work. Dating should have been as important as this all along."[105] Recast as evidence of a deep commitment to motherhood and reproductive futurity, oocyte preservation "doesn't silence the biological clock. Rather, it temporarily dulls the ticking so you can catch your breath and make good life choices . . . instead of feeling like a victim paralyzed by anxiety, you feel more in command of your own destiny."[106] The promise of egg freezing as a kind of security was imagined at the nexus of several powerful vectors—as an embodiment of US values and gendered family formation under the banner of individual empowerment.

As if to endorse this sensibility, the voices of men and industry professionals were invoked to articulate egg freezing as a signal of confidence, maternal ambition, and desirable femininity. A *Glamour* article titled, "What He Thinks about Your, Um, Eggs," was composed in the first person by Jake, "a real single guy dating in Los Angeles," who described his response to his date's frozen eggs as a mixture of intrigue and relief: "For men, women's biological clocks are like gluten-free nachos or *The Bachelor*. We know these things exist—we just prefer to pretend they don't. It's not that men are afraid of having kids (OK, we are a little afraid); it's that we don't want to be conscious of human biology forcing the issue. When that happens, romance flies out the window and we stop seeing you. Instead, we just see that clock ticking." In this masculinist response to egg freezing, complete with references to monster trucks, hot dog-eating contests, and an analogizing of cryopreservation to "Han Solo in carbonite," Jake's testimony framed egg freezing as a turn on: "men—and romance—need that space. . . . I was impressed that the Egg Lady put reality on ice, literally, not just because it took the pressure off me but because it showed me immediately that she was strong and decisive. That's part of why we made it to our second date."[107] Egg freezing is, in a word, sexy. Lest women doubt that their internal confidence and calm would translate into a relationship, the occasional punctuation of women's first-person narratives with men's voices figured egg freezing as a catalyst for heterosexual desire and romance: "many guys appreciated my frozen fertility: 'This means I can have kids whenever I want,' I told them, 'and I don't have to rush relationships.' Soon I was juggling several dates a week."[108] Industry representatives reinforced this message, emphasizing the role of advanced biotechnology in securing love and family formation: "Two months after Extend [Fertility] founder Jones froze her eggs, she got engaged. She told me of several others whose relationship moved forward after they banked their eggs. We theorized there was a 'freezing effect': When you threw The Clock out the window, you relaxed, he relaxed, and life moved along as it should."[109] The security afforded through egg freezing was at once a shrewd form of family planning for the modern sophisticated gal, as well as a means of securing relational—even marital—success in the long term. In this way, egg freezing was regularly articulated to an individual sense of security through multiple voices and contexts. It was figured as an important preventive measure—a cosmopolitan form of insurance against an aging reproductive body, a means of establishing psychological wellness in the midst of intense cultural pressures regarding motherhood and family life, and a stimulus for romance, love, and heteronuclear family formation.[110]

Preempting Infertility and Securing the Nation

The security wrought through egg freezing was not exclusively individual. The cultural promise of egg freezing was imagined along two distinct, if overlapping, vectors—written into narratives of twenty-first-century female empowerment that squared comfortably with postrecession economic realities. As popular women's magazines dedicated significant attention to the personal dimensions of fertility preservation, dominant media (including women's magazines but also media aimed at a broader segment of the population) centered on securing the productive and reproductive labor of elite women as a vital resource for the nation through the rhetoric of women's empowerment.

Egg freezing was widely lauded as the quintessential expression of twenty-first-century feminism, a claim that dovetailed conveniently with shifting trends in work and family life in the United States. On its cover, *Bloomberg Businessweek* declared egg freezing "a new fertility procedure giv[ing] women more choices in the quest to have it all."[111] Writing for CNN, Marcia Inhorn described egg freezing as a "technological game changer that enables women "to effectively rewind their biological clock, becoming mothers in their 40s, 50s and beyond. . . . [it] just might allow women to defy the notion that they can't have it all."[112] In a similar vein, Sarah Elizabeth Richards argued in the *Wall Street Journal*: "Amid all the talk about women 'leaning in' and 'having it all,' the conversation has left out perhaps the most powerful gender equalizer of all—the ability to control when we have children."[113] Once again glossing over the extraordinary wealth that egg freezing necessitates, references to reproductive control through biotechnology situated egg freezing as individual empowerment and the pinnacle expression of twenty-first-century feminism: "We are witnessing an unprecedented time in history. Women have enjoyed more opportunity in nearly every area of their lives, except the ability to have children . . . if technology can temporarily compensate by adding another layer of choice, that is a reprieve indeed."[114] In this moment, we are invited to understand egg freezing as a breakthrough feminist technology, a radical leap forward on a progressive linear narrative of women's liberation.

This sentiment was reinforced through personal narratives: "no matter how scary information was at first, it's ultimately liberating to understand my own body's reproductive possibilities—as well as its impossibilities. We have more options than ever. Understanding them can empower us and, perhaps more importantly, turn panic into peace."[115] This sense of empowerment through biological control permeated discussions of egg freezing, and was attached to cryopreservation technology itself: "On the way home [from an Extend Fertility seminar], my eyes started to water. For once, it didn't matter that I'd frittered away my 20s with a man I loved but did not want to marry. Science would save me."[116] More often than not, however, egg freezing discourses attributed agency and control to the savvy, cosmopolitan woman opting in to biomedicine: "She's about to join the vanguard of what may be the most significant social change since the advent of the Pill, taking a technological step that in just the past year has emerged as a real option for women."[117] Thus reliant on postfeminist rhetorics of choice, egg freezing was decisively figured as a means of empowerment that enabled women to govern their lives to an extent unimaginable to earlier generations.

References to oral contraceptives (the Pill) were frequent and, more often than not, used to advance an unfinished, even failed, account of feminism. The Pill was often metonymically invoked within egg freezing discourses to frame cryopreservation as a logical extension of family planning, a complimentary corrective to delayed childbearing. The *Bloomberg* article noted: "Not since the birth control pill has a medical technology had such potential to change family and career planning."[118] As patient and advocate Brigitte Adams stated: "Our lives have changed so much since our mothers' generation. . . . They had the revolution of the pill, and I really think that egg freezing is that revolution for us. It's giving us the gift of time."[119] Some references were less flattering. Simultaneously conflated with and maligned as feminism itself, the Pill was critiqued for having an injurious effect on fertility that then necessitated egg freezing as a corrective. On the fiftieth anniversary of the Pill, the cover of *New York Magazine* in December 2010 featured a close-up of a young white woman's unadorned face, her tongue stuck out in steady defiance, a round white pill placed squarely in its center. The headline declared: "Fifty years ago, the pill ushered in a new era of sexual freedom. It might have created a fertility crisis as well." Feminism and the Pill were figured as catalysts for a supposed epidemic of infertility throughout this article. Citing individual women who, in gaining "control of their bodies" were able "to forget their basic biology—until in some cases, it's too late," the author emphasized that if women remain unaware of their biological clock, then the Pill has compounded this ignorance in facilitating carefree sexual expression and childbearing delayed indefinitely. Egg freezing, then, was positioned as the solution: "There's an easy answer to this conundrum, even though it's a little weird: freezing eggs in one's twenties."[120] If, in true backlash form, feminism and the Pill were to blame for an epidemic, then oocyte preservation was articulated as the new feminist utopia, a technological horizon of hope and possibility. This logic was echoed in other outlets as well, as in a *Vogue* essay: "Stopping the biological clock through egg freezing has long been the ultimate feminist fantasy. The Pill was the first step, enabling women to delay childbearing, a revolution that profoundly altered society. But over the past five decades, the price we've paid has been age-related infertility, on an epic scale."[121] Rendered commonsense by the mobilization of a mythic narrative of skyrocketing infertility—and in a bizarre postfeminist twist—feminism was figured as both *the impetus for* and *the logical outgrowth of* egg freezing.

It was precisely in this relationship to feminism (and postfeminism) that egg freezing discourses echoed those surrounding the opt-out revolution. Moreover, each was imagined to bolster a sense of security by offering elite women greater clarity regarding their relational lives and underscoring motherhood once more as the pinnacle expression of white womanhood—and, importantly, in a manner strikingly consistent with the economic realities and ideological desires of the nation. And yet, unlike the opt-out revolution, egg freezing was publicly promoted for facilitating participation in the professional workforce. Headlines in dominant outlets included "Egg Freezing Puts the Biological Clock on Hold," "DNA on Ice: The Next Step in Women's Equality," and "Freeze Your Eggs, Free Your Career."[122] In a 2014 *Bloomberg Businessweek* feature, egg freezing was lauded for its potential to integrate love, family, and work: "Like many others who've frozen their eggs, Emily uses the word 'empowered' to describe the experience. She thinks it will allow her to date without radiating the desperation of someone who has to have a baby right this very second. And now she doesn't feel as guilty about dedicating most of her time to work."[123] A woman interviewed in *Cosmopolitan* reported feeling "a new peace of mind. 'This was something that helped me take control of my life,' she says. 'I can continue to focus on my company now and let love happen in its own time.'"[124] This refrain was contradictory and twofold. It hinged on mythic notions of women's liberation gone awry, evidenced in the familiar caricature of the neurotic, single thirtysomething woman who pursues professional success to the detriment of her personal life. But concurrently, egg freezing was publicly promoted as an extension of lifestyle feminism, as yet another "choice" for the independent postfeminist career gal who withholds social critique as "a condition of her freedom."[125] Feminism was thus imagined as the cause of infertility as postfeminist consumption was enlisted as its purported solution, emerging precisely at the moment when "having it all" was consonant with the needs of the nation.

The profound economic precarity engendered by the pursuit of egg freezing was largely absent from these discussions. Egg freezing requires considerable wealth and scheduling dexterity. A single cycle of egg retrieval ranges from $10,000 to $15,000; most women undergo multiple rounds of egg retrieval in order to store the number of eggs recommended by fertility specialists. Unlike the Pill, which is comparatively affordable and democratic (insofar as it suggests the possibility that women's reproductive control might reside in their own hands), egg freezing relies on significant personal wealth and medical intervention, relocating reproductive control to fertility specialists and clinics. These are issues rarely interrogated within mainstream egg freezing narratives. Thus, in a moment remarkable for its candor and anomalous character, Richards observes in her memoir, "it began to sink in that I had left myself financially vulnerable. I had traded my financial backup for a fertility backup."[126] The rarity of this reflection underscores both the quality and kind of security afforded through egg freezing. In the context of global economic uncertainty and employment scarcity, egg freezing is touted as an act of feminist empowerment and independence *in spite of* the significant financial insecurity it likely engenders; it is imagined as a desirable form of security because it preserves the possibility of motherhood no matter the cost, but particularly for an exclusive demographic of women with access to significant wealth.

As such, egg freezing is promoted as a technological panacea for a narrow demographic—the tool for early twenty-first-century women of means to single-handedly level the playing field. Egg freezing discourses relentlessly reify postfeminist femininity, fetishize individual consumption as a vehicle of women's empowerment, and reduce feminism to personal decision making. This kind of "choice feminism," as Michaele Ferguson explains, "is radically depoliticizing . . . it shuts down critical discussion about which choices should be valued and which choices are mere illusions, it uncritically embraces consumerism, and most problematically for the future of feminism, it deters women from being active in politics to improve childcare, public schools, and working conditions."[127] And indeed, as postrecession economic conditions rendered opting out obsolete, gendered inequities within organizational settings began to register within mainstream public discourse. "Leaning in" was questioned for its elitist individualism, the inordinate demands of working motherhood began to make headlines, and the Obama administration pushed for paid family leave during the economic recovery.[128] It was precisely in this moment that egg freezing was widely touted as *the* twenty-first-century feminist revolution, the most radical innovation since the Pill. In short, just as broader public debates surrounding gendered workplace inequities surfaced, egg freezing was imagined as the neoliberal substitute for structural redress, all in the name of feminism.

This is perhaps most clearly evidenced not only in the timing of egg freezing's mainstream embrace, but also in the temporary backlash against it. A momentary rupture within this laudatory narrative emerged in response to two major tech companies' decisions to offer egg freezing as a health care benefit, as a part of comprehensive "reproductive insurance" plans for their employees. Following the announcements of these policies in 2014, Facebook and Apple were located at the center of a media firestorm; each company faced significant public criticism and speculations about a brave new world, evidenced by headlines that declared "Egg Freezing a Better Deal for Companies than for Women," "Egg Freezing 'Benefit' Sends the Wrong Message to Women," and "Why We Should Be Alarmed that Apple and Facebook Are Paying for Employee Egg Freezing."[129] Significant and valid criticisms, including those that discuss the absence of structural support for women in the workforce, were raised within these articles and public debates; they echo a range of concerns previously raised by feminist bloggers and policy analysts when mainstream publications began to sing the praises of egg freezing for women.[130]

What remains worthy of mention, however, is both the timing and substance of these critiques. For it is not the case that egg freezing was subject to intense forms of public criticism in general, but rather, that it was interrogated as "bad for women" at the moment of its inclusion within employee benefits packages. Unlike most workplace environments in the United States, Facebook, and to a lesser extent Apple, have institutionalized support systems in order to make the workplace more welcoming to women, families, and work-life balance; they are, in fact, giants in an industry renowned in the United States for generous workplace benefits.[131] Thus, while corporate-sponsored egg freezing is certainly worthy of feminist suspicion and critique, the fact that oocyte preservation benefits became the catalyst for public criticism in an otherwise celebratory narrative of a technological "revolution" for women affords insight into cultural attitudes and beliefs. Egg freezing, it seems, is to be celebrated so long as it is relegated to individual women's management of structural forms of gendered inequity; it is to be lauded so long as it participates in the broader narrative that elevates motherhood above all else in women's lives. It is decidedly suspect, however, when included as one of many options within workplace infrastructure. The postfeminist logic of choice is evidenced here in its most exaggerated and grotesque form—free and fully supported so long as it is made available exclusively through the market; in other words, as a luxury for elite women, predicated on a commitment to individualism, consumption, and a withholding of political critique. Egg freezing enables women to "opt in" to both work and motherhood successfully as long as they possess the capital to do so, solidifying an exclusive—and thus, for the nation, "desirable"—market for this technology.

Of course, these dominant discourses did not circulate without challenge. As egg freezing was figured through rhetorics of security and empowerment, several feminist writers and activists critiqued the postfeminist logics at work, including attempts to substitute individualism for solidarity on behalf of better working conditions for all women and their families. As a feminist scholar, I share these concerns. I would add to them a cultivated and necessary sensitivity to significant discursive consistencies across the twenty-first-century landscape of maternal and reproductive politics—in other words, a concern for the persistence of homeland maternity as a primary operating logic that fuels the valorization of elite motherhood and mobilizes various cultural forces on its behalf. Put another way, the public attention devoted to egg freezing and DIY fertility safeguards did not function in isolation, or even simply as additional examples of postfeminism in popular culture. Rather, these discourses worked in concert with broader cultural trends that bolstered national interests, promoting motherhood for women of means in homeland security culture.

Homeland Maternity: Reviving Republican Motherhood in the Early 21st Century

From the opt-out revolution to fertility preservation and egg freezing campaigns, elite professional women in the wake of national crises were publicly scrutinized for "underperforming" in the arena of biological reproduction. Across a range of discourses and settings, motherhood was reanimated as an ideal for white women of means—not simply a cultural expectation, but figured as an innate desire, one central to personal happiness, success, and security. In the aftermath of 9/11, the opt-out revolution helped to resuscitate republican motherhood for the twenty-first century, recasting domesticity as requisite to the future of the nation and as the pinnacle expression of feminism itself. Years later, in concert with a global recession, collective fears over an impending "baby bust," and the rise of lean-in feminism, the economic necessity of women's paid labor was met with a powerful surge in pronatalism that reminded cosmopolitan women to safeguard their fertility as a key dimension of personal happiness and security, both reproductive and otherwise—and importantly, in ways that aligned conveniently with the longstanding articulation of motherhood to nation. Thus, consistent with histories of antifeminist backlash and particularly salient during times of collectively felt insecurity, US mothers of means were charged with a specific form of homeland security—securing the home front through domesticity and investments in reproductive futurity.

These struggles over elite motherhood in homeland security culture reflect a range of persistent public concerns regarding work, family, and citizenship. They animate contemporary ambivalences and anxieties regarding how elite women contribute to the nation, in their dedication to labor within public and private spheres. And as republican motherhood is reinvented for the twenty-first century, feminism is insidiously, in Angela McRobbie's words, "taken into account"—incorporated into a narrative that both assumes the successes of feminist struggles as it simultaneously resists and undermines ongoing sites of feminist critique. The opt-out revolution, pre-pregnancy fertility directives, and the public embrace of egg freezing constitute specific moments with remarkable consistencies; they illustrate the cultural requirements and constraints of elite female citizenship in homeland security culture as tethered to motherhood and to reproducing the nation.

Thus, interrogating the recent history of pronatalist campaigns in US culture illuminates one of many significant dimensions of homeland maternity. It clarifies how homeland maternity bears meaningfully on elite women's status and citizenship in the early twenty-first century. Even as opting out was challenged on multiple fronts and debunked as media-driven mythology, its cultural force persisted, helping to resurrect and reinvent the archetype of the domestic goddess for the twenty-first century. And in the wake of the great recession, this archetype was recast as young cosmopolitan women were directed to opt back in, made individually responsible for juggling motherhood and employment by caring for their reproductive futurity diligently as they contributed meaningfully to economic growth. The power of these mythic norms regarding elite motherhood were, and continue to be, amplified across various cultural sites. Mothers of status are showered with public accolades and scrutiny alike, from Mom-in-Chief Michelle Obama and global mother-ambassador Angelina Jolie to Yahoo's working mother of infamy Marissa Meyer. Some women have launched lucrative careers by capitalizing on maternal cachet, cataloging daily joys and conundrums in the mommy blogosphere or securing reality star status for extraordinary fertility that garners varying degrees of public praise and ridicule.[132] Consistent across this tumultuous terrain is the mythic status of motherhood, its valorization as the pinnacle of elite womanhood and, in a postfeminist twist, the apex of women's empowerment. Indeed, the "retro wife" has been recently heralded for her return; today's feminists are (once again) allegedly "having it all—by choosing to stay home."[133]

The focus on elite women's childbearing and dedication to motherhood is but one dimension of homeland maternity. A fuller account of this phenomenon requires careful attention to its differential impacts, to how homeland maternity intensifies the requirements of motherhood while disciplining those who cannot, do not, or refuse to adhere.

CHAPTER 2

Risky Reproduction and the Politics of Octomom

Infertility treatment for an unemployed, single mother of six? Eight embryos in one womb? There must be a proper word in the medical literature to describe this achievement. I think the word is "nuts."

—Ellen Goodman, *New York Times*

All I wanted was to be a mom. That's all I ever wanted in my life.

—Nadya Suleman

On January 26, 2009, Natalie (Nadya) Suleman gave birth to octuplets in a hospital southeast of Los Angeles, assisted in conception by her fertility specialist and in delivery by a medical team of forty-six. Believed to be septuplets until the last moment of delivery, the Suleman eight were only the second set of octuplets born in US history and, within a week, were the longest surviving. When news first broke of the Suleman birth, awe and celebration reverberated through US reporting. But what was initially heralded as a story of medical miracle was not to last. As dimensions of Suleman's circumstances were revealed—a single, thirty-three-year-old woman of European and Southwest Asian descent receiving food stamps and disability payments with six young children already at home—she was quickly located at the center of a public firestorm. Questions surfaced regarding a range of concerns, from the ethics of fertility therapies—their regulation or lack thereof—to the sanity of Suleman herself. These discourses constitute the archive of this chapter, in which I trace the prominence and function of the rhetoric of risk as it constitutes another dimension of homeland maternity.

Homeland maternity is a central underlying dynamic for how some mothers are publicly venerated as others are maligned and punished; Nadya Suleman's story is exemplary in demonstrating these dynamics at work. In her attempt to wed assisted reproductive technologies (ART) with public assistance, Suleman threatened to collapse longstanding and significant cultural distinctions between "deserving" and "undeserving" mothers. Public discourse pathologized Suleman, eviscerating her claim to motherhood while lending velocity to supposedly neutral rhetorics of risk that are increasingly used to position pregnant people against the fetuses they carry in contemporary US culture. Recent scholarship has theorized risk as a socially constructed phenomenon and a mode of contemporary governance, all the more powerful for its claim to objectivity. In the case of Nadya Suleman, I argue that risk was rhetorically constructed vis-à-vis a deeply racialized and classed notion of pathological motherhood, marking Suleman as an unruly reproductive body, a perpetrator of risk, and a threat to be contained through an assertion of medical authority. As a central feature of homeland maternity, the rhetoric of risk persists as a powerful presence in contemporary reproductive politics, policing the motherhood of marginalized women in particular and asserting the primacy of medical—or even state—authorities in regulating the reproduction and motherhood of low-income women, immigrant women, single women, and/or women of color.

A critical interrogation of the public discord surrounding the birth of the Suleman octuplets thus clarifies the differential dimensions of homeland maternity. The previous chapter, focusing on the veneration of elite motherhood in opt-out discourse and the zealous marketing of egg freezing technologies to young professional women, theorizes homeland maternity as an extension of republican motherhood, anchored in recent pronatalist discourses that infuses elite motherhood with unparalleled cultural significance and contribution, aligning it with citizenship, virtue, and the security of the nation. Women of means are encouraged to pursue motherhood at any cost, to spare no expense, and to enlist extensive, even experimental, reproductive technologies as necessary in order to secure future prospects of becoming a mother. The story of the Suleman octuplets also emerged in the wake of the economic recession, but its unfolding is markedly distinct from the pronatalist discourses urging elite women to contemplate fertility preservation. As a powerful exemplar of homeland maternity that points to its uneven distribution and effects, Suleman's story demonstrates that the claim to venerable motherhood is far from universal; that reproductive technologies have never been imagined to benefit just anyone who struggled with infertility. While ART access is notoriously uneven given its steep price tag, the Suleman saga represents a unique moment of cultural rupture wherein the informal social and economic barriers to assisted reproduction were decisively breached and thus rendered visible. The public struggles that ensued in an attempt to fortify once more the borders of "legitimate" ART consumption were predicated on longstanding attitudes regarding pathological reproduction and motherhood, recast in the context of homeland maternity through the rhetoric of risk.

Scholarship concerning the Suleman case is sparse, despite the significant discord her case provoked and the centrality of public discourses in organizing its resolution. Existing scholarship is written largely from legal perspectives, responding to calls for regulation and industry reform, with little consideration afforded the communicative and cultural forces that fueled such calls for reform.[1] For years, Suleman was featured regularly in tabloid culture, mainstream media, and fertility industry and public policy disputes. Her story has inspired a musical, a doll with eight detachable babies, a made-for-television documentary, and a reality series. She was consistently depicted in mainstream media as self-obsessed and attention seeking, less routinely but not infrequently described as insane, pathological, criminal, a metonym for everything wrong with a range of institutions—California, the welfare state, the cult of celebrity, and media's reward of "unconscionable" excess. The blogosphere has proved frighteningly misogynist, containing references to Suleman as a "child hoarder," "psychotic bitch," "Octo-cu-t," and a "dirty specimen of a mammal." She and her publicists received multiple death threats; in a particularly xenophobic and racialized post, Suleman was falsely accused of getting IVF (in vitro fertilization) treatments in Mexico and "crawling across the border" to give birth.

This degree of public contempt urges careful exploration of the logics through which such fury is marshaled, how it is rhetorically deployed, and to what ends. For embedded within these public discourses are deeply ingrained attitudes regarding "legitimate" motherhood and citizenship within homeland security culture. Critical interrogation of "risk" as a mode of governance helps to make sense of how Suleman was made publicly meaningful and resonant, including her function as a fixture in popular culture, a point of contentious debate, and a reminder of the conditions of what Nikolas Rose terms biological citizenship under the guise of "responsible choice" and "risk management." Suleman is, to be sure, a complicated and sensationalized figure, but the discourses surrounding her story are instructive insofar as they reveal the borders of virtuous motherhood and medical authority, and clarify the centrality of rhetoric in policing these borders through the concept of "risk." Thus, to make sense of the Nadya Suleman story in all of its complexity and discord, I gathered and read a range of artifacts that bear meaningfully on the constituting of her case in public culture. My interest in Suleman is in exploring the process and function of her discursive pathologizing, illuminating how she is constituted as a public threat to be disciplined and contained through the rhetoric of risk.

The timing was significant. The Suleman octuplets were born in the week following the inauguration of President Barack Obama, who had been swept into office by a public beleaguered over two ongoing and distant wars and a domestic economy in shambles. By early 2009, support for the US invasion and ongoing presence in Iraq was steadily dwindling.[2] Widespread hardship hit home through shrinking paychecks, home loss, drained savings and retirement accounts, and long-term unemployment. A Pew Research report released in December 2008 detailed the extent of diminished morale—92 percent of respondents believed that the economy was in fair or poor shape, 73 percent indicated that jobs were difficult to find in their community, 63 percent expected unemployment to rise in 2009, and 35 percent reported that a household member was unemployed and looking for work in 2008.[3] The Suleman story was thus a perfect storm, as cultural critic Mark Greif astutely notes: "at the moment when American capitalism tottered under the mistakes, bad bets, lies, overconfidence, cupidity, and evil of its financial firms, the press groped at traditional scapegoats."[4] In the case of Suleman, that scapegoat was a low-income Assyrian American mother, a woman who was subsequently figured as unconscionable excess embodied—carrying high-order multiples, a single mom reliant on her parents and the state, with six children already at home, including several with disabilities. To extend Greif's insight, Suleman was not simply a convenient scapegoat, someone easily vilified through existing racist ideologies and the criminalization of poverty (although she was that). But also, in a moment of national crisis, Suleman was a simple, synecdochical site for the pathology afflicting the nation *precisely because of her reproductive decision making and mothering*. As motherhood is imagined as a vehicle for the nation, Suleman's reproduction was deemed symptomatic of the excess that threatened to undo us all.

Focused on dominant media that circulated at the height of public controversy surrounding the Suleman octuplets, I assembled a range of artifacts to trace the significance of the rhetoric of risk in constituting homeland maternity. My archive includes newspapers, magazines, blogs, television news, and talk shows, between the date of the octuplet birth in January 2009 and July 2011, when the State Medical Board of California revoked fertility specialist Michael Kamrava's medical license due largely to his role in Suleman's octuplet pregnancy, at which point public interest in the story began to dwindle.[5] These discourses are of particular interest for their prominence and circulation, for their indexing of public concern over "risky reproduction" and the role of technology in family formation in a moment of national economic uncertainty.

To explore one facet of homeland maternity's differential distribution and impact, I first examine the public pathologizing of Nadya Suleman, focusing on the merger of two culturally incompatible tropes and subsequent violations of "legitimate" maternity. I turn then to the emergence of "risk" as a rhetorical device that worked alongside cultural assumptions regarding motherhood to mobilize a contemporary mode of governance. Finally, I attend to the significance of "risk" to homeland maternity writ large, noting that as risk is rhetorically evoked to position women against their pregnancies, it works simultaneously to shift the gaze of the clinic—decentering women, elevating the fetus, and fueling the discursive conditions necessary for the deprivation of pregnant women's rights and liberties. The logic of preemption is on clear display here—insisting that some women's "risky" reproductive behaviors necessitate intervention and punishment should those women refuse to govern themselves accordingly. Thus, my critical reading of Suleman and the rhetoric of risk is situated within larger cultural trends and patterns related to homeland maternity, and specifically, that of increasing state actions against marginalized pregnant women and the uptick in legislation to authorize these actions.

Pathological Motherhood

"Octocrazy." "Tramp." "Cheap slut." "Pathological liar." "Sociopath." "Serial mom." "The poster child for immoral, unconscionable behavior." Public condemnation of Suleman was widespread, raising questions related to motherhood and its differential legibility vis-à-vis assisted reproduction. The Suleman case is, of course, nothing if not complex. To begin, I offer a brief sketch of her story, highlighting facts of significance as well as persistent tensions and complexities.

The Suleman octuplets were conceived through IVF in a manner that simultaneously challenged and corresponded with fertility industry guidelines and norms. By implanting Suleman with twelve embryos, Dr. Michael Kamrava far exceeded the number recommended by the American Society for Reproductive Medicine (ASRM). Kamrava cited Suleman's preferences and medical history as his rationale, in accordance with ASRM recommendations that prioritize professional judgment and patient history, and that explicitly refuse enforceability.[6] Compounding these peculiarities, Suleman's circumstances at the time of the octuplet birth were relatively unstable, if also preceded by general cultural support for large families and multiple births. In January 2009, Suleman was single, living with her parents, pursuing a graduate degree, and a mother to six children under the age of eight. Her income consisted of student loans, food stamps, disability payments for three of her older children, and workers' compensation from a back injury sustained during a patient riot at a state mental hospital where she had been employed. Suleman used her workers' compensation payments and a small inheritance to pay for infertility treatments; in the case of the octuplets, she had reportedly hoped for one more daughter. Her circumstances were not entirely anomalous—she was not the first to parent many children (including through ART) in the context of financial uncertainty or unemployment. Her case was, however, the first to instigate widespread outrage and legal action. Indeed, public scrutiny of Suleman's circumstances led to several anomalous events, including dissemination by the Associated Press of public records containing Suleman's medical history, the formal investigation of her fertility doctor, and heated debates over fertility industry regulations by elected officials and the press. Suleman's medical records revealed years of chronic pain from her workplace injury and infertility, resulting in bouts of depression and the eventual dissolution of her marriage. The intensity of public outrage over the Suleman story fueled a search for the doctor responsible; Michael Kamrava was publicly named, charged with gross negligence, and his medical license was revoked by the California Medical Board in July 2011.

To date, most scholarship regarding the Suleman case draws on the octuplet birth to explore ART industry regulation and render broader health care reforms.[7] Many note, however, that Suleman's story is less aberrant than dominant narratives might suggest. Citing other instances of high order multiples, Camille Davidson observes that "before the single unemployed Octomom gave birth to her eight babies, the media celebrated other multi-fetal pregnancies and rewarded the parents and children of these 'miracle births' with endorsements and television shows," footnoting Suleman's vilification as "subject for another paper. Unlike famous moms of multiples, Octomom was a single, non-Christian, woman of color."[8] Indeed, as an American of Southwest Asian descent, that is, someone categorized as white by the US Census but subject to racialized scrutiny and violence in the United States particularly since 9/11, Suleman was frequently figured through racialized scripts and thus discursively jettisoned from whiteness. In other words, as Radhika Rao observes, the perceived public crisis was fueled more by Suleman's cultural status than by her conduct,[9] animating longstanding attitudes that pathologize mothers who lack wealth, racial and ethnic privilege, and/or a husband. Deborah Forman quips that: "our common acceptance of the term 'Octomom,' is itself revealing—we have reduced her to a grotesque caricature of motherhood; she's a creature, barely human and certainly not one that in any way resembles our vision of a good mother."[10] Thus, while feminist legal scholars focus primarily on the public policy implications of the Suleman case, they also flag as critically suspect those discourses that cast Suleman as a "bad" mother.

Building on this scholarship, I argue that the discursive pathologizing of Suleman's maternity enabled the rhetoric of risk to become the salient, dominant frame for public remediation of the octuplet birth. I draw also from the work of anthropologist Dana-Ain Davis, whose early study of the Suleman case illuminates how normative discourses of race, class, and family formation shaped mainstream-mediated narratives. Davis demonstrates how Suleman became a site for the policing of motherhood and the neoliberal retooling of reproductive choice: "a casualty in the process of stratified reproduction, whereby her right to reproduce and nurture was denounced because she was single, had no verifiable source of income, and was an inadequate representative of whiteness."[11] Moreover, the public controversy was animated in part by Suleman's untenable occupation of two culturally resonant but incongruous tropes, both deeply inflected by concepts of race and nation—specifically, that of the sym/pathetic[12] infertile woman and the welfare queen. In other words, as a woman trying desperately to conceive, as well as a single mother receiving public assistance, Suleman threatened to collapse distinctions between "deserving" and "undeserving" mothers, a move deemed parasitic by some and criminal by others through a range of public discourses that coded Suleman as pathological and as a threat to be contained.

In the midst of growing criticism following the birth of the octuplets, Nadya Suleman appeared in a few televised interviews in which she attempted to recast herself as a responsible, degree-seeking woman who struggled with infertility and desperately wanted children. Talking with NBC's Ann Curry, Suleman underscored her more conventional attempts at motherhood: "I did get married. . . . I went through about seven years of trying [to conceive]. And through artificial insemination. And through medication. And all of which was unsuccessful."[13] Eventually, Suleman explained, an ectopic pregnancy revealed extensive medical complications: "I had so many reproductive problems from fibroids . . . lesions [and scars] in my fallopian tubes";[14] IVF was her only option. This history of struggle, Suleman insisted, was often neglected in the public rendering of her story: "[critics] are not taking into consideration my past history. Seven years of infertility, seven years," in addition to an IVF history that resulted in the birth of one child for every five or six embryos implanted.[15] In short, when pressed to explain her decision making, Suleman consistently referred to her troubled history with conception, drawing on rhetorics of maternal desire and the right to choose: "I feel as though I've been under the microscope because I've chosen this unconventional kind of life. I didn't intend on it being unconventional. It just turned out to be. All I wanted . . . was to be a mom. That's all I ever wanted in my life."[16]

But Suleman's attempts to situate herself within mainstream frameworks for infertility and reproductive choice proved an exercise in futility, in part because the cultural trope of the sym/pathetic infertile woman was unavailable to her. As chapter 1 discusses, cultural myths have long maintained infertility as an affliction of elite white women who delay childbearing to their own detriment. These myths are decidedly rooted in antifeminist backlash and nativist ideologies. First, mainstream narratives position wealthy white women's infertility at the center of national panic, and in an insidious inversion of correlation, faults feminism for the "epidemic" of infertility against all evidence to the contrary.[17] This is a contemporary trend with significant historical precedent. While the medicalization of infertility, and even infertility itself, is commonly believed to have originated alongside the development of ART in the 1970s, feminist scholars have traced its origins to at least the mid-nineteenth century. Put another way, infertility as a medical diagnosis emerged in the wake of early US feminisms and abolitionist struggles, as efforts for gender and race-based equity challenged white supremacist patriarchy. Infertility was explicitly connected in medical discourse and popular imaginaries to white women's "unruly" or otherwise "unfeminine" behavior; as Robin E. Jensen notes, "women's lack of success in bearing children was attributed to immorality, sexual perversion, strenuous intellectual work, and so-called masculine professional aspirations."[18] And despite alarmist narratives about recent spikes in infertility, significant shifts in the rates of infertility for married, middle-class couples have trended downward since the mid-1960s; the only demographic to experience a rise in these rates since the mid-1960s is women under twenty-four, due in large part to a rise in sexually transmitted infections that, left untreated, are linked to long-term reproductive harm. The infertility rate of the general population has fluctuated between 9 and 13 percent for over a century, and research demonstrates that greater gender equality and access to reproductive health care—in short, the gains of feminism—are positively correlated with fertility.

Moreover, contrary to popular belief, infertility disproportionately impacts women of color and low-wealth women due largely to institutionalized racism and health care disparities, yet these women remain largely ignored within dominant discussions of infertility.[19] As infertility "epidemics" are filtered through the eugenic logic of maternal worth, a multibillion-dollar industry in assisted reproduction has emerged in the last several decades that, by all available measures, both reflects and perpetuates inequities. The US Centers for

Disease Control and Prevention (CDC) reporting requirements include information regarding clinic practices, success rates, patient ages, medical histories, and reasons for pursuing ART, but demographic information concerning race and ethnicity, education, income, sexuality, and source of payment for services remains conspicuously absent. There is a comparative paucity of data regarding the use of infertility services, with the exception of the National Survey of Family Growth.[20] This survey, in all of its iterations, demonstrates that women who use infertility services are privileged by education, income, race, marital status, and age because primary barriers to access are economic, geographical, and cultural. Such are the barriers that Suleman transgressed in seeking treatment for infertility, and for which she was subject to considerable public scorn and ridicule.

The most optimistic reports on the Suleman octuplets were published prior to the release of any identifying information regarding the mother or her circumstances. The *Los Angeles Times* narrated the birth with surprise and delight: "It took only five minutes—from 10:43 am to 10:48 am—for all six boys and two girls to be delivered and processed lovingly through an assembly line of medical workers. The mother and her medical corps had made history."[21] Associated Press reporting emphasized the "rare" and "amazing delivery" and the "stable condition" of the newborns.[22] The *Today Show* featured an interview with the Chukwu family, which includes the only other set of octuplets born in the United States. The upbeat report focused on the children's current health and happiness, soliciting advice that the "First Family" of octuplets might offer the "new *parents* of eight" (emphasis added).[23] Throughout breaking coverage, Suleman was assumed to be partnered, and medical concerns were tempered with comparative optimism. But within days, as various dimensions of Suleman's social position and circumstances were revealed, the tenor of reporting shifted dramatically, featuring headlines such as "A Mom's Controversial Choice," "The Ethics of Octuplets," "When Eight Is Seven Too Many," and "Where in the World Is Octodad?"[24]

This public refrain proved caustic and unyielding, drawing on the contemporary trope of the "welfare queen." Figured as lazy, promiscuous, excessively fertile, unruly, of color, and even criminal, the trope of the welfare queen masks the structural origins of poverty and is implicated in eviscerating low-wealth women's reproductive rights and claims to motherhood.[25] A single, low-income mother who lacks a formal or sufficient relationship to the labor market is marked as an illegitimate consumer and choice-maker—an undeserving beneficiary of public assistance. The "welfare queen's" childbearing is deemed parasitic for society as a whole; as a result, Rickie Solinger writes: "many Americans have been increasingly unwilling to acknowledge the rights, the motherhood status, or the citizenship status of poor mothers. Instead, most have chosen to support public policies designed to be ever tougher on incorrigible women bent on taking the taxpayer for a ride."[26] Thus, the image of the welfare queen as a public pariah—an illegitimate consumer who cheats the system and is a poor parent to her children—stands in direct opposition to the figure of the sym/pathetic woman who struggles with infertility. Each becomes the site for the naming of a public crisis; indeed, the collectively imagined crises are two sides of the same coin, as each is predicated on the same socially unbalanced reproductive equation. On one side resides a well-to-do white professional unable to conceive and, on the other, an unruly breeder who bears children to avoid employment and abscond with public resources.

Nadya Suleman was aggressively articulated as the latter. Rhetorics of irresponsibility, sexual excess, mental illness, poverty, and criminality coalesced to publicly pathologize Suleman, casting her as an illegitimate mother (and ART consumer) and eclipsing any claims she might make to access or choice. Under the guise of "responsibility," Suleman was interrogated for her failure to adhere to normative maternity, as decisively wed to the labor market if not to a man. Despite Suleman's insistence she was neither dating nor sexually active, despite the fact that her children were conceived through IVF with donor sperm, the specter of sexual excess became a subtext for her pathology, a clear marker of the trope of the welfare queen at work. Reports surfaced regarding adult film offers, fueling rumors of a history of sex work, and Suleman's resemblance to Angelina Jolie provided fodder for much debate—noting Suleman's sex appeal while mocking her as a fake and disturbing celebrity wannabe.[27] Her mental health was under relentless scrutiny, her medical records obtained from the State of California and released to the press.[28] Referred to as "insane," "disturbed," "a self-obsessed, publicity-driven lunatic," or simply "off her fucking rocker," speculations concerning Suleman's mental health ranged from depression to psychosis, from pregnancy "addiction" to "body dysmorphia. Where [the individual] just want[s] more and more of the surgeries to feel better."[29]

A particularly insidious rhetorical device coded Suleman as criminal, a move striking for its candor and cultural context, one in which pregnant and parenting women—and particularly those of color and/or low-income—are increasingly subject to state policing and violence.[30] The public reveal of Suleman's marital and employment status prompted a swift and decisive turn in public opinion; her lack of class standing assumed to indicate criminality (vis-à-vis citizenship) or used to fuel racist caricatures of single motherhood. Absent additional information, rumors regarding Suleman's race, ethnicity, and national belonging flew through the blogosphere, some questioning whether Suleman was "legal" and others claiming that she was African American, and later, Palestinian.[31] An early report featured an interview with Suleman's parents in which her father was twice described with reference to "his native Iraq,"[32] underscoring Suleman's ethnicity in a post-9/11 era in which South Asian, Southwest Asian, and North African[33] communities in the United States increasingly are targets of public hostility, discrimination, hate crimes, and state violence.[34] Thus, as a more complete picture of Suleman emerged in the days and weeks following the octuplet birth, racist, classist, and xenophobic caricatures persisted, a cacophony of discourses that raised the specter of criminality in dominant imaginaries.

Metaphors of addiction and dependence codified Suleman's criminality, as evidenced in the following quotation from CNN talk-show host Jane Velez-Mitchell: "she is addicted to having children. And the one thing that we know about addicts, it's progressive. It only gets worse."[35] Referred to as a "resource hog," a "baby addict,"[36] a "baby junky,"[37] and even a "serial mom,"[38] Suleman's desire for children was deemed illicit, compulsive, and potentially lethal, the trope of the welfare queen taken to its logical extreme. Her childbearing was, in some instances, infused with xenophobic paranoia regarding the "alien" maternal body as a threat.[39] As one blogger writes: "There is no difference between the 'octomom' deliberately producing children that taxpayers have to take care of and illegal alien women producing children as 'anchors' for us to provide education, health care, and welfare."[40] Evoking a slur that undercuts the belonging of US citizens born to undocumented parents, Suleman was criminalized by proxy. As debates over immigration raged in Washington and the public perceived tensions between native and nonnative US residents as greater than those related to generation, race, and class,[41] Suleman's reception tapped into a range of Othering registers. Maternal citizenship and national belonging remain predicated on class standing and economic self-sufficiency—so much so that in this case, citizenship and wealth became inextricably enmeshed, the requisite condition for the right to bear children.

Indeed, Suleman's criminality is compounded by frequent indictments for lack of sufficient resources, as Whoopi Goldberg asserted on *The View*: "Just because you wanna have fourteen kids—doesn't mean [you should] unless you've got the dough."[42] References to the taxpayer monies Suleman received in food stamps, student loans, and disability became commonplace, framed by allusions to her aberrant standard of living and parenting: "Her family lives in a ramshackle house—the only one on the well-kept block—with a barren front yard. A front window is held together with electrical tape, and toys, a stroller and a tricycle are strewn around."[43] Similarly noted in *People*: "Inside . . . two cribs were strewn with clothes and towels, and the window was covered by a bedsheet; another bedroom, equipped with bunk beds, showed knee-high mounds of clothes tumbling from a closet."[44] Suleman's lack of wealth and her defiance of middle-class norms of domesticity mark her as unworthy not only of public assistance, but of maternal status as well. Appearing on HLN, psychologist Brian Russell suggested hosting an "Adoption Idol" in which "good parents from around the country compete to adopt this woman's kids. You can be a judge. I'll be a judge. She gets her show. She gets her money. The kids end up with parents who aren't complete loons. Everybody wins."[45] Russell prefaced his comments by acknowledging their shock value but, regardless, comments such as these reflect a history of reproductive politics in which the motherhood of marginalized women is discursively challenged and subsequently denied through a range of legal, medical, economic, cultural practices. Here, the trope of the welfare queen was rhetorically evoked to fix Suleman in public discourse as deviant and criminal, a mother whose childbearing constituted a drain on taxpayer resources and the nation itself.

Thus, the initial embrace of the octuplet birth as a spectacular feat of modern medicine quickly dissolved as aspects of Nadya Suleman's circumstances were revealed. A woman who dared wed public assistance to IVF, she came to represent the uncomfortable articulation of two incongruous tropes that led to a series of assumed paradoxes—a low-income woman struggling with infertility? A welfare recipient able to gain financial access to IVF? The strict social and economic barriers to assisted reproduction were simultaneously revealed and decisively breeched—the modern miracle transformed into monstrosity. Suleman's story suggested the possibility of single, low-income women reproducing themselves, the possibility that ART had fallen into the "wrong" hands. Indeed, Suleman signaled a public crisis because her actions threatened to collapse distinctions between deserving and undeserving mothers, to disappear significant cultural categories that have long fixed motherhood as an individual privilege that reproduces the nation as white, wealthy, and self-contained. Thus, the rhetoric of risk was afforded velocity through the crisis signaled by Suleman's "unruly" reproductive body. Masking the racist, classist, and xenophobic overtones of pathological motherhood, the rhetoric of risk functioned to sanitize public dialogue through the ethos of expertise.

Governing Reproduction in an Era of Risk

In an interview with NBC News in the weeks following the Suleman birth, director of the New York University Fertility Center Dr. Jamie Grifo expressed a sentiment widely reported among medical professionals: "she obviously [was not] behaving rationally. . . . She risked her life and those babies' lives. She didn't fully understand [the risks], apparently."[46] Similar assessments of Suleman prevailed, incredulity and outrage tempered in part through the rhetoric of risk. As previously noted in the theorizing of homeland security culture writ large, the naming of risk is an act of power, one that sets in motion the compulsion to act and to preempt. As a culturally specific and rhetorically constituted phenomenon, risk is definitively normative; it reflects the investments of elite actors and is discursively deployed under conditions of cultural desire or distress. It names some practices excessive or unconscionable, and others ideal or otherwise necessary. The rhetoric of risk is thus powerful—a vehicle for world making, for policing boundaries, defining normativities, and shaping cultural practices and beliefs. Risk exists in the realm of imaginative speculation and the plausible, authorizing any number of preemptive strikes in its wake.

Moreover, the rhetoric of risk has been named central to the ideology of intensive mothering. "Good" mothers are those who manage to anticipate and avoid *all possible* risks to their children—those seen and unseen, those present and future—by mastering a complex calculus for all aspects everyday life.[47] Tending to rhetorics of risk in the case of Nadya Suleman clarifies how risk governs women differentially. Here, the rhetoric of risk is predicated on pathological motherhood as it simultaneously assumes the objectivity of medical expertise. Put another way, Suleman's "risky reproduction" builds on racist and classist cultural assumptions regarding motherhood while denying the force of these assumptions through claims to medical expertise, a site frequently coded as politically neutral.[48] As Carolyn Miller writes, risk effectively marshals the ethos of expertise as "an ethos that denies the importance of ethos . . . [and] is all the more powerful for its self-denial."[49] Thus, the rhetoric of "risky reproduction" sanitizes public anxieties provoked by Suleman's "pathological motherhood," and, as a grammar of neoliberal governance, functions to restore the ART industry as a responsible steward of health and progress.

Animated by the threat of Suleman's "unruly" reproductive body, medical authority was quickly assembled to assert the risks of high-order multiple births, risks that built on ableist norms regarding human wellness and worth. Significantly, these risks were neither new in their discovery nor in their documentation, but rather, regularly overlooked in a culture of enthusiastic reproductivity. The risks of multiples garnered unprecedented publicity, however, as the Suleman story unfolded, drawing heavily on the ethos of established medicine. The *New York Times* foregrounded extensive interviews with infertility specialists, noting "the disastrous health consequences that sometimes come with multiple births—infant mortality, low birth weights, long-term disabilities and thousands of dollars' worth of medical care."[50] The *Washington Post* concurred, articulating fetal health risks to Suleman's circumstances as it distanced established medicine from the octuplet event: "The birth of eight babies to a woman who becomes responsible for 14 children is attracting a different set of worries from the medical community, particularly fertility doctors, who say it goes against the mission of their work: to minimize high-risk, multiple-birth pregnancy and safely provide a woman with a single healthy baby."[51] Citing ASRM, coverage of the Suleman eight in *People* magazine included a sidebar titled "When More Isn't Better," which stated that "multiple-birth babies run higher risk for cerebral palsy and breathing and vision problems."[52] While discussions focused largely on infants, the risks for expectant mothers were occasionally included, if diminished in comparison: "For the mother, [the risks are] less severe; diabetes and hypertension . . . months of bed rest with clots and embolisms. For the infant, the risks are lifelong: prematurity, cerebral palsy, blindness, months in intensive care."[53] Thus, the intense focus on "risk" directed public concern to questions of infant health and safety, issues of deep cultural salience that remain largely immune to critique despite trafficking in ableist, even eugenic, logics.[54]

The risks became such a pronounced feature of the Suleman saga, in fact, that the "ethics" of multiples drew extended consideration in reporting that followed birth of the octuplets. In *People* magazine, Suleman's story was aptly described as "the focal point of an intense national debate about whether doctors have an ethical responsibility to safeguard against what might be considered 'extreme' multiple births, which can imperil both mother and babies."[55] An *ABC News* headline declared that the "lesson" of Octomom was the frequency with which "couples pressure doctors," positioning the "ethical choices" and "professional judgment" of infertility specialists against "patient autonomy" and desire for children.[56] Responding to inquiries about the lack of consistent regulations governing the ART industry, ASRM was forced to defend its "strong ethical process" and professional guidelines as benefitting providers and patients.[57] The question of ethics and medical intervention quickened as reports noted Suleman's refusal of "selective reduction," which was framed not only as standard practice but also as a moral imperative. A National Public Radio broadcast evidenced this trend, including this assessment: "That [Suleman] did not elect what is referred to as 'selective reduction' surprised many within—and outside—the medical community. And when a local news station revealed she was already the mother of six, critical chatter spiked: 'What *was* she thinking?'" (original emphasis).[58]

Discussions of "selective reduction" remained remarkably bereft of abortion politics, eclipsed by the focus on Suleman's pathological motherhood and the risks she took in carrying her pregnancy to term. The tensions between reproductive and disability politics evidenced here are worthy of note. As a form of pregnancy termination that leaves one or more fetuses undisturbed but is frequently compelled by the risks of high-order multiples, selective reduction tends to generate far greater public sympathy than it does controversy. Much like the termination of a pregnancy with diagnosed fetal abnormalities, selective reduction is a form of abortion that is often framed less as a "choice" and more as an imperative—a set of circumstances that compels an agonizing decision. To be clear, I do not take issue with the framing of pregnancy termination as a difficult decision in any circumstance, and certainly in the context of a pregnancy both very much desired, and simultaneously, atypical and/or high risk. Nonetheless, in a cultural climate of relentless hostility toward abortion rights and minimal support for people—including children—with disabilities,[59] it is worth noting the set of circumstances that publicly render abortion a moral choice—even a moral imperative—in the Suleman saga. In this moment, abortion as a moral imperative collides in a disturbing manner with eugenic logics that include the pathology assigned to Suleman's motherhood as well as mythic norms that frame the prospect of disability as a tragedy, or even as a form of harm to children, that should be avoided by any means necessary.[60] In short, the arguments advanced in favor of selective reduction simultaneously inverted and deployed antiabortion logics, authorizing abortion as a moral decision while constituting Suleman's "risky" reproductive body as a threat to her unborn children and to herself.

Feminist scholars have interrogated how prenatal health and its myriad diagnostics often position women against their pregnancies,[61] eclipsing a defining characteristic of pregnancy as nourishing another being, and articulating pregnant individuals instead as threats to their potential offspring. Risk aversion in prenatal contexts is intimately tethered to disability/ability, urging women to submit to screening and genetic testing in order to exercise "responsible" decision making.[62] This exacts what Silja Samerski terms "compulsory self-determination" under the guise of improved reproductive choices: "the call for responsible decision making under the shadow of genes and risk must be understood as a social engineering technique . . . [making] women powerless while holding them responsible."[63] Following the birth of the Suleman eight, various reports relied on medical experts to assert multiples as inherently risky, few marking any distinction between twins and higher-order multiples.[64] An *ABC News* headline declared: "Octomom Lesson: More Couples Pressure Doctors," followed by the reading line "Transferring more than one embryo puts mothers and babies at risk for twins, triplets."[65] Multiples become "risky" in and of themselves; as women and fetuses are positioned as "at risk" for multiples, pregnant women are chastised for their lack of knowledge and inadequate "risk prevention": "Many are so keen to ensure the health of their future child that they overhaul their diets and cut out all caffeine and alcohol. Yet they remain under the impression that it is okay to allow their fetus to do one of the most dangerous things possible: share a crowded womb."[66] As pregnant people are understood in opposition to their pregnancies, a risk assumed by an expectant parent is rhetorically situated at the expense of the fetus or fetuses. Figured as ignorant at best, if not also self-absorbed or even criminal, the carrier of multiples-to-be abandons the fundamental requirements of contemporary "total motherhood," as "a moral code in which mothers are exhorted to optimize every aspect of children's lives, beginning with the womb."[67]

The figure of Suleman, rigorously articulated against virtuous motherhood, fueled the rhetorical construction of "risky reproduction." In other words, it is hardly coincidental that the medical risks of multiples gained recognition and popular traction in the wake of the Suleman story. The degree of resonance did not reflect concern for the risks engendered by *any* set of multiples; rather, the emergence of risky rhetoric was predicated on the existence of a *risky maternal body*—one imagined to parent against the norms and interests of the nation. Moreover, this rhetoric called on medical expertise to contain the risky maternal body, as evidenced in a *Los Angeles Times* editorial that declared: "now that more has come to light about the octuplets' family situation, medical authorities would be right to look into the mother's in vitro treatment."[68] An editorial titled "Mothers Gone Wild" in *MacLean's* posited that "mega-multiple births create substantial risks for the unborn children. That, and [Suleman's] precarious home life, suggests a failure by the medical community to actively protect the best interests of potential children—and a reason for society to be involved."[69] Widely cited in this case, Arthur Caplan, director of bioethics at the University of Pennsylvania, proposed fertility screenings akin to adoption procedures as he rhetorically sutured health, risk, and social position: "The right to reproduce isn't unlimited. You can't put children at risk. The field of reproductive medicine and fertility treatment has an absolute responsibility to look out for the children it is creating in new ways. And in this case it seems to have failed."[70] Clarifying the responsibilities of fertility specialists to discern and contain risky reproductive bodies, Caplan concluded: "With all due respect, the idea that doctors should not set limits on who can use reproductive technology to make babies is ethically bonkers."[71] In a move that reflects the precarious fusion of surveillance and policing in the homeland security state, pregnant individuals are held relentlessly responsible for reproductive decision making in strict accordance with dominant norms and expectations, and the state—or other forms of (biomedical) authority—will be invoked should they fail.

While some rhetorics of risk implicate Kamrava and the fertility industry, medical expertise was deployed in ways that consistently assigned risk to Suleman herself. In an interview with *ABC News*, ASRM spokesperson Sean Tipton argued that "a patient's [*sic*] does not have the right to demand the physician practice dangerous medicine." Similarly, *USA Today* showcased new and improved IVF procedures to reduce the "risk of multiples," underscoring this necessity vis-à-vis Suleman: "Carrying so many fetuses brings massive health risks to the mother and children, and Suleman's irresponsibility places a burden on society."[72] Articulations of Suleman's social and economic burden tapped into endemic anxiety as global markets continued their descent, redirecting public rage away from those culpable for the economic crisis and aiming it instead at a low-income single mother, as Mark Greif deftly argues.[73] Assumed to be utterly dependent on the state and thus a "drain" on the system, Suleman became the representative anecdote that signaled widespread moral decline, faulting poverty- and working-class peoples for their economic conditions despite clear evidence to the contrary. An editorial in the *Wall Street Journal* titled "Where in the World Is Octodad?" quipped that "our equivocation about paternity is finally untenable. Out-of-wedlock birth rates in the U.S. are now 38%; among African-Americans the figure is 70%. . . . Children who grow up without their fathers experience more poverty, have more problems at school, more trouble with the law—and more single motherhood in the next generation."[74] In lieu of examining a range of critical factors that might constrain the lives of working-class peoples and mothers in particular, such as livable wages, educational opportunity, or the accessibility of health care, single motherhood itself is positioned as the fountainhead of profound national ills.

This positioning of particular (low-income, unwed) maternal bodies as "risky" reflects the differential valuation of motherhood and marshals the cultural capital of health and medicine to reassert these assumptions through the rhetoric of risk. As J. Blake Scott argues, risky rhetoric is predicated on the existence of a deviant or "risky" body, stigmatizing particular (and often already marginalized) populations by conflating risk with identity. As such, certain communities are positioned "more as *risky* or threatening than as *at risk*, facilitating policies that primarily seek to detect and contain rather than engage and empower" (original emphasis).[75] Understanding how risk is rhetorically constituted as identity, in lieu of as a set of behaviors or environmental conditions, illuminates a critical dimension of its resonance in the Suleman case and its subsequent reverberations across the contemporary landscape of maternal and reproductive politics, a matter to which I return in the conclusion of this chapter. In the case of Nadya Suleman, the rhetoric of risk was mobilized by pathological motherhood and the cultural crisis assigned to her excessive and "risky" reproductive body. Figured as a threat to her children, the fertility industry, and the nation at large, the rhetoric of risk emerged to mark Suleman, not as *at risk*, but as a *perpetrator of risk*, a threat to be contained.

Suleman's threat, and the cultural response to it, reflects the conditions of contemporary biopolitics under late capitalism, which is, in Nikolas Rose's words, "concerned with our growing capacities to control, manage, engineer, reshape, and modulate the very vital capacities of human beings as living creatures." Thus, contemporary biopolitics are relational, administered through personal responsibility, and guided by new forms of authority and expertise: "The role of biomedical authority here is not to encourage the passive and compliant patienthood of a previous form of medical citizenship. Citizenship is to be active . . . to work with doctors to obtain the best program of medical care." It is a form of governance steeped in an ethic of autonomy and individual responsibility, masking overt directives and reigning instead through related logics of "informed consent" and "choice."[76] Reproductive decision making is particularly implicated in this model of medical citizenship, as developments in assisted reproduction are accompanied by technologies of the self that carefully delineate the borders of legitimate, "responsible" choice for both doctors and patients. It is a trend evidenced in the prosecution of Kamrava for failure to refer Suleman to a mental health professional, as well as in fertility specialists' comments that blurred the boundaries between informed and coerced consent: "When given the data [by medical professionals], most people make the right decision [regarding multiples]."[77] Put another way, medical expertise, properly exercised and dispensed, inches closer toward medical dictate under the guise of greater freedom and autonomy.

Understanding contemporary biopolitics in this way strengthens our ability to understand both the significance and vilification of Nadya Suleman in public discourse. For it is not simply that she threatened to collapse significant cultural distinctions between "deserving" and "undeserving" mothers, between the trope of the sym/pathetic woman and the welfare queen, although this did lend considerable fuel to the fire. Suleman's violation was much more substantial than this. Not only did she gain access to the infertility clinic, as a space of reproductive choice never intended for her, but once there, she proceeded to make all of the "wrong" (unruly and undisciplined) choices, to violate the conditions of biological citizenship as tied to "responsible" decision making consonant with the interests of the nation. Thus, Nadya Suleman's story functions as a logic through which new forms of citizenship are made visible and exigent, underscoring the strict requirements of reproductive decision making in an era of homeland maternity. At the same moment in which assisted reproductive technologies are discursively wed to an expansion of choice, so too are they accompanied by new forms of governance, that which is exercised by individuals but invariably shaped by medical "experts." In other words, greater choice through ART is accompanied by a more expansive set of imperatives to avoid and manage risk, to govern reproduction so as to optimize life in ways that are culturally sanctioned. Thus, the high-profile treatment of the Suleman case becomes valued as a popular heuristic, her figure a reminder of gendered and racialized biopolitical responsibility under the banner of responsible choice and risk management.

Octomom and Risky Reproduction in Homeland Security Culture

In response to public outrage over the Suleman octuplets, several states considered legislation to regulate the fertility industry, as federal law tends to limited matters.[78] A bill proposed in Georgia would have limited the number of embryos transferred per IVF cycle to two for any woman under the age of forty, and three embryos for women over the age of forty. In Missouri, proposed legislation would have mandated that all ART clinics and specialists comply with ASRM guidelines or risk losing medical licensure.[79] But despite overwhelming public anger and express calls for industry reform, legislative redress met significant resistance from fertility specialists, professional organizations, and clients, and failed to gain traction. In lieu of legal reform, the rhetoric of risk emerged as the dominant frame through which the Suleman birth was discursively managed and collectively assuaged, building on "pathological motherhood" as it concealed cultural attitudes regarding family formation, race, and class. Sifting through this moment of public discord, I offer two distinct but overlapping provocations in order to clarify the significance of Suleman to homeland maternity. I first attend to the specifics of the Suleman case and its implications for ART use, noting how risky rhetoric functioned on several levels—drawing on medical expertise to mask differential valuations of motherhood, enforcing neoliberal governmentality through an emphasis on proper risk "management," and demonstrating industry discipline and capacity for self-regulation and rule. Turning then to broader context, I consider how rhetorics of risk shape reproductive politics in homeland security culture writ large, its role in the policing of those pregnant and parenting, and how it might be made available to discursive intervention and redress.

This investigation of the Suleman story illuminates the role of risk in masking reproductive stratification. Tasha Dubriwny's study of the "vulnerable empowered woman" is instructive here for theorizing of the figure of the monstrous maternal and its role in demarcating acceptable from unacceptable risk. She notes that while risk may be strategically embraced by "good" mothers to resist the madness of intensive mothering, the "risky mother" identity has distinct implications for women already marked as "bad mothers" due to social location or circumstance. As a single mom on welfare, racialized as an ethnic Other, Suleman was always already imagined as a "risky" reproducer, always already imagined as monstrous in her femininity and motherhood.[80] Thus, risk functioned in this instance as a means of marking pathological motherhood while denying the force of that pathology through a reliance on the ethos of expertise. Tending to the Suleman story extends Dubriwny's work, illustrating how the rhetoric of risk functions as a form of governance that is unevenly distributed among women and mothers, and most significantly, in such a way that it often obscures the role of race, class, and family formation in its functioning. Thus, even as assisted reproduction continues to be culturally venerated for expanding "choice" and "self-determination" in motherhood, the differential assignment of risk evidenced in the Suleman case suggests a clear delineation between biological enhancement and distortion; a designation that hinges less on biological or technological capacity than it does on cultural legitimacy. The public discord provoked by Suleman's story, her intolerable linkage of infertility and public assistance that fueled her figuration as a pathological mother, signal the strict cultural requirements and responsibilities of legitimate "choice" in homeland security culture.

This case offers a clear example of how culturally legible motherhood remains a privilege of income, class, marital status, race, and other markers of cultural capital, perhaps differently, but no less now than ever before. Prior to the Suleman octuplets, the birth of high-order multiples to married, middle-class, and typically white couples typically resulted in warm public reception, large-scale donations including houses and cars, and (lucrative) media opportunities. The Gosselins of the wildly successful *(Jon &) Kate Plus Eight* were both unemployed when they brought home the sextuplets, which proved to be neither a point of public contention nor an impediment to their success.[81] In a far cry from condemnation, Michelle Duggar of *19 Kids & Counting* was awarded "Arkansas Young Mother of the Year" in 2004, when she and her husband had fourteen children and the fifteenth on the way.[82] The public treatment of phenomenal fertility in the Suleman case was decidedly distinct, working to reinscribe the differential valuation of motherhood that has historically exacerbated and made possible a host of reproductive injustices.[83] In this way, the silence surrounding this case from feminist scholars and activists is both remarkable and profound. To the extent that feminists are concerned that motherhood be neither scripted as the pinnacle of virtuous and white womanhood, nor used to criminalize marginalized women and communities, the Suleman case deserves feminist contemplation and intervention.

Significantly, beyond the specifics of this case and its implications for Suleman and her doctor, this story compels us to consider how rhetorics of risk in homeland security culture enable a mode of neoliberal governance that is at once distant but also authorized to intervene in more direct and juridical ways. Risk is relentlessly directive and normative; it strips individuals of agency as it saddles them with liability and duty. This is particularly evidenced in the context of reproductive decision making, as rhetorics of risk simultaneously render women powerless and yet responsible.[84] Risk guides individual decision making under the banner of personal "choice" and "responsibility" but also, significantly, authorizes intervention by state and/or medical authorities (on behalf of the fetus) when women refuse to act in accordance with its dictates. And as risk is increasingly rhetorically evoked to position women against their pregnancies, antiabortion logics of fetal personhood are bolstered in contemporary imaginaries. This gross inversion of the dynamics of pregnancy and reproduction—the misogynist dismissal of women's lives as lives that matter—fundamentally shifts the gaze of the clinic. It decenters women, elevates the fetus, and fuels the discursive conditions necessary for the deprivation of pregnant individuals' rights. This trend is not entirely new but rather draws on the powerful discourse of risk to rationalize an uptick in state surveillance and policing of pregnant peoples.

Tamara Loertscher's unjust incarceration by the State of Wisconsin provides one example, but her story is tragically familiar. Christine Taylor, a single and pregnant mother of two, was arrested for attempted feticide after passing out and falling down a flight of stairs in Iowa.[85] Alicia Beltran was involuntarily committed by the state of Wisconsin for disclosing a former addiction at a prenatal appointment.[86] After suffering a pulmonary embolism that left her brain-dead, Marlise Muñoz was forced by the State of Texas to remain on life support against her advance medical directives and the express wishes of her family in order to maintain a pregnancy with no chance of fetal survival.[87] Bei Bei Shuai, a Chinese immigrant and resident of Indiana, was incarcerated without bail and charged with murder and attempted feticide after a failed suicide attempt resulted in the loss of her pregnancy.[88] Women have been forced to undergo Caesareans, held criminally liable for negative pregnancy outcomes, incarcerated for seeking medical assistance following a miscarriage, and threatened with jail time for alcohol or drug use.[89] They have been denied due process, stripped of medical confidentiality, and refused critical prenatal and maternal care while in state custody. In other words, pregnant women have been targeted for state punishment that, under any other set of circumstances, would constitute egregious violations of their constitutional rights. While some stories made national headlines, these represent a small fraction of the women across the country recently deprived of fundamental human rights in the name of fetal health and protection, a logic that is afforded velocity through rhetorics of fetal risk that position women as threats to the pregnancies they carry. Significantly, state actions against pregnant women are disproportionately inflicted on low-income women, immigrant women, and women of color—women far more likely to be imagined as "unruly" or "risky" reproducers.[90]

Moreover, women are increasingly policed through the concept of risk in homeland security culture, not only during their pregnancies, but also, alarmingly, for their *potential* to conceive. In 2016, for example, the US CDC issued the following warning: "An estimated 3.3 million women between the ages of 15 and 44 years are at risk of exposing their developing baby to alcohol because they are drinking, sexually active, and not using birth control to prevent pregnancy."[91] The broad spectrum of fetal risk in this example compels discipline for women deemed "pre-pregnant"—in short, for anyone who dares to be both female and fertile simultaneously. In order to prevent fetal alcohol spectrum disorders (FASDs), the CDC committed to reducing "risky alcohol use" by "tracking alcohol use among women of reproductive age in the United States" and advised health care providers "to assess a woman's drinking habits during routine medical visits; advise her not to drink at all if she is pregnant, trying to get pregnant or sexually active and not using birth control; and recommend services if she needs help to stop drinking." Putting aside the fact that women like Loertscher have been subject to involuntary commitment for refusing care providers' "recommendations," warnings such as these also fail to address related structural concerns that include, for example, legal, economic, and cultural barriers that restrict access to birth control for many women. Moreover, the CDC warning focuses exclusively on policing women's behaviors, ignoring other significant factors in FASDs such as nutrition, levels of stress, access to prenatal care, genetic factors, and the influence of male partners.[92] Thus, rhetorics of risk draw on the concept of fetal health and warrant increased surveillance of women's lives, whether those women are pregnant, trying to conceive, or simply happen to be of reproductive age. In summation, from agency guidelines to legislative directives and state intervention, women are increasingly subject to surveillance, coercion, and violence, a troubling trend predicated on a concept of fetal risk that positions women at odds with their pregnancies and consistent with a broader cultural context in which preemption through surveillance and policing rules supreme.

The Suleman case is thus instructive on many levels; it frames the critical feminist work that remains undone and urgently begs attention to rhetorical deployments of "risk" and their centrality to the treatment of those pregnant and parenting within homeland security culture. We might begin by taking seriously Dubriwny's provocation: "what might be different if a feminist perspective were more available?"[93] While Suleman's story raises several concerns that warrant extended consideration, I argue that in lieu of decrying Suleman's personal decision making through racialized tropes and demonizing her desire to be a mother, we are better served in thinking broadly through these concerns with a steadfast orientation toward reproductive justice and an affirmation of family formation in its myriad forms as a dimension of human rights and dignity.

This might include, for example, extended consideration of the ethics and politics of assisted reproduction, particularly as it relates to multiple births, as well as the long-term implications of high-order multiples for mothers, families, and communities. For example, are there limits to reasonable uses of assisted reproduction, and what are the roles of individuals, professionals, states, and/or markets in determining those limits? In the United States, ASRM guidelines are increasingly rigorous, but they remain unenforceable, and clinic compliance rates are low. The expense of infertility treatments and lack of consistent health care coverage for procedures encourage women and couples to pursue higher rates of embryo transfer to increase their odds of conception. If we are to take seriously the concerns engendered by high-order multiples, then we might adopt recommendations from legal scholars and advocates who promote just access through careful industry regulation, comprehensive coverage for services (including for individuals and couples on public assistance), and dedicated support for families both in their formation and in their ongoing health and well-being. In this sense, we have a long way to go. Simply in terms of ART access, even in the sixteen states that mandate infertility coverage, access to services is often precluded by state regulations that cap expenditures or procedures, bar sperm or egg donation, and/or require the patient to be married.[94]

Considering these questions might also prompt an interrogation of reigning logics of choice that affirm markets as the arbiter of ART access, wherein supply is bracketed largely by clinic policies and demand is curtailed by individual wealth. This is precisely the problem that the Suleman saga reveals—nonnormative choices are deemed monstrous when made by women culturally excluded from "legitimate" consumption. In this way, "choice" prohibits our capacity to critique excess use or misappropriation of resources by women of means and, simultaneously, bars public defense of the reproductive self-determination of low-income women. In short, the pathologizing of Suleman and punishment of her doctor, in lieu of a more substantive inquiry into medical practices and regulations, reinscribes the status quo—with one troubling exception. In the wake of Kamrava's professional disciplining, fertility specialists are likely more reticent in treating any patient who resembles Suleman. While there are no formal prohibitions that prevent them from doing so, legal scholarship suggests that the threat of professional sanctions creates a climate of uncertainty and fear in which the likelihood of refusal for services is higher.[95] And the problem with current regulatory regimes (or lack thereof) is not simply concerned with low-income communities. Absent regulations that would bar clinics or practitioners from discrimination, single women and LGBTQ communities are often subject to exclusionary practices by private clinics afforded freedom to determine which clients are worthy of care.

Beyond questions of access to technologies of family formation, a robust understanding of reproductive justice necessarily includes a critical approach to disability, with heightened awareness of and resistance to public attempts to pit one against the other. While feminists have struggled to meaningfully engage the complex intersections of reproductive and disability rights, affirming ability and disability as social constructs—and disability rights as central to human rights and dignity—does not imply a diminished claim to reproductive rights. As Alison Piepmeier notes, shifting our attention to social context clarifies how disability itself is far less constraining than "the larger set of social contexts that establishes our understanding of and approaches to disability."[96] In this sense, disability advocacy and reproductive justice share much common ground. For example, many women and couples facing an atypical prenatal screening or test report feeling less, as opposed to more, empowered in their decision making as they attempt to navigate the world of reprogenetics.[97] Misinformation about the challenges and realities of parenting a child with a disability, or of living with a disability, infuse cultural and medical contexts alike and compound efforts to make "informed" decisions.[98] A profound lack of resources and support to parent a child with disabilities in dignity compounds the trepidation and uncertainty of an unexpected diagnosis.[99] And once again, a reproductive justice framework invites us to take a broader view, to affirm the right of pregnant persons to make personal medical decisions—regardless of circumstance—while also advocating accuracy in health care provider-led discussions of fetal abnormalities, as well as systems of support for families and children across the ability spectrum. As ability is both socially constructed and invariably in flux over the course of a lifetime, this orientation shifts our gaze from prenatal decision making to a much broader set of concerns, widely applicable to families at various stages of life—from the care of children to elders, as well as care for adult partners navigating serious medical conditions of their own over the course of a lifetime.

Thus the capacious project of reproductive justice is invested in the social, political, and economic empowerment of women, families, and communities.[100] In an era of homeland maternity, an era in which motherhood is differentially constrained and enabled through the logics of homeland security culture, critical interrogation of the rhetoric of risk is central to reproductive justice. As rhetorics of risk are used to mark certain bodies as threats to be contained while masking dominant logics of race, class, and family formation through a reliance on the ethos of expertise, feminists are uniquely (and centrally) positioned to challenge mythic notions of maternal worth and its boundedness to the concept of nation. The stakes are not small. The rationale that pits expecting individuals against the pregnancies they carry, wherein pregnant persons are constituted as threats to their unborn children even as they offer up their bodies and lives to bring a pregnancy to term, distorts prenatal care by elevating the fetus above the wellness and even survival of the pregnant person. To be sure, fetal health is not inconsequential. But its prioritization has undoubtedly come at the expense of those who carry and birth children. The United States claims the worst maternal mortality rate in the industrialized world—a shameful and appalling distinction.[101] And the situation is getting worse. Maternal mortality in the United States has more than doubled in the last twenty years; researchers note that the focus on infants at the expense of women is a primary contributing factor to this disturbing trend.[102] Moreover, these facts underscore another way in which maternal mortality reflects cultural assessments of which lives matter—data from the CDC indicate that black women are nearly four times as likely as white women to die of pregnancy or childbirth-related complications,[103] a figure that cannot be fully explained without accounting for the persistence of racism that informs black mothers' treatment by the US health care system.[104] Thus, a reproductive justice ethic calls for explicit attention to race and racism, as well as the relentless reimagining of fetal and infant health as inextricably reliant on the health of the adult human that carries it. To isolate the fetus, to articulate concepts of "fetal personhood" and "fetal risk" as discrete entities, fuels anti-abortion logics and lays a foundation for the discursive conditions that authorize state actions against those pregnant and parenting, including egregious forms of reproductive violence.

We might begin by considering the well-being of expecting parents as simpatico with the pregnancies they carry, even in instances where that framework is challenged in contemporary public imaginaries. Take, for example, a woman recently prosecuted for delaying a Caesarean, or women charged with murder after stillbirths.[105] The concept of risk is central to such state actions, as women have been held responsible for a series of events that lead to compromised or even tragic birth outcomes—even if that outcome was less determined by her decision making than by a confluence of forces leading up to the moment of delivery. But even in the event that a woman's reproductive decision making directly informs a negative or unanticipated birth outcome, it is worth noting that birth is unpredictable and that no "choice" is free of risk. Specific to the examples listed above, Caesareans carry risks that include premature birth, breathing problems, or lower Apgar scores for baby, as well as the maternal risks of infection, hemorrhage, injury to organs, and a higher maternal mortality rate than that associated with vaginal delivery. And while maternal mortality is on the rise in traditional US health care settings, a study on home birth in the United States published in 2014 demonstrates that "among low-risk women, planned home births result in low rates of interventions without an increase in adverse outcomes for mothers and babies."[106] Likewise, when it comes to childbirth and the politics of reproduction, legal abortion is far safer than childbirth—the risk of death in childbirth is fourteen times greater than that associated with abortion.[107] These statistics suggest that, when it comes to reproduction, there are no risk-free choices available. How might we challenge, then, recent and alarming trends in coerced reproductive decision making and state actions against women when they refuse to submit to surveillance, medical expertise, or contemporary reproductive and maternal normativities?

The issues we are invited to contemplate in the wake of the Suleman octuplets necessitate ongoing feminist consideration and struggle. The case of Nadya Suleman sharpens our focus on how rhetorics of homeland security culture fuel reproductive stratification and violence in the early twenty-first century. Building on discussions of security and risk, I turn now to the politics of emergency.

CHAPTER 3

Post-Prevention?

Conceptualizing Emergency Contraception

> Amy Cappiello was 24 years old the night the condom broke. She sat up in a panic, thought about her job on Capitol Hill and her grad school commitments, and cried. Then there was the fact that she and her boyfriend had only been seeing each other for two months. It was just not the time for her to become somebody's mom. With her boyfriend, Cappiello went right to the emergency room at George Washington University Hospital. There, a doctor and nurse introduced her to the concept of emergency contraception . . . [which] Cappiello took. To her relief, she didn't become pregnant. "Not being married, making less than $30,000 a year and going to grad school, having a baby would have been a nightmare," Cappiello says now, a year later. "Not only was I not physically ready in terms of being able to provide a stable environment for a baby, but emotionally I was nowhere near ready to have a baby thrust upon me. We would have handled it, but it would have been devastating.
>
> —Suz Redfearn, *Preparing for a Mistake*

Penned in May 2002 for the *Washington Post*, Suz Redfearn's report on the politics and promise of emergency contraception (EC) noted the increasing entanglement of EC "in one of the most sensitive debates of our time—the nature of life's beginning."[1] As debates over the accessibility of EC accelerated in the years following 9/11, Redfearn's focus on personal experience was exceedingly rare. Indeed, Cappiello's story was a narrative respite in a sea of politically contentious disputes over scientific evidence, religious beliefs, and so-called family values. What, then, did this story reveal? Cappiello signaled, in many ways, the twenty-first-century American dream for women, made possible by the gains of first- and second-wave feminisms. Young, upwardly mobile, pursuing higher education and a career in government, Cappiello seemed steady on a path toward success. As Cappiello herself was clear to note, however, her circumstances barred her from parenting in accordance with dominant cultural norms. She was not in a long-term relationship, made less than $30,000 annually, and was still pursuing her education. Thus, the emergency remedied here was not simply a broken condom. The emergency was also the potential pregnancy under Cappiello's circumstances—a clear threat to the American dream and its attachments to white, middle-class heteronuclear family formation. The use of the term "nightmare" was both fitting in its candor and revealing in its broader cultural context.

Homeland maternity provides a critical framework for understanding the political tensions and cultural stakes that animated public struggles over the availability of EC in the early twenty-first century. These public struggles were nearly nonexistent when EC was approved for US sale in 1997, but they intensified quickly and considerably in the early years of the George W. Bush administration—fueled by the rise of "family values" politics, abstinence culture, and the swift return to conservativism that articulated traditional gender roles (and femininity specifically) to the interests of nation in the wake of the 9/11 terrorist attacks. Within homeland security culture, the concept of emergency acquired a new meaning and traction and, consequently, reshaped birth control politics. This becomes clear through the public discourse concerning EC between 1997 and 2006, when EC was formally approved by the US Food and Drug Administration (FDA) but available only by prescription. A coalition of feminists, medical professionals, and public health organizations launched a campaign for over-the-counter (OTC) EC; in April 2003 the manufacturers of Plan B® (the most well-known brand of EC) submitted an application to change its status. While the requirements for nonprescription drug status are straightforward—and Plan B seemed a textbook case—contentious debates raged for years, ensnaring public health officials, advocacy organizations, medical associations, FDA commissioners and committee members, media outlets, members of Congress, the Government Accountability Office, and even the Bush administration itself. These debates reside at the heart of this chapter. What follows is a close investigation into the origins of the public debates circulating around EC, to elucidate how early debates shaped how it would come to be understood in dominant imaginaries for years to come. My analysis reveals how the unorthodox reclassification of EC was uniquely tethered to a dispersion of reproductive surveillance and control—an impact felt more acutely by some of the most vulnerable women, those already subject to increased surveillance in homeland security culture.

Although EC was not necessarily new at the start of the twenty-first century, its polemic function was invigorated through FDA deliberations on OTC status and intensified through its location within homeland security culture. As FDA officials wrestled with the parameters of EC's availability, the perceived significance of an "unprecedented" means of managing pregnancy prevention—and specifically, a means of *preventing* pregnancy *after* sex—provoked a range of responses that both stoked and aimed to assuage cultural panics regarding young women and sexual expression. More specifically, as a reproductive technology imagined to disrupt normative sexuality and pregnancy prevention, EC was discursively domesticated through related logics of "exception" and "emergency" that bolstered conservative cultural beliefs. Rhetorics of emergency circumscribed EC within the bounds of normative contraceptive use. More specifically, in the midst of heightened cultural anxieties regarding the sexual "excesses" of women, what became necessary was not a defense of reproductive choice, but a demonstration of reproductive discipline. The 2006 FDA decision that followed years of public controversy was alarmingly unorthodox—never before had the agency assigned age as the factor that determines the prescription status of a medication.[2] Placing EC behind the counter and subjecting women to pharmacist refusal clauses, state identification, and age requirements, the reclassification of EC fueled an uneven distribution of reproductive choice and coercion, reflecting the disparate conditions of life in an era of homeland maternity.

The EC debates are explicitly rhetorical; they are best critically interrogated as a set of forces that shape the role of this contraceptive technology in women's lives. Mapping how dominant discourses operate alongside one another both ideologically and materially, I illuminate significant collective investments in how emergency contraception was made meaningful—including its imagined "legitimate" use (and users). I assume that technologies like EC are neither inevitable nor predetermined in their cultural force, but that they function instead, in the words of Andrew Feenberg, as "scene[s] of struggle"[3]—sites of cultural anxiety onto which codified social roles are projected and played out.[4] Foregrounding the complex and mutually constitutive relationship between culture and technology, I am less interested in the mechanical function of EC than in its cultural import and epistemological function, in how it was discursively imagined to reshape individual agency as well as collective values. Of course, EC undeniably enables a particular physical effect on the reproductive body; in fact, it may offer much promise to those who advocate birth control methods that place the locus of control in the hands of women in order to guard against reproductive coercion and abuse. Most often, EC is self-administered and, in a significant departure from other contraceptives, designed to be taken *after* unprotected sex. That said, I argue that EC also engenders another set of material effects that rely on its discursive figuration—that is, an expansion (and subsequent contraction) of possibilities through which women's reproductive rights and choices—their experiences of sexuality, maternity, indeed of the body itself—are negotiated and constrained. In this way, the debates over EC function as a clear representative anecdote for homeland maternity, as a set of discursive alignments between motherhood and nation that draw on the logic of homeland security culture to govern women's sexual and reproductive lives.

A number of sources would provide insight into an exploration of EC's discursive figuration, illuminating how EC is imagined to negotiate relationships and identities. To the extent that mediated accounts provide access to public voices and cultural sentiments that substantively inform public policy decisions regarding the use and regulation of EC, my focus here is on dominant media coverage of the EC debates.[5] In the critical reading of these popular discourses, I explore how EC occupies contested and unstable ontological ground, transgressing the borders and chasms between birth control and abortion and fueling cultural panics regarding sexual purity. In response to this instability, I argue that EC is discursively managed through rhetorics of "emergency" that draw on the ethos of science, emphasize normative family planning and sexual restraint, and discipline women differentially. I note how advocacy for EC access ultimately reinscribes antiabortion cultural sentiment and racialized understandings of sexual "purity," particularly for young and/or single women. Finally, I turn to the peculiarities of the FDA decision to place EC behind the counter for women eighteen and older. Age and point of sale restrictions remained formally in place until 2013; a convoluted history of shifting restrictions has resulted in uneven access and availability to this day. Significantly, FDA restrictions were both forecasted by and resulted in the uneven intensification of control over young women's sexual and reproductive lives in the early twenty-first century.

Nebulous Conceptions for Emergency Contraception

Prior to disentangling the "emergency" from the "contraception," some historical and factual information is of critical note. Postcoital contraception, now commonly referred to as EC, is a concentrated dose of birth control that can prevent pregnancy up to five days after unprotected sex. The only forms of EC available on the market during the OTC debate—and the only forms available OTC today—are time sensitive, meaning that effectivity declines significantly as days pass. Importantly, these forms of EC cannot harm or terminate an existing pregnancy. Perhaps contrary to popular belief, EC is not a recent development,[6] and its complex history continues to shape its use and availability to this day.

The practice of combining regular birth control pills in order to prevent pregnancy after unprotected sex dates back almost to the inception of hormonal birth control itself. In the mid-1960s, two of the scientists credited with the development of the pill initiated research on a "morning-after pill" that would prevent conception by reducing the chance of ovulation and/or fertilization. Scientists' uncertainty over the naming of this contraceptive—early considerations included "morning-after pill," "week-later pill," and even "second-thought pill"—foreshadowed struggles over the meaning of EC in the early twenty-first century that constitute the focus of this chapter. In the late 1960s, physicians began to offer patients off-label[7] combinations of regular birth control pills in order to prevent pregnancy in what they would deem "emergency" circumstances—mostly in cases of sexual abuse and incest; simultaneously, postcoital contraceptives were folded into burgeoning contraceptive activism on college campuses.[8] In 1974, A. Albert Yuzpe published the first scientific study of EC; the standard regimen that ensued bore his name and consisted of a series of regular birth control pills taken twelve hours apart.[9] The Yuzpe regimen and related forms of postcoital contraception, however, remained obscure and largely inaccessible for decades despite the promotional efforts of health care providers and organizations.[10] During this time, mainstream media coined the term *morning-after pill* to describe postcoital contraception. The colloquialism remains a common descriptor to date, despite that its effectiveness for up to five days after unprotected sex renders the title a misnomer. Advocates adopted the term *emergency contraception* in the 1990s in an attempt to define EC as a form of contraception intended for use in exceptional circumstances,[11] a rhetorical shift that indicates, as I argue in this chapter, the rootedness of recent EC struggles in the politics of sexual purity and abortion.

In 1997, the FDA officially sanctioned the Yuzpe regimen and, in an unprecedented move, solicited pill manufacturers for a new drug explicitly designed for "emergency" use, one that could be easily administered and would avoid the side effects associated with combining regular birth control pills.[12] While major pharmaceutical companies refused, citing concerns over profitability and potential liability, two companies formed with the explicit objective of creating a dedicated postcoital contraceptive pill—Gynétics, the manufacturer of Preven®, and the Women's Capital Corporation, the manufacturer of Plan B.[13] While Preven was removed from the market in 2004, Plan B proved successful in its safety, effectivity, and ease of use, with minimal side effects or complicating factors. The FDA approved Plan B for prescription use in 1999, but as many health professionals noted, EC easily fulfilled the requirements for OTC availability. As David Grimes, clinical professor of obstetrics and gynecology at the University of North Carolina, explained, EC should be made available over the counter because "it's not dangerous, addictive, or complex."[14] In 2001, the Center for Reproductive Law and Policy submitted a citizen petition on behalf of a large coalition to make EC available over the counter; the manufacturer of Plan B followed in 2003 with a formal application to the FDA for OTC consideration.[15]

The formal approval of prescription-status EC by the FDA was greeted with little political fanfare and an emphasis on scientific progress and technological promise. In 1997, even prior to the introduction of Plan B and Preven, *Time* was quick to celebrate the implications of the FDA's decision to approve the Yuzpe regimen. "The Good News" section of a regular health update declared that "America wakes up to MORNING-AFTER PILLS" (original emphasis). "The FDA has okayed the use of megadoses of ordinary birth-control pills, taken within 72 hours of sex, to prevent pregnancy. The regimen, which is 75% effective, is already widely used in Europe."[16] Other early headlines broadcast the news in similar, fairly neutral terms, proclaiming "New Access to a Range of Contraceptives" and "Emergency Contraceptive Gives Women a Second Chance to Prevent Pregnancy."[17] And echoing this sentiment on the heels of the FDA announcement, EC was featured on the popular prime-time television series *ER*, sympathetically written into the narrative as a key element of compassionate care for victims of sexual assault.[18] Thus, much of the public discourse surrounding EC at its official entry onto the US market reflected similar emphases on Western innovation, medical progress, and compassionate care; it also assumed, for the most part, political neutrality. These assertions were relatively short-lived, however, quickly eclipsed by moral panic and public disputes regarding EC's use and function.

Emergency contraception filtered into public consciousness in the early years of the twenty-first century, as conservativism was enthusiastically revived in the social and political fabric of US life. Conservativism stoked public controversy over EC considerably and, complicating matters, the FDA was deliberating the status and availability of EC just as another pill was making headlines: medication abortion (commonly referred to as mifepristone, RU-486, or the abortion pill).[19] While entirely distinct from one another in their use and function—again, EC cannot compromise or terminate an existing pregnancy—this coincidence accelerated existing confusion and anxiety over EC. For example, even early celebrations of EC as a "new and improved" technique were tempered by discordant explications of its functioning: "Preven's dose of hormones keeps a fertilized egg from implanting in the uterine wall. It's available only by prescription, but it'll stop a pregnancy 72 hours after sex."[20] The use of the word "stop" is peculiar in this context—it does not quite refer to pregnancy prevention, but neither does it refer to pregnancy termination. Thus, as this quotation suggests, one of the fundamental tensions marking the discursive entry of EC into US life at the turn of the century was its tenuous and unstable location within reproductive politics. EC was regularly articulated as both, but not quite either, abortion or birth control. Nonetheless, it was frequently positioned as a defining issue within contemporary abortion politics: "the abortion pill and the emergency contraception pill—because of their ease of use, the mechanisms by which they work and the fact that they are taken after sex—have blurred the line between contraception and abortion and have added a new wrinkle to the traditional anti-abortion movement."[21] This fundamental conflation quickly became the site for the expression of various cultural anxieties, including those related to sexual purity and abortion. If EC was to be publicly justified for OTC use, these collective fears demanded discursive negotiation and redress. In short, EC became a flashpoint for abortion politics in homeland security culture; as a result, an exceptional means of negotiation emerged to assuage public fears.

Post-Prevention Contraception

EC occupied unstable ground within an increasingly hostile anti-choice environment. As President George W. Bush's 2000 campaign slogan "compassionate conservativism" gave way to post-9/11 security concerns and the resurgence of "family values" politics, the so-called culture wars ignited, locating issues such as abortion and same-sex marriage at the heart of social, political, and legislative struggle. In the wake of the terrorist attacks, the Reverend Jerry Falwell famously blamed feminists and other progressives for 9/11 and more general US decline: "the pagans, and the abortionists, and the feminists, and the gays and the lesbians. . . . I point the finger in their face and say, 'You helped this happen.'" Pat Robertson was quick to agree with Falwell: "I totally concur, and the problem is we have adopted that agenda at the highest levels of our government."[22] While Falwell faced public censure as a result of these comments and eventually issued an apology, his sentiments were echoed by other conservative leaders such as Karen Hughes, senior advisor to President Bush, Focus on the Family founder James Dobson, and conservative journalist John O'Sullivan. As Susan Faludi explains, "post-9/11, feminism's defense of legal abortion was accordingly deemed a Benedict Arnold act."[23] In concert with the veneration of white, middle-class motherhood that functioned as a collective salve in a post-9/11 world (see chapter 1), abortion was figured as contrary to the "culture of life" valued anew in the months and years following the terrorist attacks.

As pro-natalist, opt-out culture surged, so too did anti-choice legislation. According to the Guttmacher Institute, "the number of states considered hostile to abortion skyrocketed between 2000 and 2014."[24] Severe legislative restrictions enacted in states across the country more than doubled the number of states considered hostile to abortion rights; of the twenty-seven considered "hostile" to abortion rights in 2014, eighteen were considered extremely hostile, up from zero in 2000.[25] In the same period of time, "the number of states supportive of abortion rights fell from 17 to 13 . . . [and] the proportion of women of reproductive age living in supportive states fell from 40% to 31%."[26] These statistics reflect a steady erosion of abortion rights across the country due to policies that, for example, severely restrict minors' access to services, mandate waiting periods, and/or state-scripted counseling designed to deter women seeking abortion, and target abortion providers with unnecessary regulations that threaten their capacity to provide care. Thus, at the turn of the twenty-first century, abortion was increasingly targeted by legislators and figured within dominant US culture as one of the defining moral crises of the time, an issue to which I return in the next chapter. For now, I note that EC was quickly folded into the factious politics of abortion as struggles over EC's function frequently, and erroneously, conflated EC with abortion (both in general and with medication abortion specifically). At the very least, EC was frequently imagined as not quite preventive enough—an imagining read against the grain of the preemptive paradigm arresting the homeland in the early years of the twenty-first century.

One of the fundamental questions animating public debate centered on making sense of EC, on determining whether this technology was a method of birth control, a form of abortion, or not quite either. This question was raised in both implicit and explicit terms, as EC was regularly positioned in the unsettling space *between* contraception and abortion. Imagined as *post-prevention* contraception, EC was simultaneously defined *as* birth control while disarticulated *from* birth control. It oscillated between the new and the familiar, the exception and the rule, with regularity but little ease. Its apparent instability as a reproductive technology was a site of continual rhetorical struggle. First, EC was regularly asserted as a method of contraception, but continually circumscribed by the logic of emergency: "Plan B, as the name implies, is the backup when Plan A fails. It's the second chance to avoid pregnancy after sex. It's what you can do instead of waiting in a high state of anxiety."[27] The notion of exception permeated this imagining. EC was figured as post-prevention contraception—an opportunity to eclipse fear and distress by preempting the possibility of unintended pregnancy when typical preventative practices have failed. The use of EC is clearly the exception, as opposed to the rule—or more precisely, it is an addendum to the rules: "And if the condom breaks? Or a woman forgets to take her pill? There's something for emergencies now, too, a last stop before pregnancy."[28] This was, then, *not* your everyday birth control.

And yet, at times EC was figured as precisely that—an ordinary, commonplace, and otherwise unremarkable method of pregnancy prevention. Particularly for advocates in favor of loosening restrictions, aligning EC with everyday birth control was used to compel legitimacy. A medical director for Planned Parenthood stated that "[EC] is one of the safest medicines we have available, and it can prevent unplanned pregnancies."[29] EC's hormonal constitution was often cited as evidence of its normalcy: "The pills are essentially birth control pills in higher doses. But as their name suggests, they are not intended as regular birth control. They are for what advocates say they hope are rare instances of unprotected sex, or when, say, a condom breaks."[30] This delicate dance elides clear definitional categories. Here, and in much of the public discussion regarding the ontological location of emergency contraception within reproductive politics, there was a clear conflation of terms. EC was simultaneously figured as not-at-all birth control and just like birth control; it was both unremarkable and everyday, extraordinary and exceptional. It was rigorously positioned as preventive, but simultaneously situated as an atypical form of prevention.

The exception that continually marked and legitimated EC was, in part, affectively mobilized by the medication's (imagined) tenuous relationship to abortion itself. At times, medication abortion functioned simply as a counterpoint to distinguish emergency contraception and clarify its use: "unlike Mifeprex or mifepristone, previously known as RU-486, which can induce an abortion safely during the first 49 days of pregnancy, morning-after pills do not cause abortion, advocates say."[31] Citing "advocates" in this way questions the distinction between EC and mifepristone, even as it was asserted. And indeed, the differences between these two medications were not always entirely clear; at times they were thoroughly confused. Summarizing noteworthy medical advances in 2003, an article in *Time* magazine stated that "Plan B, as the two-pill regimen would be called, would enable women to end pregnancies within 72 hours of unprotected intercourse."[32] Wording that referred to "ending" pregnancies clearly marked EC as a method of termination, and implicitly invoked the abortion pill. While the technical language in *Time* was corrected in a later issue, the original description exemplified a common conflation of terms that tended to muddle EC's meaning. Moreover, antiabortion advocates regularly drew on common misunderstandings of EC to advocate against its increased availability. Drawing on the logic of emergency for anti-EC advocacy, President of the American Life League Judie Brown stated to the *New York Times* that "the pill acts to prevent a pregnancy by aborting a child . . . the emergency in this case is a baby."[33]

Thus, in attempts to anchor EC in public discourse, the specter of abortion was continually invoked. Abortion was simultaneously *conflated with* and *disarticulated from* EC in a series of rhetorical struggles over how to locate EC within reproductive politics. The instability of EC, however, was not solely linked to an environment increasingly hostile to abortion rights, but it also signaled significant cultural anxieties regarding a perceived excess of choice and sexual freedom in young women's lives. Thus, and significantly, the public reception of EC was also tied to the purity politics that were steady on the rise in homeland security culture.

Purity and the Morning-After Problematic

Amid heated debates surrounding EC and its location within reproductive politics, anxieties began to surface regarding women's supposed "excess" sexuality, anxieties fueled by heightened attention to sexual purity in homeland security culture. The premium placed on purity targeted young white women and girls in particular, and has been interrogated by scholars and activists alike across a range of public controversies, movements, and popular trends.[34] While the debates over EC accessibility have been largely overlooked in interrogations of purity culture, I argue that dominant understandings of EC were fundamentally shaped not only by homeland security abortion politics, but by its attendant politics of purity as well.

A few examples clarify the significance of "purity" in homeland security culture writ large, and particularly at the time that EC's availability was hotly contested. First, the debate over sex education policy is decisively linked to the politics of purity. While abstinence education is not exclusive to the homeland security state,[35] funding for abstinence programming grew exponentially under the two-term Bush administration, with total expenditures exceeding $1.5 billion by 2010, when its funding was significantly curtailed under President Obama.[36] A 2004 report by US Representative Henry Waxman revealed federally funded abstinence curricula to be riddled with factual inaccuracies, dangerous omissions, and discriminatory content.[37] Medical misinformation included egregious claims regarding the ineffectiveness of condoms and the transmission of HIV through sweat and tears; popular curricula used shame and blame to promote conservative gender ideologies, encouraging male dominance in interpersonal relationships while maligning LGBTQ peoples and condemning sex outside of (heterosexual) marriage.[38] Studies of abstinence education have consistently demonstrated that it fails to significantly delay sexual activity and may increase the incidence of unprotected sex at a time when US youth continue to be burdened with one of the highest rates of sexually transmitted infections (STIs), abortions, and unintended pregnancies in the industrialized world.[39] In short, abstinence education is both failing and harmful, but remains championed by social conservatives—and this was particularly true of the George W. Bush administration—under the banner of youth protection and purity.[40] President Obama's proposed 2017 budget would have eliminated federal funding of abstinence education, but the Trump administration reversed course—increasing abstinence-only funding by 50 percent to total $90 million in 2017.[41]

The premium placed on sexual purity is not limited to dangerous public policy or educational curricula, however. As many cultural critics note, abstinence was (and to some extent remains) a powerful pop culture phenomenon and conservative social movement with ties to evangelical Christianity that not only endorses but also fetishizes virginity and sexual inexperience.[42] Abstinence advocacy was popularized in the early twenty-first century by teen celebrities like Britney Spears, Jessica Simpson, Selena Gomez, and Miley Cyrus. As Casey Ryan Kelly notes, abstinence is a mainstay in popular cinema and is marketed to girls and young women, quite literally, in the form of sexy virginity apparel.[43] For example, the Candie's Foundation partnered with *Seventeen* magazine to "educate America's youth about the devastating consequences of teenage pregnancy," designing tank tops and T-shirts that proclaimed "I'm SEXY enough . . . to keep you waiting" (original emphasis), draped on models in provocative poses and captioned "be sexy, it doesn't mean you have to have sex."[44] In rendering chastity "sexy," abstinence advocates proffer "a contradictory series of messages that both admonishes adolescent girls for their sexual desires and valorizes their inexperience as 'worth the wait.'"[45] The virginity fetish has translated also into the sexualization of teens, tweens, and even toddlers—from high heels and bras marketed to preschoolers in mainstream stores like Target, to the popular, if also controversial, reality program *Toddlers in Tiaras*. These disturbing trends reflect what Gigi Durham terms "the Lolita effect," the sexualization of girls in popular culture that insists, simultaneously, on sexual allure and naïveté.[46] The effects reverberate across age—just as the childhood of girls is under relentless assault, so too are women bombarded with messages that their postadolescent bodies are grotesque, from the demonization of fat to the insistence that women rid themselves of all body hair (save that on their head). Sexiness is equated with youth and innocence—in other words, women are desirable when they are inexperienced objects of desire, not when they insist on sexual agency and/or pleasure on their own (adult) terms.

Lastly, the rise of evangelical abstinence campaigns such as True Love Waits, Pure Freedom, and Silver Ring Thing amplify the purity premium. In sex-segregated forums, young women are encouraged to harness the power of modesty, as young men are instructed in containing their "natural" sexual urges.[47] But even as evangelical abstinence campaigns advocate resistance to sex-saturated popular culture, so too do they use sex as a vehicle for the promotion of purity—events feature risqué "second-virginity" testimonies and personal conversion narratives, and borrow on sex positivity to recast "just say no" as "'just say yes' to great sex within marriage."[48] While fairly popular around the turn of the twenty-first century—by 2005, 2.5 million US teens had pledged abstinence through the True Love Waits Campaign alone,[49] and an estimated 10 percent of teen boys and 16 percent of teen girls in the United States had signed virginity pledges by 2007[50]—studies demonstrate that pledging, much like abstinence education, has had no lasting effect on teen abstinence and has fueled a rise in unprotected sex, unintended pregnancy, and increased STI transmission among young people.[51] The efforts of evangelical abstinence campaigns also target younger audiences through father-daughter purity balls, which draw on rituals of marriage to publicly commit the virginity of girls—some as young as four years old—to their fathers until their wedding day. Over 1,400 federally funded purity balls were held in 2006.[52] These events have been extensively—and rightly—critiqued elsewhere by feminist critics for trafficking in antiquated notions of female sexuality as male property as well as what Jessica Valenti describes as "pseudo-incestuous" references to daddy-daughter dating.[53] Here I simply note the presence of purity balls as yet another site where abstinence culture reigns supreme, and where the sexual agency of girls and young women is subject to overt patriarchal control.

Thus, as conservativism flourished in the months and years following 9/11, so too was purity promoted, rendered desirable, and persistently racialized in dominant imaginaries as a means of protecting white womanhood. Put differently, securing the virtue of white female youth was rendered a collective imperative as white motherhood was imagined as a vehicle for the nation. The politics of sexual purity in homeland security culture provides an important contextual framework for understanding how EC was discursively imagined as a form of contraception that provoked promiscuity and evacuated sex of "consequence." As one FDA official infamously wrote in an internal memo (released to the public in 2006 through a lawsuit over undue political influence in the FDA's decision making), making EC OTC might instigate "extreme promiscuous behaviors such as the medication taking on an 'urban legend' status that would lead adolescents to form sex-based cults centered around the use of Plan B."[54]

Such crazed speculation over teen sexuality mimicked a similar impulse in response to the introduction of the birth control pill in 1960,[55] and even anticipated the cultural backlash against the HPV vaccine that Monica Casper and Laura Carpenter trace to the politics of purity.[56] However, to the extent that EC poses the unique capacity for individuals to prevent pregnancy after sex, the belief that this contraceptive fueled sexual excess was particularly acute and invited a new logic—namely, that of emergency—to manage female sexuality. Assumed to encourage casual sex through heightened convenience, EC fueled existing public concerns over sexual purity and youth culture. EC was thought to be too easy and expedient; its consideration for OTC status, the fact that EC "would not only be sold in drugstores, but could also be as available as aspirin [is], on supermarket shelves or in convenience stores or gasoline stations,"[57] rapidly accelerated the circulation of these concerns. To the extent that a morning-after pill might "encourage" sexual pleasure and independence through a proliferation of reproductive choices and the removal of "consequences," EC was imagined to threaten the purity of young white women at the moment that purity itself filtered into the new reproductive regime of the homeland security state.

The "problem" of women's sexual excess was explicitly wed to age. Young women's sexual expression quickly became a volatile site for debate regarding the moral dimensions of EC: "If Plan B goes over the counter . . . what stops teenage girls from using these pills as regular birth control? Will we get to the point where 14-year-old girls are feeding quarters into restroom vending machines for something other than tampons? Will we see a rise in sexually transmitted infections?"[58] OTC EC was figured as access to excess—the impending seduction of too much choice. Indeed, increased availability of emergency contraception was thought to rival, perhaps even eclipse, the pill in validating irresponsible sex and rewarding "deviant"—or otherwise undisciplined—sexual behavior by evacuating it of "consequence" (in other words, diminishing the threat of pregnancy as a punishment for sexual activity) and by removing young women from the medical gaze altogether. As the president of conservative Christian public policy organization Concerned Women for America queried, "How can you make it available OTC for most women and not have it get into the bodies of girls for who it has not been approved without prescription?"[59] In the midst of heightened neoconservatism and the resurgence of the religious right, this explicit reference to young women's (or "girls") bodies positioned EC as a direct threat to white, middle-class purity and virtue. Drawing on common representations of girls in postfeminist culture, girls at the center of the EC debates were rhetorically figured as "at risk." They were "endangered by the world around them (including the proliferation of choices in part provided by feminism and postfeminism) and their personal choices within this context."[60] EC threatened young women in positing the possibility of unprotected sex without material (or, more specifically, maternal) consequence. It seemed to offer superfluous choice and to warrant sexual excess; in other words, it provided young women the opportunity to make "bad" choices.

Moreover, single women in general were figured as "at risk." Reporting on public response to the FDA's eventual easing of restrictions on access to EC in the *New York Times*, journalists noted that one woman "could not decide whether she was glad the morning-after pill would soon be more readily available. Several of her friends have already used the pill multiple times." Throughout much of this discourse, there seemed an unspoken categorical limit that differentiated an authentic emergency from assumed carelessness. EC was regularly faulted for encouraging frivolous and irresponsible sex: "Knowing a backup is available over the counter . . . might make [women] more likely to have unprotected sex. 'Some girls are probably going to get careless. . . . If I didn't get so sick I would use it more often.'"[61] Young women, in other words, were not to be trusted with this kind of decision making. These attitudes anticipate in many ways the FDA decision to place EC behind the counter, transferring and dispersing supervision of women's reproductive lives from doctors to pharmacists who are, significantly, less likely to be favorable to EC access. This is a matter to which I soon return; for now, I note that, according to dominant cultural wisdom, left to their own devices and without the supervision of a medical professional, women might overuse—or even abuse—this method of contraception.

And in some ways, how could they not? The name "morning-after pill" evokes and substantiates fears surrounding the threat of sexual excess: "No more trauma over 'Am I or am I not?' No more decisions on whether to abort, adopt, or go ahead and raise a child you can't afford. The morning-after pill, known as Plan B, erases the night before."[62] In a rare moment of candor and clarity, this reporter for the *Washington Post* underscored a profound source of cultural distress. The "morning after" implies a "night before"—a euphemism for sexually adventurous, even lascivious, behavior. The "morning after" assumes shame, guilt, and regret for actions in violation of normative codes of feminine conduct. Thus, any "morning after pill" was always already constituted through social and moral aberration. Supposedly well-behaved women don't have a "morning after" because they never had a "night before." Thus, how can a pill, imagined to alleviate ills brought on by one's own undisciplined behavior, be properly coded as a rightful choice? This is, of course, precisely the problem—it cannot. Instead, rhetorics of emergency and exception worked to domesticate the meaning of EC. The discursive force of "emergency" was, in fact, disciplinary, mobilizing a politics that hailed immediate action and tightly circumscribed the boundaries of EC's acceptable use.

Science, Purity, and Abortion Politics on the Morning After

In order to refute concerns related to abortion and sexual purity, science became the broader discursive terrain within which claims regarding the proper, "emergency" use of EC were situated so as to compel EC's contraceptive legitimacy. Despite its strategic potential to secure reproductive rights, the discursive mobilization of science and related rhetorics of emergency ultimately reinforce, rather than challenge, the conservative politics of purity and antiabortion sentiment that continue to reign supreme in homeland security culture.

First, advocates for OTC access rely on science to challenge the allegation that EC promotes promiscuity. Rather than questioning the cultural premium placed on purity, repeated scientific accounts of women's sexual and reproductive discipline became a common refrain: "Studies indicate that improving access to emergency contraception neither encourages sexual activity by adolescents nor causes women to abandon their regular methods of contraception."[63] Hard data were offered in support of these claims: "studies showed that making [EC] available did not prompt women to use it repeatedly. Of 540 women in one study . . . 10 used it more than once."[64] Another report drew a parallel between EC-inspired anxieties and those that circulated around other dimensions of sexual health and rights: "When sex education was introduced in schools, some Americans predicted that young people would start copulating like rabbits. Talking about sex would make kids have sex. Carefully controlled studies showed that hasn't been the case for the current generation. . . . It looks as if young women have learned something about abstinence and sex, and they don't make decisions about either because of what they can buy."[65] Thus, scientific demonstration of women's sexual restraint—their adherence to EC as a method of exception and only in cases of emergency—becomes the primary avenue through which EC was made palatable to broader US publics, which were already primed to accept frameworks of emergency and exception as both logical and warranted. Research studies are regularly cited to counter the fear that the increased availability of EC would encourage women's sexual impulses. In an attempt to counter purity panics through empirical evidence, rhetorics of science ironically fix EC within the moral conceptual terrain of purity and sexual restraint. Arguing that women remain sexually disciplined despite ease of EC access, their behavior quite independent from the relative convenience of contraceptives, only functions to reinforce the premium placed on purity in homeland security culture.

Moreover, rhetorics that revert to the "exception" discipline reproductive bodies into traditional feminine sexuality and domesticity. As EC is rhetorically framed as a form of birth control for *extra*ordinary circumstances and scientific evidence marshaled on behalf of these claims, purity panics are tamed by figuring EC within familiar, heteronuclear understandings of family planning. As a method of *exception*, this positioning of EC allows for a circumvention of the imagined threat of "sex cults" or other forms of casual sex, rendering EC consonant with homeland maternity writ large. In a particularly explicit example, EC was declared "not a form of birth control. It is there in case the birth control method fails. The condoms breaks, the diaphragm slips. A woman forgets to take her pills. Or she has sex when she wasn't planning on it."[66] Here, the use of EC signals neither carelessness nor a shirking of responsibility, but rather, *extra* care and diligence in pregnancy prevention efforts, a kind of preemptive preventive preparedness. Simultaneously, in this same example, a variety of exceptional circumstances are identified so as to underscore the compatibility of EC with mainstream family planning measures, consequently recasting women's use of EC as thoroughly responsible, disciplined, and perhaps even unremarkable. Implicit is the suggestion that EC functions as the "non-choice" between the practice of ordinary birth control and the politicized right to an abortion—in other words, EC becomes the inevitable (and *responsible*) middle ground between one choice eclipsed and another suspended altogether. The discourse of emergency, then, articulates EC to extraordinary circumstance and, in so doing, disciplines its use—and women themselves—into normative codes of sexuality and "responsible" decision making.

Rhetorics of science and emergency were also inflected by reproductive stratification and the differential valuation of motherhood. Science was deployed not only to deflate or minimize fear of sexual excess, but also in the circulation of a related, differentiated fear—that of reproductive excess. In other words, in addition to demonstrating women's sexual restraint, scientific studies of EC focused specifically on the potential of EC to address the structural dimensions of so-called unwanted pregnancies and abortion, as reported, in this example, by the *Washington Post*: "advocates of wider use say [EC] would result in a decline in unwanted pregnancies and abortion."[67] While offering women another preventive safeguard against unintended pregnancy remains a laudatory goal, throughout this discourse there exists a troubling slippage between how individual women may feel about their pregnancies (i.e., as desirable or not), and social attitudes about "unwanted pregnancies" and who is "fit" for motherhood. For example, a *New York Times* reporter noted that opponents of EC were not convinced of the drug's safety, but "others argued that for teenagers pregnancy was a far worse alternative."[68] In this moment, drug safety and teen pregnancy were positioned as mutually exclusive and of equal concern; implicit was the suggestion that teen pregnancy could lead only to undesirable outcomes (viz., teen parenting or abortion, a matter to which I return to more fully in the next chapter). In a similar example, prior to the arrival of the OTC debate in the United States, early reporting focused on the loosening of restrictions to EC access in Europe and was framed in this manner: "In the last decade, Britain has experienced a steady increase in the number of teenage pregnancies, unwanted pregnancies and abortions. In 1998, the last year for which figures are available, 22 percent of pregnancies ended in abortion. In addition, in a country struggling to promote a family-based agenda, 51.2 percent of new babies were born to unwed mothers."[69] While this statistic was corrected a week later (the correct percentage of single mothers being not 51.2 but 37.8), the anxiety expressed here was palpable; EC was explicitly imagined as a means of managing the reproductive "excesses" of particular women. In this example, teenage and single mothers are isolated demographics among otherwise "unwanted" pregnancies and the overall rate of abortion; indeed, single motherhood was cast in glaring opposition to family—and, by extension, the nation.

These repeated scientific emphases on reducing "unwanted" pregnancies play on longstanding race and class bias regarding the politics of motherhood, effectively relocating cultural concern from the *sexual* excess of some women to the *reproductive* excess of other women—namely, young, unmarried, and/or low-income women. Consistent with a history of reproductive politics in which young women, low-wealth women, racialized immigrant women, and women of color are figured as "unfit" mothers, EC became another site where longstanding cultural bias was enacted on a twenty-first-century stage. Thus, scientific arguments for EC that focus on women's sexual restraint and reproductive discipline reinforce conservative purity politics at best, but also offer more insidious endorsements of the differential valuation of motherhood and racist, heteronormative conceptions of nation.

Second, in addition to shoring up purity politics, EC advocates' use of science frequently draws on antiabortion cultural sentiment as a primary rationale for increasing access to EC. This is evidenced in earlier examples wherein the specter of teen pregnancy was raised to marshal support for preventing the possibility of abortion (or teen parenting). But antiabortion sentiment is also a touchstone of EC advocacy, which emphasizes Plan B as a "middle ground" in the divisive politics of abortion: "The decision is by far the most politically contentious that [the FDA] has confronted in a decade. Whether to provide easier access to the pill has become a pivot point in the debate on abortion rights. Some conservatives say the pill, viewed by the drug agency as a contraceptive, is really an abortion pill. Liberals respond that easier access to it would actually reduce the 800,000 abortions a year in the United States."[70] Similarly, in an editorial titled "A Workable Plan for Fewer Abortions," syndicated columnist Ellen Goodman wrote: "our country still has 3 million unintended pregnancies per year, the highest rate in the industrialized world among adults and teens. Half of them end up as abortions. This is where pro-life ought to meet pro-choice. This is where we should get the politics out of the science and get Plan B on the drugstore shelf."[71] Karen Judd Lewis, a board member of the Wish List organization supporting pro-choice Republican women, concurred to the *Washington Post:* "This is a bridge issue; one in which reasonable people on both sides, those who support abortion rights as well as those who oppose, can find common ground because Plan B can reduce the number of abortions in this country."[72] And Dr. Susan Wood endorsed a similar sentiment in her public resignation as director of the FDA Office of Women's Health: "I feel very strongly that this shouldn't be about abortion politics. . . . This is a way to prevent unwanted pregnancy and thereby prevent abortion. This should be something that we should all agree on."[73] This rhetorical move seemed to address public concerns directly and with expediency, as arguments centered on reducing the incidence of abortion had the potential to placate those who oppose abortion rights and curry favor with mainstream publics who continue to support abortion rights but also register discomfort with the issue.

The focus on abortion, however, specifically elides other ways in which EC might be publicly legitimized. For example, in lieu of anchoring the distress of unintended pregnancy in the fact of unintended pregnancy itself and the limited possibilities that it infers (i.e., adoption, abortion, or parenting), reliance on antiabortion sentiment reinforces figurations of *abortion* as that which is always already tragic and undesirable. EC in many ways makes a unique contribution to reproductive justice advocacy—for instance, in its capacity to offer some relief to survivors of assault, and in its potential to locate reproductive control more squarely in the hands of women. EC might have been discursively justified as such, or even simply as yet another method for pregnancy prevention. Mainstream advocacy efforts on behalf of EC, however, regularly emphasize a predicted reduction in the US abortion rate. While these attempts to position EC as a "middle ground" in the politics of abortion eventually proved politically expedient, they nonetheless acquiesce to increasingly mainstream conservative values. Put another way, in lieu of a political defense of reproductive justice in all of its forms, the science marshaled on behalf of EC access bolsters antiabortion sentiment as both reasonable and mainstream. EC, it would seem, could not escape the politics of abortion that informed much of the initial public discord over its availability and use.

The discursive figuration of EC is also notable for what remains absent. Significantly, rhetorics of choice were largely removed from the debates that ensued over Plan B in the early twenty-first century. This departure from what was then, and to a certain extent remains, a mainstream rhetorical framework for reproductive rights was precipitated by the reinforcement of purity and antiabortion politics in EC advocacy efforts. "Choice"—not to mention something as radical as reproductive justice—was rendered politically incompatible with a "morning-after" contraceptive that was imagined to encourage casual sex and muddy the border between pregnancy prevention and termination. Thus, in the midst of heightened cultural anxieties regarding the sexual and reproductive excesses of women, *what became necessary was not a defense of choice, but a demonstration of discipline*. This was precisely what the rhetoric of emergency works to do—it builds on reigning logics of purity and antiabortion sentiments to properly circumscribe EC within the bounds of "acceptable" use. To the extent that EC is constituted through a logic of exception and emergency, as a reasonable and responsible attempt to avoid abortion, EC is disciplined and legitimized as a "choice." At best, then, choice remains defensible only to the degree that it was, and is, wed to normative sexuality, reproduction, and motherhood. Or perhaps, more insidiously, the logic of exception mobilizes a *suspension* of reproductive freedom and autonomy insofar as it assigns duties that women avoid unintended pregnancy, and the specter of abortion, at all costs. EC is then subsequently ontologized within this space as the nonnegotiable *non-choice of necessity*.

Importantly, the fundamentally conservative ideological terms of the EC debates remain unchecked and unchallenged; they are, in fact, fortified through repeated scientific demonstrations of women's sexual restraint and predicted declines in the rates of unintended pregnancy and abortion. This conservative deployment of science and attendant politics of emergency and purity assembled a horizon of unprecedented possibilities for the ruling on EC. The rhetorical insistence on demonstrating discipline, restraint, and preemptive action, as opposed to defending contraceptive access or reproductive justice, enabled a peculiar set of FDA regulations to unfold regarding Plan B. What followed, consistent with the modes of governance most central to homeland security culture, was an uneven, heightened surveillance and policing of women's sexual and reproductive decision making by their local pharmacists.

Behind the Counter

The early years of struggle over the function, use, and availability of EC has had a lasting impact on policy and public attitudes. Indeed, these debates resulted in a form of regulation that amplified the surveillance of the most vulnerable women's reproductive decision making. In 2006, after protracted public debates, excessive requests for additional research on the safety of EC for minors, lawsuits over and government inquiries into the Bush administration's political interference in the process, the FDA finally approved Plan B for nonprescription sales, but with two significant restrictions related to age and point of sale. Plan B was made available in pharmacies and health clinics "behind-the-counter" to those eighteen and older with a valid form of identification.[74] Advocates challenged this ruling in court. In 2009, a federal judge ordered the FDA to lower the age restriction to seventeen; the FDA complied but did not reevaluate the age restriction more broadly, as per the court order. Lawsuits continued; the manufacturer of Plan B submitted more data on the safety and effectiveness of EC for younger teens. Given clear and resounding scientific evidence, the FDA was prepared to lift all restrictions on EC. But in December 2011, less than one year prior to the 2012 presidential election, then-secretary of Health and Human Services Kathleen Sebelius overruled the FDA commissioner. The move was stunning—never before had HHS overruled the FDA. Echoing the ideological insistences of their administrative predecessors, and despite all scientific evidence to the contrary, Sebelius cited concerns about inadequate data on adolescent use of EC, and President Obama concurred publicly. Another lawsuit ensued. In 2013, a federal judge ordered the FDA to lift age and point-of-sale restrictions, noting that prior FDA decisions regarding Plan B had been "arbitrary, capricious, and unreasonable."[75] The Obama administration appealed the ruling but was denied. Thus, in the summer of 2013, Plan B was finally made available over the counter. Related generics were quick to follow.

The impact of the behind-the-counter ruling was, and remains, complex and differential. Studies demonstrate that the change in status increased the availability of EC and bolstered its use as well; between 2002 and 2011, the number of women who reported using EC at some point in their lifetime more than doubled.[76] As advocates predicted, increased access has not fueled "risky" sexual behavior, but interestingly, studies suggest that neither has EC's behind-the-counter status decreased the incidence of unintended pregnancy.[77] Young women, Spanish speakers, and women in rural communities continue to face greater obstacles in obtaining EC. Studies have repeatedly demonstrated that teenage girls and women face significant bias in their attempts to access EC from pharmacists—research has revealed that young women are more likely to be given false information about parental consent, age restrictions, and availability than their male peers or physicians.[78] Research on language and geography reveals that Spanish-speaking women and women in rural communities are more likely to be refused access to EC from pharmacists than their English-speaking or urban peers.[79] The costs associated with EC bar some low-income women from access in the absence of consistent Medicaid coverage,[80] and misinformation about EC availability is more common in pharmacies located in low-income neighborhoods.[81]

Compounding these concerns, the fluctuating rules and regulations surrounding EC's availability have proven a barrier to accessibility. A 2014 report revealed that Indian Health Services (IHS) denied Native American women consistent access—20 percent of IHS clinics did not carry Plan B and, despite regulatory changes, 11 percent demanded a prescription and 72 percent imposed age restrictions.[82] IHS clarified its policy in 2015, resulting in significant improvements,[83] but similar trends persist in dominant health care settings as well. A national survey in 2015 demonstrated that only two-thirds of pharmacies stock EC; of those that do, almost half place EC in a locked box or case that requires the involvement of a store employee and draws attention to the purchase.[84] Moreover, the study revealed that "misinformation about age restrictions and ID requirements continues to be widespread"; 38 percent of pharmacies surveyed required an ID to purchase EC, and 39 percent of participants were erroneously informed by pharmacy staff that there was an age restriction to purchase.[85] The result is uneven and unpredictable OTC access that tends to work against the most vulnerable women and communities.

In addition to numerous scientific studies that have accounted for the uneven effects of the FDA rulings, the discursive dimensions of the initial decision to place EC behind the counter and its aftermath are worthy of interrogation. Consistent with other troubling aspects of homeland maternity, the behind-the-counter ruling drew on the logic of purity and antiabortion cultural sentiment, ultimately subjecting women to public layers of surveillance and policing, from pharmacy personnel to the publicity of the pharmacy itself. Indeed, the ruling places women directly in the crosshairs of contentious disputes over EC and health care refusal. In lieu of standard OTC availability, the FDA decision requires women to consult with pharmacists in order to purchase Plan B in a political climate enamored with purity, hostile to reproductive rights, and increasingly supportive of pharmacists' right of refusal based strictly on personal beliefs (as opposed to reasonable medical or professional concerns that center the health care rights and needs of patients). Persistent debates over EC's status—as birth control, abortion, or not quite either—emboldens conservative movements' attempts to deny women access to EC at the pharmacy counter under the banner of personal conscience and freedom of religion. In short, despite regulatory shifts aimed at ease of access, pharmacies retain immense influence over the availability and accessibility of emergency contraception, and public struggles over right of refusal have curtailed the ability of those seeking EC to expect decent and dignified treatment in the process.

Health care refusal is not limited to EC, but rather it is rooted more broadly in opposition to reproductive rights. "Conscience clauses" or "right-of-refusal clauses" target reproductive health care specifically as "the only field in medicine where societies worldwide accept freedom of conscience as an argument to limit a patient's right to a legal medical treatment."[86] In the United States, after Supreme Court rulings in *Roe v. Wade* and *Doe v. Bolton* struck down laws banning abortion nationwide, state and federal governments enacted legal, financial, and professional protections for health care workers and institutions that refused to provide reproductive health care based on personal conviction. On the federal level, most laws guarantee a right of refusal to medical professionals for abortion or sterilization, and the vast majority of states have passed companion legislation at the state level. Public controversies over EC at the turn of the millennium, however, fueled an alarming expansion of "religious and moral objections to providing [reproductive health] care . . . beyond doctors, nurses and hospitals to include pharmacists and pharmacies."[87] Thus, as the EC debates raged, the right to deny reproductive health care based solely on personal belief—even if that belief refused science in asserting, for example, that EC was an abortifacient—was increasingly mainstreamed in homeland security culture, and was thus consonant with a broader context that increasingly authorizes invasions of citizens' privacy and lateral modes of surveillance.

In the early 2000s, state assemblies across the country began to legislate pharmacist refusals. As of this writing, 22 percent of states protect individual pharmacists or pharmacies who refuse women EC, while 10 percent of states require pharmacists to fill all legal prescriptions; some states explicitly name EC as subject to refusal, and others cover EC in refusal clauses related to reproductive health more broadly.[88] In states that lack clear legislative directives, women remain subject to the whimsical judgment of whomever they encounter behind the counter; formal reports of refusal have surfaced in at least twenty-five states.[89] They include horrific accounts of pharmacists refusing to dispense EC despite it being stocked in the pharmacy, confiscating women's prescriptions without filling them, and shaming women loudly and in public. In a particularly egregious example in 2006, a pharmacist in Milwaukee screamed at a mother of six in a crowded waiting room: "You're a murderer! I will not help you kill this baby. I will not have the blood on my hands." The woman reported feeling so embarrassed that she did not attempt to fill her prescription elsewhere and, weeks later, discovered she was pregnant.[90]

Research suggests that these are not isolated incidents. Despite the fact that pharmacists in some locales remain strong proponents for EC, women—and particularly teenagers—report experiencing greater bias, stigma, and judgment from pharmacists than they do from their primary care provider in attempts to obtain EC.[91] These reports cohere with disparities noted between doctors and pharmacists, as studies suggest that the former tends to be more knowledgeable about and supportive of EC than the latter.[92] Corporate and managerial policies provide another layer of complexity, as certain pharmacies refuse to stock EC. Thus, the legal architecture that enables EC refusal is tethered to gendered attitudes regarding sexual and reproductive agency that inform a wide range of cultural practices, and constitutes yet another dimension of the increasingly hostile environment in which women are forced to negotiate their reproductive lives.

Situating our understanding of the EC controversy—and its attendant cultural politics of emergency and purity—within the framework of homeland maternity clarifies the currents and stakes of the struggle. First, homeland maternity draws our attention to how the logic of homeland security culture shapes attitudes and practices related to reproduction and motherhood in contemporary contexts. In the case of the EC debates, the rhetorics of emergency that both authorized and constrained EC's use circulated within a discursive economy of "emergencies" in the homeland security state. In airports, schools, workplaces, and homes, whether instituted through official readiness protocols or suggested via preparedness guidelines on Ready.gov, the discourse of emergency places a premium on preemptive, immediate action. It carefully delineates that which is exceptional from that which is ordinary, suspending normative practice in favor of exceptional practice in moments of perceived rupture or disruption. In the EC debates, the "exception" becomes sex that is unplanned or unprotected—shoring up purity culture and circumscribing "respectable" sexual expression—and particularly for women—as that which is wed to planning, predictability, and heteronuclear family formation. Relatedly, the so-called right to refuse to dispense EC was offered legitimacy through the logic of exception, which quickly eclipsed normative codes of conduct governing relationships between patients and pharmacists. Put another way, as EC was figured a form of birth control for exceptional circumstances, so too did pharmacists claim an exception of their own—that which nullified the mandate to fill women's prescriptions or otherwise provide reproductive health care.

Second, this particular form of dispersed surveillance and policing—located in the hands of individual pharmacies and pharmacists—reflects the logic and modus operandi of homeland security culture writ large. It calls attention to how reproduction and motherhood are increasingly governed from a distance, but governed intensely and differentially nonetheless. The behind-the-counter ruling resulted in increased access for a relatively privileged demographic—namely, adults possessing state identification and insurance or financial security—but shifted the locus of authority from the clinic to the pharmacy. In a context evacuated of privacy and intimacy, and despite a lack of consistent training and education regarding EC, pharmacists were newly anointed gatekeepers, able to determine individual access to a time-sensitive contraceptive on a case-by-case basis. Thus, those able to seek emergency contraception over the counter were caught in a web of cumbersome and misunderstood regulations, inconsistent stocking on pharmacy shelves, as well as pharmacist insensitivity and refusals. In this way, the reclassification of EC both relocated and intensified surveillance of women's reproductive lives and decision making. While visiting a pharmacy is certainly more convenient than visiting a doctor, the mandated involvement of the pharmacist complicated the arrangement considerably—relocating authority to a health care professional less likely to be supportive of EC and in a far more public setting.

Thus, the initial FDA ruling complicated access by creating different sets of barriers for EC access. Prior to 2006, access to EC was largely inhibited by a ticking clock—in other words, access pivoted on finding a doctor and obtaining a prescription as quickly as possible, a process that advocacy groups eased by forming EC hotlines staffed by medical personnel. As the point of access shifted, making pharmacists and pharmacies the ultimate arbiter of EC access, so too was there an escalation of documented pharmacist hostility to dispensing this medication.[93] The pharmacy thus marked a kind of liminal space between the convenience store and the doctor's office—a space of access that was neither speedy nor slow, one that traded both anonymity and confidentiality for an ambivalent space of access. At best, this ruling offered more timely access to a supportive, knowledgeable health care provider who would assist women with care and expediency; at worst, the pharmacy fractures both speed and confidentiality, offering instead a health care professional to stand in the way, publicly, and in some cases, with unduly expressed malice. Much like in the case of Nadya Suleman, the initial FDA ruling on EC mobilized a mode of governing from a distance, a mode that promised intervention when women refused to govern themselves in accordance with heteronuclear norms. And indeed, the negative consequences of this decision have been most acutely felt by women already subject to increased surveillance in the homeland security state—teens, immigrants, low-income women, and women of color. Subsequent rulings have eased legal access considerably, but have also resulted in confusion and uneven availability in ways that continue to compromise access for vulnerable populations.

The behind-the-counter ruling that rendered EC accessible only through a convoluted chain of command was, in many ways, the logical outgrowth of the conservative rhetorical framing that anchored EC in mainstream imaginaries. This case thus points to technology's rhetoricity, to how, in Casper and Carpenter's words, "sexualised technologies (e.g. Viagra, male contraception) . . . cannot be understood outside gender relations and attendant cultural politics."[94] My analysis demonstrates that as a contraceptive technology EC is, indeed, rhetorical, rendering material effects on the world as it is simultaneously made meaningful through public discourse. The cultural ambivalence about EC's effects, the perception of its proximity to abortion and casual sex, and the overreliance on scientific demonstrations of sexual and reproductive discipline all functioned in concert to solidify EC within conservative purity and antiabortion frameworks that were on the rise in homeland security culture, even as its use was authorized in "exceptional" circumstance (notably, under circumstances that privileged the needs of adult women of means). This conservative imagining of EC bolstered arguments in favor of restrictive points of access and tacitly authorized new forms of reproductive surveillance, as EC's placement behind the counter proved particularly insidious in a cultural climate of sexual purity and abstinence.

Thus, much like other instances of homeland maternity traced throughout this book, the discursive figuration of EC fueled a simultaneous dispersion and intensification of discipline in the early years of the twenty-first century. While more recent FDA rulings have undoubtedly improved access to emergency contraceptives, the process has been slow, hampered by this early history—in other words, by the weight of purity politics and antiabortion cultural sentiment that continues to fuel pharmacist refusals and, more broadly, in a context marked by the steady erosion of reproductive rights and dignity in homeland security culture. With varying impact on many US women and disproportionate burdens placed on young women, low-income women, immigrant women, undocumented women, women of color, and rural women, this chapter highlights once again how homeland maternity carries with it differential implications for women that turn on capital, status, and means. While EC advocates' use of conservative frameworks led to some limited success, the relocation and intensification of surveillance is only one consequence of note. The failure to advance a comprehensive defense of reproductive justice in this context—and the implicit support for antiabortion cultural sentiment—renders abortion rights in homeland security culture ever more vulnerable. In the next chapter, I turn to the treatment of teen pregnancy in dominant media, elaborating on purity culture and the "problem" of youth sexuality, and its connection to the increasing colonization of reproductive health clinics in the United States.

CHAPTER 4

Crisis Pregnancy and the Colonization of the Clinic

Yet fiction, the zone where objective truth is not told, paradoxically becomes the site where one specific kind of truth is best articulated.

—Susan Merrill Squier, *Liminal Lives*

I'm like a legend. They call me the Cautionary Whale.

—Juno MacGuff, *Juno*

In the late 2000s, the cautionary "whales" were everywhere. Between 2007 and 2009, as federal funding for abstinence education soared and the pregnancies of celebrity teens Jamie Lynn Spears and Bristol Palin made headlines, a series of films and television shows, including *Juno*, *Glee*, and *The Secret Life of the American Teenager*, premiered to much acclaim and controversy. These narratives, although varied with regard to plot lines and characters, shared a fixation on white teen pregnancy and postfeminist articulations of its proper care and negotiation. Not to be outdone in shock-and-awe programming, reality television quickly followed suit, placing the so-called crisis of teen pregnancy at the center of MTV series *16 and Pregnant*, with spin-off *Teen Mom* premiering shortly thereafter to record-breaking viewership.[1]

Homeland maternity undergirds dominant beliefs about the centrality of motherhood and reproduction in performing citizenship, and popular film and television function as powerful vehicles for this "cultural training."[2] Thus, the pop culture fixation on unintended pregnancy among white teens offers an exemplary site to investigate how young pregnant and parenting women are uniquely governed by and through homeland maternity. Indeed, the proliferation of representations of white teen pregnancy in popular media prompted significant debate. Film critics marked the emergence of a "pregsploitation" subgenre, while scholars named a "Juno effect"[3] and studied points of postfeminist articulation among films like *Juno, Knocked Up*, and *Waitress*.[4] Much ado was made of the "glamorization" of teen pregnancy and motherhood, particularly in the wake of Spears and Palin, the Gloucester 18 "pregnancy pact,"[5] and maternity lines launched by popular teen clothing stores.[6] Most studies of teen pregnancy entertainment media have focused on questions of media effects, debating how films like *Juno* and reality programs like *Teen Mom* influence the sexual and reproductive decision making of teenagers.[7] While these are important sites of scholarly inquiry, this chapter does not engage questions related to teen behavior and its causal forces. Rather, I extend a smaller body of critical scholarship, which tends to focus *either* on representations of teen pregnancy in reality programing *or* unintended pregnancy in film regardless of age.[8] I argue for sustained engagement across genres, with an explicit focus on *teen* pregnancy, in order to examine how young pregnant and parenting women are folded into homeland maternity.

The paucity of attention to young women of color in the midst of this cultural zeitgeist does not necessarily signal their absence. References to youth—and teenagers in particular—in the context of reproductive politics have long functioned as discursive shorthand, voicing national anxieties over race, class, and family formation while denying their significance. From cultural panics over unwed motherhood in post–World War II containment culture to the "epidemic" of teen pregnancy declared decades later, young, unmarried mothers have long been imagined to threaten the "ideological and material production of the nation."[9] Homeland security culture offers a new context, but proves no exception in exhibiting these patterned alignments between nation and motherhood. The racialization of so-called teen pregnancy sculpts how *all* teen mothers are read to a certain extent and, as such, renders whiteness a condition of possibility for resolving the "crisis" in popular media narratives. As yet another site of interest for exploring the form and function of homeland maternity, the recent history of teen pregnancy in popular entertainment media coincides meaningfully with pronatalist fertility panics, as well as recent public struggles over teen sexuality and access to contraception; moreover, they emerge at a unique moment within the history of US adoption and abortion politics.

In this chapter, I trace the proliferation of teen pregnancy in popular entertainment media of the late 2000s, analyzing how rhetorics of crisis anchor the meaning and salience of teen pregnancy and motherhood in dominant imaginaries. The texts of interest include a full-length feature film (*Juno*), a critically acclaimed television show (*Glee*), and two hit reality series (*16 and Pregnant* and

Teen Mom).[10] This does not exhaust the presence of crisis teen pregnancy in popular entertainment media. It does, however, study those narratives that share three primary features; first, that of cultural salience, evidenced through critical acclaim, a widespread audience, and powerful presence in popular culture. Second, each scripted text relies on comedy to shape the meaning of crisis and its resolution, which dovetails with the makeover impulse of reality programming in ways that prove significant to representations of race and class. Finally, these narratives emerge at a significant moment in US reproductive politics. Between 2007 and 2010, teen pregnancy garnered a wealth of public attention—not only for its ubiquity in popular culture, but also because the teen birth rate spiked in 2006, briefly reversing a decades-long decline as federal funding for abstinence education neared its zenith. Concurrently, international adoption rates fell to historic lows due to increased regulation and oversight under the Hague Convention. Given the expansiveness and diversity of the selected texts, my focus is less on providing a detailed analysis of each than it is on charting their coherence with one another and their connection to homeland maternity.

To begin, I situate teen pregnancy historically and elaborate on related contemporary phenomena that include adoption, purity politics, and the overt sexualization of girls and young women in popular culture. I then turn to a critical reading of the aforementioned texts, noting how crisis teen pregnancy entertainment media manage anxieties over motherhood and nation by offering teens neoliberal risk tutorials—tools for self-governance that emphasize postfeminist empowerment through (pre)maternal prudence and responsibility. Finally, I explore how the logic of crisis resonates beyond entertainment media to shape contemporary US reproductive politics, with specific attention to the crisis pregnancy center movement led by the evangelical right and the colonization of comprehensive women's health clinics across the country.

Figuring Crisis Teen Pregnancy, Then and Now

Teen pregnancy is in many ways a fiction, an "epidemic" invented in the late twentieth century that rewrote concerns related to race and class through the prism of age. Raced and classed figurations of single mothers and their families in the early twentieth century serve as powerful historical precedents to the invention of teen pregnancy as an epidemic. In the early twentieth century, single motherhood was defined as a social problem, and white unwed mothers in particular were imagined as fallen women who passed along their "inferior" moral fiber along to their children.[11] Still, their motherhood, though sharply criticized, was neither questioned nor denied. But as the nation recovered from the Great Depression and entered another world war, the rise of youth culture fueled the invention of the teenager as a liminal space between childhood and adulthood, and various changes took hold in the postwar era that followed. Dominant media figured adoption as child rescue, piquing public interest as the number of nonfamily adoptions rose precipitously and hopeful couples outnumbered healthy (and thus desirable) available infants ten to one.[12] Moreover, as childless white couples were recognized as a significant market, Freudian theories achieved increasing resonance and thus the biological pathologies attributed to white single motherhood ceded to psychology and were reimagined as reparable. As a result, white babies born to unmarried women were newly defined as both desirable and adoptable, despite the stigmas stubbornly attached to their mothers.

At the same time in the postwar era, premarital sex and unintended pregnancies were on the rise as birth control was tightly restricted, sex education nearly nonexistent, and abortion often illegal and life threatening. Many young women—mostly, but not exclusively, white—were caught in the midst of these tensions, as strict codes for middle-class conformity evicted unwed pregnant teens from their families, schools, and communities.[13] Kicked out of school, shamed by religious leaders and family members, young women were exiled to maternity homes—forced to wait out their pregnancies, give birth, surrender their babies, and return home months later sworn to secrecy. Based on extensive interviews with the "girls who went away," Ann Fessler concludes that the expectation that women "move on as if [their pregnancies] never happened caused many irreparable harm. Rather than being prepared during their residency either for mothering or for the feelings that would follow relinquishment, the women were made to feel like something was wrong with them for loving and mourning the loss of their child." Even those who exerted extraordinary effort were rarely successful in keeping their children, as social, economic, and legal structures disempowered unwed mothers and all but ensured child transfer into "normal" white, nuclear families. From 1945 to 1973, 1.5 million newborns were adopted in the United States,[14] a significant number of them forcibly surrendered by young white middle-class women who found themselves pregnant and powerless.[15]

By the early 1970s, however, major second-wave feminist victories led to better reproductive health care, increased educational and workplace opportunities, and delays in marriage and childbearing for women of means in particular. In 1972, the passage of Title IX prohibited sex discrimination in federally funded educational institutions, and thus barred public schools from the common practice of expelling pregnant students. In addition, two landmark US Supreme Court decisions established a woman's constitutional right to privacy with regard to reproductive and childbearing decisions: first, the 1972 ruling in *Eisenstadt v. Baird* affirmed a right to birth control for single women; second, in 1973, *Roe v. Wade* overturned state and federal restrictions on access to abortion. These court decisions related to teen pregnancy and motherhood in at least two ways. Perhaps most obviously, young single women gained access to effective contraception and were able to terminate unintended pregnancies. But *Eisenstadt* and *Roe* encouraged women to assert reproductive autonomy in a more wholistic sense. Empowered by the rising tide of feminism and legally recognized reproductive rights, most young women were simply less likely to allow parental or governmental authorities to exert influence over their childbearing and parenting decisions. In short, when teens decided to carry their pregnancies to term of their own volition, free from the threat of expulsion and forced disappearance into maternity homes, they were much less likely to offer their babies for adoption.[16] As historian Rickie Solinger explains, "dignity and independence are, in fact, the life-enhancing ingredients that tend to be incompatible with relinquishing a child."[17]

Teen pregnancy emerged as a "problem" in the wake of these seismic cultural shifts, but interestingly coincided with a steady *decline* in the teen birth rate. By 1979, the birth rate for women under the age of twenty had dropped 45 percent from its peak in 1957.[18] But even as the teen birth rate diminished overall, the proportion of unmarried women within this population increased—between 1960 and 1980, nonmarital births rose from 15 percent to 48 percent of the total teenage birth rate.[19] Moreover, the 1970s witnessed steep declines in the number of white babies eligible for domestic adoption and, relatedly, the growing number of young white women who rejected adoption in favor of single motherhood.[20] Put another way, while teen pregnancy was in decline overall, an increasing number of single teens began to embrace motherhood; more specifically, the reproductive decisions of young, middle-class, white women began to resemble more closely those of their working-class peers and peers of color. Cultural anxieties over teen pregnancy were thus far less tethered to age than to race, class, and marital status.[21] The problem was, it would seem, less the fact of teen pregnancy than the audacity of teen motherhood, particularly among white and middle-class teens.

These challenges to white, middle-class normativities were amplified alongside other cultural transformations of the mid-twentieth century, including large-scale movements for racial justice at home and abroad, substantive economic restructuring, and immigration reform that loosened racist restrictions on US entry through the elimination of national-origin quotas favoring applicants from Western and Northern Europe. These shifts fueled deep-seated anxieties regarding racial purity, national identity, and belonging that shaped dominant understandings of teen pregnancy; as Clare Daniel astutely observes, "age became a politically acceptable index for concerns about race and class."[22] Teen pregnancy proffered coded terminology, constructing a "universal" transgressive maternal body that was relentlessly articulated against middle-class heteronuclear family formation and discursively aligned with racialized understandings of poverty (i.e., "urban decay" and "welfare dependence").

Moreover, these changes catalyzed shifts in the geopolitics of adoption. As domestic adoption plummeted in the early 1970s, a global industry soared in its stead.[23] As if to echo Solinger's observation above, research indicates a strong correlation between social, political, and economic powerlessness and high rates of child transfer abroad. Transnational adoptions to the United States began in response to political conflicts of the early- to mid-twentieth century—for example, the fostering of refugee children from Hitler's Europe.[24] As US (and eventually other Western nations') interest in international adoption grew precipitously in the postwar era, a lucrative and demand-driven industry emerged, often functioning in tandem with US military interventions and efforts at nation building.[25] In some cases, the incidence of international adoption reflects dire social and political circumstances that have left children institutionalized—although, significantly, many were neither abandoned nor orphaned as dominant US narratives suggest.[26] Governmental agencies, NGOs, and scholars have documented fraud, coercion, kidnapping, and other forms of serious, systemic abuse in adoptions originating from a number of popular sending countries such as Cambodia, Ecuador, Ethiopia, Guatemala, Liberia, Nepal, Peru, Samoa, and Vietnam.[27] Some of this exposure has resulted in moratoriums on child transfer abroad. These occurrences are diminished in dominant US discourse as isolated events, and narratives of child rescue continue to be rigorously marketed to hopeful, affluent citizens of the West and the Global North. But much like domestic adoption in the United States, demand far exceeds the number of healthy infants orphaned or voluntarily surrendered, thus creating a climate vulnerable to corruption and abuse.

While a complete history of adoption exceeds the scope of this study, the symbioses among adoption, human rights, and cultural figurations of motherhood are of note. Despite some of the more radical potentialities of adoption on an individual level, its structural dimensions are particularly germane to unpacking the significance of representations of crisis teen pregnancy in homeland security culture—its function as a demand-driven industry, the unequal access to resources and political power across parties, its relationship to white and Western capitalist accumulation, and its history of dividing low-wealth families and families of color.[28] Since peaking in 2004 at 22,989, the number of international adoptions to the United States has declined; in 2017, the most recent year for which data are available, the number of adoptions fell to 4,714.[29] This figure has been impacted not only by criminal investigations of human trafficking and fraud, but also by the Hague Convention, an international agreement designed to set standards for intercountry adoption and to safeguard against unethical practices. The United States joined the convention in 1994 and the regulations took effect in mid-2008, at which point the number of international adoptions to the United States fell to its lowest point in over ten years.[30] The precipitous decline in international adoption coincided with renewed public interest in the "problem" of teen pregnancy and the proliferation of representations of white teen pregnancy in entertainment media.

Moreover, these representations unfold in a context wherein teen pregnancy and motherhood remain deeply stigmatized—racialized in dominant imaginaries and positioned as the root of myriad problems from poor health to poverty, marital instability, educational curtailment, limited employment opportunities, and state dependency. These correlatives are certainly disturbing. But much of this literature reverses cause and effect.[31] Mounting evidence suggests that teen motherhood is *preceded* by socioeconomic and educational disadvantage: "the age of the mother is not a determining factor for the 'negative' social consequences attributed to teen parenthood but is instead a marker of the conditions of poverty and social marginalization that already affect the lives of many youths."[32] Put another way, poverty is far more likely to lead to teen pregnancy (as well as poor health, limited employment prospects, and so on) than the other way around. Some evidence suggests that young motherhood functions as an adaptive response to poverty, allowing young women in particular to focus on parenting when they are most likely to have good health and strong family networks. As Dorothy Roberts writes, "it is fairer to say that poverty makes pregnancy a more rational option.... Having a baby is [typically] a response to poor achievement in school and little hope for a decent job."[33] This sentiment is reflected in the testimonies of young low-wealth mothers themselves, who describe motherhood as motivating them to pursue education and meaningful employment, and as a means of giving value to their lives and making life more fulfilling.[34]

Research that blames teen childbearing for negative outcomes not only fails to attend to young women's experiences in its inversion of cause and effect, but it also ignores significant structural barriers to teen mothers' well being and achievement.[35] As Teresa Younger, president of the Ms. Foundation for Women, stated at the release of a landmark report on teen pregnancy authored by Young

Women United: "the current frame of teen pregnancy prevention only results in starving young people from access to the appropriate resources so that they can make their own informed reproductive decisions."[36] Recent studies demonstrate that when teen mothers have access to material resources, support, and community, they (and their children) thrive in no uncertain terms—including in terms of infant health and development, parental skills and knowledge, as well as maternal wellness, educational success, and advancement in earning potential.[37] Particularly for young women who lack other environmental motivators, becoming a parent can fuel individual motivation in pursuing educational and professional opportunities.[38] Figuring teen pregnancy as an epidemic obscures the conditions of socioeconomic hardship that incentivize motherhood for young women as it simultaneously deprives them of critical resources and support.

The media narratives of interest in this chapter also emerged at a significant moment in sexual and reproductive politics. Between 2007 and 2010, teen pregnancy not only was ubiquitous in popular culture, but it also garnered attention because, as already noted, the US teen birth rate spiked in 2006, briefly reversing a decades-long decline. This is usefully read against the backdrop of the cultural premium placed on purity in homeland security culture and attendant "family values" politics. Examples abound—they include the growing popularity of teen virginity pledges and father-daughter "purity balls" in the early to mid-2000s,[39] age requirements for emergency contraception (see chapter 3), and significant federal spending on abstinence-only education despite overwhelming evidence of its inaccuracy and harm.[40] Parental-consent laws constraining minors' access to abortion exist in thirty-seven states at the writing of this book (by comparison, only five states require parental involvement for minors who wish to place a child for adoption), and each year state legislators across the country aim to intensify surveillance of minors, from notarized parental consent to the criminalization of state border-crossing for abortion services.[41] Most public-school-based health centers are barred from dispensing contraceptives, and recent cultural panics over "sexting" signal yet another site where teens—and particularly, girls and young women—are harshly censured for sexual desire and expression.[42]

And at the very moment that teen pregnancy entertainment media took flight, we were witnessing the slow, spectacular implosion of the Queen of Teen—the public figure who had managed, for years, to stitch the contradictory and misogynist demands of purity culture into a coherent and captivating whole: "Virgin and pin-up, wide-eyed innocent and worldly temptress, icon of cool and conservative Christian role model,"[43] Britney Spears and her meteoric fame indexed the desires and anxieties of the early twenty-first century. So, too, did her demise—relentlessly, viciously maligned for transgressing gendered norms that included consensual sex with her boyfriend, weight gain, inadequate undergarments, shaving her head, and poor parental decision making. In short, as the paragon of fetishized teen purity was trapped in a vortex of public shame, the crisis of teen pregnancy—a convenient collapsing of concerns over youth, sexuality, gender, race, class, and nation—echoed across the media landscape.

Without laying claim to a linear causality, it is fair to say that these teen pregnancy narratives resided at the center of a constellation of forces. They inherited the weighted history of adoption and single motherhood; in other words, they reflect longstanding investments in regulating young—often powerless—women's reproductive choices in concert with national anxieties and desires. Simultaneously, these forms of entertainment media circulated alongside broader cultural phenomena—amplified in their proximity to newsworthy teen pregnancies, public debates over abstinence education, the rise of teen purity culture, the brief 2006 spike in the teen birth rate, and the sensationalized train wreck of a global teen idol. Moreover, these narratives function as another example of reproductive politics in the context of homeland maternity—yet another moment in which the responsibilization of the self was paired with an uptick in surveillance and policing as powerful mechanisms of control over pregnant and parenting women.

Pregnant Teens on Display

The stories told in *Juno*, *Glee*, *16 and Pregnant*, and *Teen Mom* are distinct, yet share a fixation on white crisis teen pregnancy and postfeminist articulations of its proper care and negotiation. In what follows, I trace how these popular forms of entertainment circulate what Laurie Ouellette and James Hay refer to as "informal 'guidelines for living,'"[44] specific to the requirements of motherhood in homeland security culture. Reinventing the "girls who went away," crisis teen pregnancy narratives in the late 2000s offered the pregnant teens on display, a transformation that retooled secrecy into hypervisibility, private shame into public moralizing and "securitainment."[45] To begin, I offer a brief introduction to each text.

Juno is an independent film about a middle-class white teen in small-town Minnesota, Juno MacGuff, who got pregnant after having sex with her best friend Bleeker out of boredom. Released in late 2007, the film boasts an indie rock soundtrack and a cast of cult favorites, including Ellen Page, Jason Bateman, and Michael Cera. The Juno character is quirky and endearing—she dons eclectic clothing, shrugs at typical high school sociality, and trades almost exclusively in witty repartee. The film was a stunning success. A breakout hit for screenwriter Diablo Cody, *Juno* toured the international film festival circuit and was showered with nominations and awards, including an Oscar for Best Original Screenplay and nominations for Best Actress, Best Director, and Best Picture.[46] Film reviews from the *Wall Street Journal* to the *Village Voice* hailed *Juno* as "crisp" and "mordant," "a thing of beauty and grace." Ellen Page ("Juno") appeared on *Saturday Night Live*, the *Ellen DeGeneres Show*, and the 2008 pre–Oscar Awards *Barbara Walters Special*. In the genre of crisis teen pregnancy media, *Juno* was undoubtedly the most critically acclaimed and popular film of its time.

Glee, a musical television series about a high school glee club, earned similar critical accolades and at its apex commanded an unparalleled presence in pop culture. Airing from 2009 to 2015, the show and its cast members won seventy-two awards and received 176 nominations, including Emmys, Golden Globes, People's Choice Awards, Teen Choice Awards, GLAAD Media Awards, and even a Grammy.[47] Celebrated early on as "bold," "transcendent," and "thrilling," *Glee* defied precedent not only in its successful integration of musical theater and choreography into primetime television, but was also credited with helping to redefine the scope of television as an enterprise. Boasting its own clothing line, beauty products, and, in early 2011, the most popular iPad app in the country, *Glee* was not only a show but a brand.[48] At the peak of the show's popularity, *Rolling Stone* critic Rob Sheffield asserted that *Glee* had "taken its place at the heart of pop culture, where radio and MTV used to rule supreme."[49] Central to the plot of the first season was high schooler Quinn Fabray and her unintended pregnancy. If Juno is the endearing teenage outcast, Quinn is the opposite—a petite blonde, captain of her high school's nationally ranked cheerleading squad, dating the quarterback of the football team, and president of the school's celibacy club.

While *Juno* and *Glee* enjoyed remarkable success, both faced public scrutiny for being unrealistic and facile, for normalizing premarital sex and glamorizing teen pregnancy. These media depictions followed a brief spike in the rate of teen childbearing in the United States. While this rise was both slight and anomalous,[50] the media attention that ensued was considerable. MTV executive producer Liz Gateley stated that these trends encouraged the network, in partnership with the National Campaign to Prevent Teen and Unplanned Pregnancy (NCPTUP), to create programming that told "the honest, unpleasant truth of teen pregnancy in America."[51] While NCPTUP maintains that *16 and Pregnant* and *Teen Mom* are important educational tools in reducing rates of teen pregnancy and childbearing, this claim remains contentious.[52] *16 and Pregnant* premiered in 2009 with mixed reviews, variously described as another instance of reality programming's "working-class voyeurism," "reputable, well-intended and potentially helpful," and the most controversial programming in MTV history.[53] Nonetheless, *16 and Pregnant* delivered ratings and viewership far beyond expectations and was quickly parlayed into the record-breaking spin-off series *Teen Mom* (retitled *Teen Mom OG* in its fifth season).[54] In *16 and Pregnant*, each documentary-style episode chronicles the trials and tribulations of a pregnant teen, from the second trimester through the first few months of parenthood. The first season of *Teen Mom* follows the lives of four of the stars of *16 and Pregnant* through their first year of parenting. For this chapter, I focus on the first season of both series and the moms who bridge them—Maci Bookout, Farrah Abraham, Amber Portwood, and Catelynn Lowell. Their early stories are of particular interest for their cultural salience and timing—these four teen moms launched a wildly successful franchise as the visibility of teen pregnancy in public culture was soaring. Their shows have translated into numerous tabloid covers, book deals, and additional television appearances.[55] *Teen Mom OG* is in its seventh season at the writing of this book, starring all four original cast members.

Reality programming has been theorized as a form of governance uniquely suited to homeland security culture for its steady integration of surveillance and security into the fabric of popular culture and everyday life.[56] Specific to teen pregnancy and motherhood, reality television is figured "as birth control." As Ouellette notes, it conveniently functions "as a technology of citizenship"[57] that emphasizes personal responsibility and self-sufficiency while obscuring structural impediments to actual contraceptive technologies. Building on Ouellette and others that have studied teen pregnancy in reality programming, I argue that reality television coincides meaningfully with other moralizing and instructive media narratives that offer teens tutorials of (pre)maternal citizenship. Building on critiques of crisis teen pregnancy media for its promotion of conservativism,[58] in what follows I examine the logic of crisis as it shapes teen pregnancy politics in entertainment media more broadly, with specific attention to its animation of historical tensions between unwed motherhood and nation. The stigma attached to white, middle-class teen pregnancy may have shifted since 1945, but the framing of crisis in contemporary teen pregnancy narratives indicate significant continuities with an earlier era marked by secrecy and maternity homes. In homeland security culture, the containment era "girls who went away" are resurrected with a postfeminist, neoliberal twist—teens may no longer be subject to exile but rather are subjected to exhibition and surveillance; their crises are no longer silenced but given amplified voice in service of mythic norms of motherhood and family.

Crisis, Choice, and the Paradox of Teen Motherhood

These crisis teen pregnancy narratives privilege whiteness and class mobility, and promote "good" choice making and motherhood to mitigate the crisis of teen pregnancy (and relatedly, the infertility of elite women). Abortion, when referenced at all, is figured as a crisis incomprehensible. Unlike adoption or parenting, abortion is rarely mentioned, let alone positioned as a real option for young women facing unintended pregnancy.[59] *Juno* dedicates more screen time to abortion and its adamant refusal than does *Glee* or either reality show. The attention is brief and facile, as the development of the Juno character hinges on recoiling from a visit to an abortion clinic; as Kristen Hoerl and Casey Kelly note, "sex may not be shameful, but the decision to terminate a pregnancy is; to maintain her moral virtue, Juno decides to carry her unplanned pregnancy to term."[60] Through a series of burlesque performances that parody contemporary abortion politics, Juno is terror stricken in the clinic by the choice she has almost made. Before the receptionist can call for a "Miss MacGoof" (a moralizing mispronunciation of Juno's name), Juno has flown out the door and down the street. The clinic scene proves pivotal to the storyline. It is the catalyst for both character development and the overall plot, figuring abortion as an intensification of the crisis of teen pregnancy.

This characterization of abortion is consistent throughout teen pregnancy entertainment media. Quinn Fabray of *Glee* provides an additional example—as the president of both the Christ Crusaders and the Celibacy Club, she leads peer workshops on chaste forms of intimacy, or "immaculate affection."[61] Quinn's screen time is minimal in the first several episodes until she discloses her pregnancy to her boyfriend, Finn. The moment unfolds from Finn's perspective; his initial confusion obscures Quinn's tearful explanation, a narration that underscores a common affective experience of unintended pregnancy as personal crisis. Finn recovers, stammering, "are you gonna . . . ?" Before the question can escape his lips, Quinn interjects with a resolute "no." The circumstances of her pregnancy are complicated: the father of her child is actually her boyfriend's best friend, Puck. Quinn attempts to maintain that Finn is the father, telling Puck: "I only had sex with you because you got me drunk on wine coolers and I was feeling fat that day."[62] The unsettling question of consent goes unaddressed. But the suggestion of assault performs rhetorical labor, as Quinn's adamant refusal of abortion is assigned greater significance. Her commitment to carrying her pregnancy to term is, like Juno's, framed as a reassertion of moral fortitude and reclamation of virtue in the face of potential shame.

The specter of abortion in crisis teen pregnancy narratives fuels the crisis at hand. This is a common characterization of abortion in mainstream media—often unnuanced, frequently rejected outright or otherwise figured as horrifying and traumatic, with few exceptions.[63] The taboo nature of abortion may inform its glaring absence in media.[64] Although approximately half of all unintended pregnancies in the United States are terminated, this particular reality does not seem to make for good television. Thus, crisis teen pregnancy narratives synecdochically extend the affective experience of unintended pregnancy as personal crisis to refigure abortion itself as a collective crisis (a move embraced also by the crisis pregnancy center movement, a claim to which I return). Not only does this conflate personal and political exigencies, but in so doing, it sanctions public investment and intrusion in individual reproductive decision making. This blurring of boundaries both fuels and is fueled by an understanding of motherhood as a vehicle for citizenship, metonymically sutured to the nation.

If abortion is coded as a crisis intensified (or even inconceivable), then teen motherhood is figured a crisis without end. *Glee* and *Juno* underscore this point by proxy, as neither of the pregnant characters decides to parent her child. Instead, these narratives highlight adolescent immaturity and position adoption as crisis resolution, a point to which I return. For now, the unending crisis of teen parenting is most clearly expressed in reality programming, which, in keeping with the generic tendencies of the medium, functions as a pedagogy of citizenship and risk tutorial in a post-9/11 world. While reality programming may, as critics claim, normalize teen sex and pregnancy, *16 and Pregnant* and *Teen Mom* consistently frame teen parenting as difficult, compromising, and paradoxical.[65] Presented in documentary form, each teen's story is told through an assemblage of vignettes that highlights struggles with education, relationships, and economic security. The narration is punctuated by animation featuring adolescent doodles and voice-overs culled from the teens' video diaries. As an anchor to each storyline, the voice-overs offer insight into the teens' thoughts and curate tools for managing crisis pregnancy. The take-home message is resounding and clear—mothering involves a level of hardship and sacrifice that teens are ill equipped to manage or meet.

Each teen's story is filtered through the lens of crisis, rendering the notion of teen mothering itself a contradiction in terms.[66] Take Maci, a white, middle-class teen mom from Chattanooga, Tennessee, who wistfully observes her high school friends leaving for college as she focuses on parenting, struggles to pursue education, and fields parental pressures to form a lasting relationship with her disinterested boyfriend, Ryan. As if in summation of the entire series, Maci muses in her video diary: "Today it's good; tomorrow it might fall apart again," and later, "I'm starting to see how much I've given up to be a mom."[67] Many moments within the series recall these familiar refrains, from the voice-over narration to animations that depict a baby bottle destroying a stack of textbooks or a family portrait shattering over a hearth while a storm brews outside a window. In aggregate, the narratives are structured through each teen's negotiation of persistent stressors and turmoil. Crisis is the narrative engine, persistently present as the narrative undercurrent that informs a series of hardships—from education and independence to teen relationships and social lives.

Educational disruption is depicted as a perpetual site of crisis, with difficulties that reflect fluctuating levels of familial support. Noting that her "due date was on a collision course with graduation,"[68] Maci enrolls in an accelerated high school program; the series highlights how her postsecondary educational aspirations have been stymied by the realities of parenting and a lack of support from Ryan. Farrah, a suburban teen from Council Bluffs, Iowa, opts to complete high school online after a series of hardships that include her expulsion from the cheerleading team and the cruelty of the teen gossip mill. Farrah's pursuit of a culinary education relies on continued financial support and free childcare from her parents. But the clearest example of educational struggle is Amber, a working-class teen from Anderson, Indiana. After dropping out of high school to have her daughter, Amber seeks out a career counselor for guidance in earning her diploma. This desire is tempered by a reality check—unemployed and economically dependent on her boyfriend, Gary, she cannot afford enrollment fees for online high school coursework and is advised to seek a GED instead. Amber dissolves into tears at this suggestion, but in postfeminist style quickly resigns herself to this fate because she "screwed up" her life and will have to make do. The compromise does not lessen Amber's burden—the first season of *Teen Mom* chronicles her failed attempts to persuade Gary to "watch" their child so that Amber can attend a GED class. Even when able to secure childcare, she struggles with an unreliable car that prevents her from attending classes. Amber's voice-over highlights frustration and despair: "It's not as easy to leave when I have to think about [daughter] Leah too."[69]

Relational distress and sacrifice is another significant theme in teen pregnancy reality programming. Maci's relationship with her baby's father is tumultuous despite her best efforts. Ryan ignores Maci and their son, parties all night with friends, and refuses to seek employment after losing his job—all of which compound Maci's difficulty in juggling school, work, and (for a brief period) wedding planning, while taking sole responsibility for their child. After Maci withdraws from her online college coursework, and in a rare moment of uttering more than a few syllables in a row, Ryan offers his unsolicited opinion. He calls Maci "lazy as fuck"[70] and declares that she probably will not finish college for lack of effort. His behavior is, at best, immature and diminishing, but is perhaps more accurately described as delusional and abusive. Farrah's story also includes relational sacrifice. The father of Farrah's daughter is absent, so Farrah lives with her parents while completing school.[71] The first season of *Teen Mom* centers on Farrah's pursuit of a social life despite family objections. Her voice-overs routinely reference this dilemma: "I wish my parents would stop telling me to a be a better mom and let me be a normal teenager"; or, more optimistically, "being a mom while going to school and working makes it hard to have a social life, but I'm determined to make it work."[72] Regular conflict between Farrah and her mother, Debra, is captured on screen as Farrah pursues romance while leaving baby care to Debra. Farrah is accused by her family of "farming out motherhood," "acting unmotherly" and being "irresponsible";[73] footage of Farrah's nights out on the town, dating drama, and sleeping through morning baby care bolsters these accusations. The season evolves with Farrah's lessons in responsibility; she eventually agrees to dedicate more energy to parenting, education, and economic self-sufficiency. What is figured as "typical" teenage behavior is culturally coded as unacceptable for a mother; in other words, "good" mother and teen are rendered mutually exclusive identity categories.

If reality television, as a whole, offers governing technologies of self-help and DIY possibilities for transforming productive citizens, then *16 and Pregnant* and *Teen Mom* are markedly successful in their craft. Each episode offers a set of what has been called "televised tutoring"[74] in which the crisis of teen pregnancy is the consistent catalyst and teen mothers are made responsible for the crises they face, from poverty and educational disruption to intimate partner violence. Emphasizing personal choice and responsibility, the tutorials offer lessons in neoliberal citizenship through the surveillance of teen mothers trying to negotiate the complexities of parenting, cataloging their missteps and struggles so as to offer a cautionary tale: "don't let this happen to you."[75] The framing of teen motherhood emphasizes sacrifice and hardship, unfolding in a context affectively structured through (and mobilized by) serial crises. It is, of course, difficult to deny the challenges that teen parents—and particularly teen moms—face. Those are substantive and real. But what becomes exceedingly apparent over the course of these series is the *untenable paradox that is teen motherhood*. No amount of sacrifice is enough. No matter how many educational opportunities are foregone, social outings eliminated, relationships surrendered or maintained through sheer willpower, the protagonists of *16 and Pregnant* and *Teen Mom* frequently fall short of the requirements of "good" motherhood as self-reliant, privatized, contingent on delayed childbearing[76] and, thus, consonant with the interests of nation.

Lest the paradox of teen motherhood be unclear as the first seasons of *16 and Pregnant* and *Teen Mom* drew to a close, the season finales underscore this theme. Hosted by celebrity psychiatrist "Dr. Drew" Pinski, each finale consists of a teen mom panel, a live audience, and a question-and-answer session. Dr. Drew previews each interview with a video montage tailored to each teen that recaps the season, followed by a discussion of their struggles and hardships. Highlighted throughout is the inability of these moms to sacrifice enough. Despite routine depictions of Ryan's appalling behavior, Maci is lectured on how "men are different" (read: inept) when it comes to parenting and relationships, and chastised for not trying hard enough to make things work "for [baby] Bentley's benefit."[77] Farrah is told that she lost the privileges to her carefree life when she decided to have a child. Amber's public shaming is more complex, as MTV aired a fight during which Amber shoves, slaps, and chokes her boyfriend, Gary, and for which she was charged with domestic battery. While troubling indeed, I am less interested here in the differences between the teens' individual struggles than I am in the series' clear depiction of continuity. Whether victim or perpetrator of violence, these teen moms are figured as indiscriminately at fault. Amber and Maci are offered as polarities on a singular continuum of teen motherhood that is *defined through* crisis. As an extension of the crisis of teen pregnancy, the decision to raise a child is to dwell in an endless state of personal, financial, and relational crisis. Teen motherhood, itself, becomes a contradiction in terms.

The extraordinary visibility of white teens in this genre is significant. Neither *16 and Pregnant* nor *Teen Mom* engage race or ethnicity in any meaningful way in its first season. Maci, Amber, and Catelynn are white; after much internet speculation, Farrah confronted questions about her ethnicity in a 2014 interview with Starcasm, stating that she is Syrian, Italian, Sicilian, and Danish.[78] Much like Ebony, the only teen of color featured in the first season of *16 and Pregnant*, Farrah is narrated in close proximity to her white mother and extended community. Racial or ethnic difference is thus minimized through the silence accorded to how it might matter. One might argue that the erasure of teens of color loosely reflects the fact that most pregnant and parenting teens are white. But accuracy is not quite the metric for inclusion, as demonstrated by the paucity of attention to abortion—which as already noted is sought by approximately half of all women (regardless of age) facing unintended pregnancy in the United States—as well as by the fact that a near-exclusive focus on white teens obscures the disparate impact that early pregnancy and motherhood has on black, Latina/o/x, and indigenous teens.[79]

Rather, the whiteness of teen pregnancy in entertainment media both plays on and compounds racialized pathologies assigned to teen motherhood in various ways. First, whiteness renders teen pregnancy a crisis that contains its own tidy resolution (through adoption, as we will see), or at least one less tethered to perpetual hardship, as some teen moms successfully channel race privilege alongside other forms of cultural capital—physical attractiveness, class status, wealth, and the high profile acquired through the show—into mainstream celebrity. Whiteness, put another way, lends itself well to the makeover genre of reality programming, as well as to the generic conventions of comedy in scripted media. In both *Juno* and *Glee*, whiteness undergirds the premise of a crisis that assumes the availability of breezy narrative resolution. For example, in a remarkable embrace of fantasy that fulfills the generic conventions of the rom-com, Juno's pregnancy was ultimately figured as the catalyst for—if also a light-hearted hurdle to—an innocent teen romance. As teen pregnancy and motherhood function as racialized tropes in dominant discourse, whiteness then constitutes a powerful condition of possibility for managing teen pregnancy in a way that disrupts assumptions about teen moms, while advancing normative visions of nation and heteronuclear family formation.

Second, centering whiteness obscures the structural dimensions of teen pregnancy, substituting individual work ethic for systemic challenge and critique. As popular media locates white teens at the center of crisis pregnancy narratives, social and economic mobility are hitched to personal choices in mainstream imaginaries, fueling mythic notions of self-help, hard work, and individual responsibility. It is a narrative that skirts the politics of teen pregnancy and its links to racism, sexism, classism, and poverty. It is a narrative that champions personal "solutions" to injustice, inverting causality as it blames teen motherhood—and teen mothers themselves—for social and economic precarity. In later seasons, as the script for crisis teen pregnancy in reality programming becomes rote, the genre is perhaps more able to accommodate teens of color without adapting its content and narrative structure considerably, as is suggested by subsequent seasons of *16 and Pregnant* that feature a few teens of color. Nonetheless, subsequent *Teen Mom* spin-offs (*Teen Mom 2* and *Teen Mom 3*) remain overwhelmingly white. In this way, reality programming dovetails with the comic-crisis impulse of *Juno* and *Glee*, both of which center white teen pregnancy to advance a freewheeling narrative dramedy that refuses engagement with the structural forces that shape the conditions of early childbearing.

Indeed, in the sea of whiteness shaping crisis teen pregnancy entertainment media, the exception marks the rule. In 2009, the unanticipated mainstream success of the film *Precious* ignited fierce public debate. While some applauded the film as brave, necessary, and ultimately hopeful, others sharply critiqued its trafficking in racist stereotypes and noted its remarkable success as yet another example of the insatiable appetite of dominant US culture for postracial narratives of black pathology and white innocence.[80] The film is an inappropriate and incongruous comparative on many registers—most significantly, the sixteen-year-old protagonist, Precious, is repeatedly raped by her otherwise absent father, bearing two children as a result. This detail alone renders any attempt at comparison repugnant—this is not a film about teen sexual and reproductive decision making, but rather about the horrific abuse of a teenager who tearfully confesses to her teacher that she has never even had a boyfriend. And yet, to ignore its presence would be irresponsible. As the sole representation of black teen pregnancy that captured the limelight in this moment of manic attention to teen pregnancy, *Precious* clarifies how whiteness matters. In *Precious*, teen pregnancy is figured not as *the* crisis but rather as the *symptom* of crisis. While teen pregnancy is often symptomatic of profound social and economic injustice, *Precious* refuses any such sustained engagement. Pivoting from the structural to the individual, *Precious* constitutes its crisis as the physical, emotional, and sexual brutalities inflicted on a minor by her parents. In short, the crisis constituted through *Precious* is not teen pregnancy itself but rather the pathology ascribed to the African American family.

Teen pregnancy thus operates differently outside of whiteness in dominant media. Within narratives that assume race privilege, teen pregnancy can function as a temporary, even comic, threat to the ideal family form—and importantly, a threat that contains the possibility of its own tidy resolution. This is particularly true for poor and working-class white teens like Amber or Catelynn, who are invited to imagine their reproductive decision making as either solidifying their socioeconomic status or, conversely, as a route to a middle-class life. Indeed, my analysis thus far neglects one teen mom in popular entertainment media who, like Maci, Farrah, and Amber, bridged the first season of *16 and Pregnant* and *Teen Mom*. What Catelynn's story suggests, however, is the possibility that teen moms might resolve crisis pregnancy by making the greatest sacrifice of all—choosing adoption.

Adoption and the Politics of Good Motherhood

Adoption is consistently figured as the only lasting resolution to crisis teen pregnancy. Catelynn's story on *16 and Pregnant* and *Teen Mom*, widely lauded by bloggers and critics, underscores this point. A white teen from a rural, working-class community in northern Michigan, Catelynn and her unfailingly dependable boyfriend, Tyler, seem to exemplify a real-life *Juno* story, if only intensified by their remarkable resilience in the face of adversity. Many features of their story are distinct. First, despite the strain of unintended pregnancy, Catelynn and Tyler are never shown in serious conflict with one another. In striking contrast to their peers, their relationship is the singular aspect of stability in these teens' lives. The young couple demonstrates unconditional love and support for one another, even amidst regular geographic upheaval (Catelynn notes that she has moved thirteen times in her short life)[81] and strained familial relations, as much of the screen time for Catelynn's mother (April) and Tyler's father (Butch) shows them antagonizing and berating their children.

Catelynn and Tyler's decision to give up their baby for adoption is the most pronounced distinction between their story and those of their peers in both series. It also inspired their embrace by multiple blogging audiences, from skeptics of *16 and Pregnant* that claimed Catelynn and Tyler's story "totally redeemed" the entire series, to one blogger's review that captures much of the popular sentiment: "Catelynn and Tyler are the only ones who seem to understand the gravity of their situation . . . it quickly becomes apparent that these two teenagers develop a deep love for their child, and *that* is why they're giving her up. At times their journey is so brave and raw and touching, it is almost unbearable to watch. But it is worth it."[82] The first season of *16 and Pregnant* captures a series of heartfelt dialogues between Catelynn and Tyler as they consider the options available to them. While they meet significant resistance from family and friends, Catelynn and Tyler return to the same refrain—they want to provide their child with a life they feel ill equipped to offer; as Catelynn explains it to her friend, "how am I supposed to raise a kid when I'm a kid myself?"[83]

In opting for an open adoption, and with far greater numbers of hopeful adoptive families than available infants, Catelynn and Tyler are able to select the family they want for their daughter. They choose a couple that reflects the demographic most privileged by formal institutions of child placement—a mid-thirties, white, educated, traditional, Christian couple named Brandon and Teresa, who have struggled for years to have children. In a poignant first meeting, Catelynn tearfully restates her decision to Brandon and Teresa: "I just want her to have better than what I had, and I know that I can't do that. So I'm just doing the thing that I think is the best. I know that you guys can provide for her a lot more than I can."[84] As the adoptive parents, Brandon and Teresa are given more screen time over the first seasons of the two series; their relationship to Catelynn and Tyler grows closer in unexpected ways, if also constrained by the complexity of circumstance.[85] In this way, Brandon and Teresa possess a rhetorical function within the narrative. As one of two sets of adults in Catelynn and Tyler's life, they are juxtaposed with April and Butch, and work synecdochically to reinforce Catelynn and Tyler's decision to relinquish their daughter as the best form of crisis management.

Indeed, the adoption is affirmed by the stubborn refusal of Catelynn's and Tyler's parents to accept it. This fundamental disagreement might have afforded an opportunity to work through the emotional and political complexities of adoption, and yet the portrayal of this conflict functions instead as a foil that bolsters the validity of Catelynn and Tyler's position. Throughout the series, April and Butch are cast as caricatures of the working poor—depicted as uneducated and even abusive parents, unfit to advise their children—or anyone else for that matter—on parenting. We are introduced to April in a scene where she slams the door on her daughter, calling Catelynn a "bitch."[86] She refuses to stand up to Butch as he attacks Catelynn's decision to relinquish her baby, at times joining in the chorus. Butch, a sinewy figure with a long, graying mullet and lively moustache, is a recovering addict who has been in prison for most of Tyler's life; he admits to Tyler, in one of their many altercations regarding the adoption, his own shortcomings as a parent. April and Butch's staunch opposition to adoption—insisting on the immorality of surrendering a child and urging Catelynn and Tyler to "buck up" to responsibility—serves a burlesque function. It parodies the argument in defense of teen parenting and, ultimately, affirms Catelynn and Tyler's decision through hyperbole.

This take-home message echoes across teen pregnancy entertainment media. The favorable positioning of adoption in *Glee* is constituted through a complex web of stories. Initially, Quinn plans to raise the baby with her boyfriend, but decides to pursue adoption instead. A series of moments affirm this decision—from repeated emphasis on avoiding geographic stasis—a "Lima [Ohio] loser," "caged with no future"—to a scene in which Quinn is lectured on proper prenatal care, lest her "baby will be ugly."[87] But Quinn's decision is largely extolled by proxy, through a storyline emerging as she nears her due date. The story features star Glee-clubber Rachel Berry, and rival club coach, Shelby Corcoran. Although Rachel's home life is largely peripheral to the show, she occasionally refers to her gay dads who had her via surrogate. Rival coach Shelby, seeing Rachel on stage, recognizes her as the child she gave birth to many years ago. Bound by a surrogacy contract prohibiting initiation of contact but desperate to connect, Shelby implores her star pupil to befriend Rachel. Once Rachel learns Shelby's identity, she decides to reach out. Their meeting is difficult. Sitting several rows from one another in an empty auditorium, Rachel asks Shelby if she ever regretted her decision. Shelby replies: "Yes, then no . . . so much." After a brief, stilted conversation, Shelby hastens to leave; Rachel's face betrays rejection and disappointment. Still, Rachel pursues a relationship until Shelby explains: "It's too late for us. Anything that we share is going to be confusing for you. I'm your mother, but I'm not your mom."[88]

This narrative is distinct, of course, in that Shelby was a surrogate—purposefully inseminated and legally bound to surrender. And yet, surrogacy is rarely mentioned by name; when it is, the distinctions between it and adoption are minimized throughout the narration. Shelby is continually—and by a number of characters—referred to as Rachel's "mother," as opposed to a surrogate or birth mother. Rachel's dads fail to appear on screen throughout most of the first season, an absence that renders Shelby a more plausible parental figure. As Shelby narrates her own experience, she emphasizes deep remorse in missing out on a relationship with Rachel. The brief and complicated encounters between Rachel and Shelby illustrate, on the one hand, dimensions of the emotional terrain of surrogacy and adoption that are too often overlooked—the struggles of birth mothers to come to terms with child surrender and the struggles of adoptees or children of traditional surrogates[89] in particular to connect to their own sense of history, place, and identity. Even still, the narrative ultimately flattens these complexities, affirming a cultural designation of family in lieu of the biological, a noteworthy feature indeed in an age of reprogenetics and the privilege assigned to biogenetic family formation. Shelby's response to Rachel is abrasive and even childish; in it, we are metonymically reminded that Shelby is not, cannot be, a parent to Rachel. Adoption, it seems, is clear, definitive, and best left alone. In the final episode, as if for narrative reinforcement, Shelby becomes the adoptive parent of Quinn's daughter. Finally able to realize her deep desire for a child—one that Rachel could not fulfill—Shelby surrenders her career in order to embrace motherhood. Thus, the resolution to the crisis of teen pregnancy is also upheld through favorable depictions of adoptive motherhood by older, professional women.

Similarly, Juno's decision to find an adoptive home for her baby is upheld throughout the film in various ways. For example, one scene features a condescending ultrasound technician who, on learning that Juno plans to place her child for adoption, verbalizes her relief: "I just see a lot of teenage mothers come through here. It's obviously a poisonous environment for a baby to be raised in." While Juno and her friend Leah respond, it is Juno's stepmother, Bren, who has the final word with the ultrasound tech: "They [the adoptive parents] could be utterly negligent. Maybe they'll do a far shittier job of raising a kid than my dumbass stepdaughter ever would. Have you considered that?" A brief, heated exchange ensues, with Bren silencing the ultrasound tech by telling her to "stick to what she knows" and belittling her professional expertise: "You think you're special because you get to play Picture Pages up there? My five-year-old daughter could do that." The technician leaves in a huff, and Bren is congratulated by Juno for being a "dick." The response to the technician's overt prejudice is melodramatic and sophomoric. Bren's last word: "So why don't you go back to night school in Manteno and learn a real trade,"[90] synecdochically mocks the argument in defense of teen parenting altogether as outrageous and childish. While this scene plays on (and seemingly against) noxious assumptions regarding teen mothers, the ultrasound exchange functions as an overt caricature that nurtures the attitudes it nominally attempts to unseat.

Thus, the narrative treatment of abortion, teen parenting, and adoption in crisis pregnancy entertainment media promotes the decision to bear and surrender a child as the only tenable choice, particularly for young white women. Class distinctions underscore this point even more, as adoption is figured in Catelynn's narrative as a means of upward mobility, most immediately for the baby but potentially for Catelynn and Tyler as well. Offering pedagogies of citizenship that promote individual solutions to structural inequities, these narratives function on several levels to strip reproductive "choice" of its political import and significance. Powerfully at work are cultural assumptions that good girls do not need or have abortions, and that they cannot and should not parent their own children. As postfeminist texts, crisis teen pregnancy narratives delineate the boundaries of proper maternity under the banner of feminism, and many of these teen protagonists fit the profile of a "good" mother—white, straight, able-bodied, and upwardly mobile or aspirational. But to be culturally coded as maternal, a few additional social markers are necessary. As the resolution to crisis teen pregnancy is figured as adoption, these narratives suggest that not one, but *two* crises may be averted—that of teen motherhood as well as that of the delayed childbearing of elite women.

Tied to the sym/pathetic trope of the infertile woman, adoptive mothers within teen pregnancy narratives resolve an "unbalanced" reproductive equation. Their struggles are enmeshed with those of the teen protagonists; indeed, it is often difficult to ascertain just who is in crisis. Vanessa Loring, the adoptive mother in *Juno*, is a white, upper-class, thirtysomething, married woman with a successful career who struggles with infertility. Vanessa's character is rigid, uptight, and anxious throughout the film, a common caricature of an adult woman who has no children. For example, when Vanessa says good-bye to Juno after their first meeting, she poses a steady stream of questions: "So, then, you really think you're going to go ahead with this? [. . .] How sure? Percentage-wise, would you say you're 80 percent sure, 90 percent sure?"[91] If her insecurities and idiosyncrasies were somehow lost on the viewer prior to the film's close, here they would be highlighted in absentia. In Vanessa's final scene, she is cuddled up on the bed in the nursery with the baby, post-adoption. Hair disheveled, clothes notably rumpled, Vanessa exudes serenity. It is a side of Vanessa we have not yet witnessed, a side of Vanessa that is brought into being through motherhood. Adhering to traditional gendered scripts, a thirtysomething childless woman is pitiful, neurotic, and incomplete—a caricature that at once diminishes women while trivializing the profound pain and hardship that women and couples endure in struggling with infertility. Vanessa may have spent her twenties "acquiring it all," but becoming a mother is presented as the ultimate expression and fulfillment of wealthy white womanhood.

As both a birth mother and, much later, an adoptive one, Shelby Corcoran of *Glee* offers a unique opportunity to explore the character transformations that make culturally legible maternity possible. She first appears midway through the first season as the ruthless coach of the reigning national glee club champions. Her life seems quite dissimilar from that of Vanessa Loring—she has never been married and is exclusively focused on her career. However, Shelby also typifies the stereotype of single, childless women as selfish, arrogant, and aggressive. She holds rehearsals for hours on end, with students breaking away only in dire necessity (for example, to vomit from exhaustion in trash cans outside of the auditorium), and coaches her students in unapologetic terms: "Ladies, I don't want to hear complaints about chafing because you're being forced to wear metal underwear."[92] As the season continues, Shelby's dissatisfactions come into focus. They seem to hinge initially on her inability to connect with Rachel but, as noted earlier, this relationship is quickly figured as implausible and rightly distant. In the end, much like Vanessa, a child is all that Shelby needs to be complete. In the final episode, Shelby explains to Rachel that she needs a new life: "It took meeting you to realize all this stuff that I missed out on. . . . I need a house and a garden and a dog—family. I missed out on my chance with you, and it kills me. I can't let that happen again."[93] Shelby's final scene in the first season of *Glee* is remarkably similar to Vanessa's in *Juno*: Shelby stands in the hospital, transfixed by the bundle she holds in her arms as a nurse finalizes the adoption paperwork before her. Once again, motherhood is the definitive embodiment of white, class-privileged femininity, the solution to the malaise and neurosis brought on by too much independence and professional striving—in short, by too much feminism.

The resolution to "crisis" teen pregnancy, conveniently, resolves the "crisis" in infertility through child transfer. Thus, the significance of adoption within crisis teen pregnancy narratives is also concretized through its relationship to a related but differentiated crisis—the childlessness of elite white women. The juxtaposition of the pregnant teen and the aspiring adoptive mother clarifies the narrow circumference of motherhood in the context of homeland security culture. Rather than existing as a kind of biological tie, motherhood is articulated as a social status and cultural designation—an identity figured as the pinnacle expression of wealthy, white idealized femininity. In the age of the gene, as Western science invests thoroughly in heredity, and assisted reproductive technologies such as egg freezing and gestational surrogacy reinforce biogenetic family formation,[94] it may seem incongruous to posit maternity as culturally constructed and designated. Close examination of the continual presence of crisis teen pregnancies in popular culture, however, challenges us to better understand motherhood as it relates to power, cultural capital, and the significance of gender, race, class, and family formation to the imagining of the nation. What emerges from this study is a set of narrative themes and technologies of governance that plainly specify the borders of "good" motherhood as that which squares neatly with the tenets of ideal citizenship in the post-welfare, homeland security state. Those individuals determined most "fit" for motherhood inhabit myriad positions of privilege and adhere to the status quo—exhibiting self-sufficiency, discipline, and subservience to total motherhood. Biology aside, rhetorics of crisis code these women as rightful and deserving mothers for their capacity to mother in the interests of the twenty-first-century nation-state.

Moreover, the recent fixation on pregnant white teenagers in crisis signals a powerful set of cultural anxieties colliding with seismic shifts in reproductive politics. The sudden score of scripted media has reanimated longstanding beliefs while offering pedagogies of citizenship; reality programming has bolstered scripted narratives through the surveillance and exhibition of actual teenage mothers. Thus, teen pregnancy entertainment media works to resuscitate containment culture normativities with a postfeminist twist—as the pregnant white teenager is rendered hypervisible, stories of personal crisis buttress a narrow definition of motherhood in early twenty-first-century US culture. Within these narratives, adoption is figured as the means by which teens—and their adult counterparts—might manage the experience of crisis pregnancy in a manner that aligns with the interests of nation. In other words, the treatment of abortion and adoption in crisis teen pregnancy media coincide meaningfully with the post-9/11 resurgence in conservative values, increased attacks on abortion rights, and the post-Hague decline in adoption rates. "Crisis resolution" in these texts amplifies normative visions of gender, whiteness, and family formation, securing the borders of legitimate maternity under the banner of personal choice and self-determination. And when entertainment media fails to adequately counsel teens to remain abstinent or to choose adoption, then other forms of management are made available, drawing once again on the logic and discourse of crisis. My concluding remarks focus on a proliferating exemplar of such mechanisms, namely, the crisis pregnancy center.

Colonizing the Clinic

These rhetorics of crisis are not isolated, but rather persist as a more recent fixture in US pregnancy politics. The emphasis on crisis in teen pregnancy entertainment media reverberates across a broader landscape, filtering into other aspects of reproductive and maternal politics. The conservative crisis pregnancy center (CPC) movement is one of the more visible exemplars of this trend; it works to recast abortion as a collective moral crisis while colonizing women's reproductive health clinics in its wake. And in the spirit of homeland security culture, if abortion constitutes the crisis, then CPCs and entertainment media tutorials are preemptive strikes—tools through which young women's sexuality and reproduction might be governed in accordance with homeland maternity and its attendant politics of "good" citizenship.

Much like teen pregnancy entertainment media, the CPC movement discursively trades in crisis to intervene in the politics of unintended pregnancy. As the direct service wing of the evangelical antiabortion movement, CPCs boast "more volunteers, volunteer hours, and organizations than all other forms of pro-life activism in the United States combined."[95] Many CPCs are staffed exclusively by volunteers with no medical training and harbor an explicit, if often unadvertised, mission to dissuade pregnant women from abortion. CPCs frequently masquerade as comprehensive reproductive health care facilities. They attract clients by advertising "free" pregnancy testing, abortion counseling, family planning advice, maternity apparel, and baby necessities—services that are medically uninformed and paired with antiabortion evangelism as well as Christian seminars on parenting, abstinence, or Bible studies.[96] In addition to obstructing women's access to abortion care, many CPCs proselytize to their clients and promote traditional family formation—advocating abstinence until marriage, marriage and motherhood for unmarried pregnant women, and adoption for pregnant women uninterested in marriage. In the last decade, CPCs have targeted what they describe as "urban" and "underserved" communities with their missionary services.[97] A study of CPCs in North Carolina revealed in 2017 that they are largely located in "low-income neighborhoods, neighborhoods of color, urban centers, and counties with higher than average rates of racial segregation."[98] While CPCs claim a commitment to serving under-resourced communities, they do not assist women in applying for food stamps,

Medicaid, or WIC benefits; moreover, because CPCs are not staffed by medical personnel, they cannot offer annual exams, preventive care, or treatment for sexually transmitted infections.[99]

CPCs have stirred controversy since their inception in the early 1970s. They have faced multiple lawsuits over consumer fraud, false advertising, coerced child surrender, and emotional distress related to all of the above. Legal sanctions in the late 1980s forced the CPC movement to change some of their tactics,[100] but CPCs remain a threat to women's health for their misleading and deceptive tactics, obstruction of access to abortion and prenatal care, and distribution of false medical information (e.g., asserting that contraception is ineffective or that abortion causes cancer or infertility).[101] CPCs have received millions of state and federal dollars to pursue their mission, and they far exceed the number of comprehensive women's health clinics and other agencies that provide noncoercive prenatal support.[102] Recent estimates suggest that there are anywhere from 2,400 to 3,500 CPCs nationwide, outnumbering abortion clinics by at least three to one.[103]

The personal, affective experience of crisis is the lynchpin for CPC advertising. Dotting the horizon of interstate highways, nestled alongside ads for comprehensive clinics in the Yellow Pages and popular online search engines, CPC ads announce "Help when it seems like there's no hope" or "It's Your Choice/ We're Here for You," and pose questions that highlight the experiential dimension of unintended pregnancy: "Pregnant? Scared? You have options." Crisis pregnancy centers appropriate the language of comprehensive reproductive health clinics, referencing women's "options," "health," and "choice." They play on women's fears and offer lip service to comprehensive reproductive care in ways that echo crisis teen pregnancy narratives—a fabrication worth noting in both instances insofar as the choices made available are illusory, always already edited and curated in advance. CPC rhetorics thus build on the emotional terrain of crisis, amplifying the personal experience of unintended pregnancy to frame the specter of abortion as a cultural crisis. Notably, research demonstrates that the personal sense of crisis that can accompany unintended pregnancy is less tethered to abortion than it is to uncertainty, to the urgent and weighty decision making that unintended pregnancy necessitates, and to the social stigmas attached to those decisions.[104] CPCs' synecdochical amplification, however, aligns with other antiabortion discourses in public culture to figure abortion as a collective moral crisis. To do so misattributes the personal distress wrought by unintended pregnancy to abortion, conflates personal and political exigencies, and does so in the weighted vernacular of homeland security culture.

CPC framing of abortion as a cultural crisis was on crude display in a racist and incendiary media campaign first launched by white antiabortion activists in 2009.[105] Billboards across Georgia, and later in other southern states as well as in Manhattan and Los Angeles, featured black youth and were emblazoned with "black children are an endangered species" and "the most dangerous place for an African American is in the womb."[106] The campaign directed its audience to anti-choice websites and crisis pregnancy centers.[107] The response—led by black feminist bloggers, journalists, and advocates for reproductive justice—was immediate and condemning, and forced the swift removal of at least one of the billboards.[108] Stoking racist fears of the black female body as dangerous and conflating black women's reproductive autonomy with genocide, this kind of race baiting is part of a familiar antiabortion strategy that distorts and appropriates black women's history of struggle for reproductive justice—for example, by exploiting abortion statistics with reckless disregard for the disparities that undergird such figures.[109] As Akiba Solomon writes, the campaign grossly accused "black women who make the complicated, difficult, highly personal choice to end a pregnancy . . . [of] the deliberate, systematic destruction"[110] of their own people and communities, a claim as utterly preposterous as it is dangerous. As prominent abortion provider and advocate Willie Parker notes, this racist campaign bolstered efforts to curtain all women's access to abortion through stigma and shame by targeting black women's wellness and integrity specifically.[111] It is a misconstrual that seems particularly cruel and insidious in a culture that continually denigrates black women's childbearing and mothering, one in which black women bear the brunt of political attacks on reproductive health care and rising rates of maternal mortality in the United States.[112] Among the many egregious CPC strategies revealed in this moment, one in particular is rendered explicit: the attempt to recast abortion as an urgent, collective, and defining moral crisis.

If this media campaign signals one particular instance of how crisis fuels and informs the CPC movement, additional examples underscore its persistent rhetorical presence. CPCs regularly draw on rhetorics of crisis to frame their work as "life-saving" for women and children. As national CPC networks such as Heartbeat International and CareNet note, the core mission of CPCs is to reach "vulnerable" women, those labeled by the CPC movement as "abortion-minded" or otherwise "at risk" for abortion. In a shift away from more overt forms of misogynist harassment characteristic of much antiabortion activism, but in a tone that smacks of paternalism nonetheless, CPC volunteers insist that they are "protecting women from abortion as 'an adult tells a child not to touch a hot stove.'" This phrase, popular among CPC activists, is buoyed by similar expressions such as "save the mother, save the baby," a referent to ending abortion through religious conversion on a case-by-case basis. Clarifying the evangelism of the crisis pregnancy center movement, one CPC counselor noted during her workshop for the 2015 Heartbeat International conference: "We might be the very first face of Christ that these girls ever see."[113] Infantilizing women and placing embryonic life at the heart of their mission, the CPC movement echoes narratives of evangelical child rescue that have long inflected the cultural politics of reproduction.

This spirit of evangelical conversion functions as an extension of teen pregnancy entertainment media. Not only is the CPC mission consonant with other popular narratives of crisis that render abortion an unthinkable choice, but also, in the politics of crisis pregnancy, CPCs offer a more direct mode of governing women's decision making in the absence of containment-era maternity homes and pre-*Roe* legal constraints. As pseudoclinics that traffic in traditional values and normative family formation, CPCs forcefully promote abstinence, adoption, or marriage when contemporary modes of governing at a distance do not succeed. Put another way, if teen pregnancy entertainment media circulate cautionary tales, CPCs attempt to intervene when young women fail to heed. Crisis teen pregnancy narratives delineate the borders of maternity, reinforcing longstanding attitudes about what it means to be a mother and who is best able to perform maternal citizenship in the homeland security state; CPCs unequivocally fortify these beliefs as they steer women away from abortion and toward adoption or marriage and motherhood. In homeland security culture, crisis teen pregnancy is no longer hidden but exceptionally visible, no longer silenced but excessively voiced. The stories that unfold in entertainment media are normative and directive, their messages amplified by broader discourses of crisis in contemporary reproductive politics that spiral along distinct and interconnected trajectories—from the felt experience of unintended pregnancy to CPC discourses of "child rescue," from the post-Hague decline in the number of infants available for adoption to the so-called epidemic of infertility among white, middle-class women. In this way, crisis operates on distinct and proliferating registers; it provides a framework for mediated narratives that shape the meaning of motherhood in ways that square with normative understandings of citizenship in homeland security culture.

It is difficult to deny the profound reverberations of crisis rhetorics across the divisive landscape of contemporary reproductive politics. The cumulative logic of crisis has played a central role in weakening reproductive rights and colonizing reproductive health clinics across the country. At the writing of this book, safe and legal access to abortion care is under unprecedented assault in the United States. According to the Guttmacher Institute, "more than one-quarter of the 1,074 state abortion restrictions since *Roe v. Wade* were enacted between 2011 and 2015."[114] Planned Parenthood has been a unique target of state assemblies across the country; further, repeated attempts to repeal the Affordable Care Act threaten to deprive Planned Parenthood of all federal funding. While abortion constitutes only 3 percent of its services and the organization is recognized as "integral and necessary" for its provision of "compassionate and critical health care"[115] to $2.7 million annually,[116] elected officials in the Republican Party have led multiple efforts to defund the organization and reroute tax dollars to crisis pregnancy centers, which are steady on the rise but are in no way equipped to provide compassionate and comprehensive medical care.[117] Scores of entities from health care providers to human rights organizations have publicly opposed these efforts,[118] noting the profound loss of services that this would entail for underserved communities in particular. The political attacks continue nonetheless, entirely unabated.

Finally, it is a sobering fact that women's clinics are subject to regular threats, harassment, and violence from antiabortion activists. The single most deadly assault on a clinic since *Roe v. Wade* came in November 2015, when Robert Lewis Dear Jr. opened fire in a Planned Parenthood clinic in Colorado Springs, murdering three and wounding nine others.[119] In early court appearances, Dear disrupted proceedings with antiabortion sentiments, declaring that he was "a warrior for the babies." His statements participate in an escalation of war and terrorism metaphors that permeate contemporary reproductive politics, a matter beyond the scope of this chapter but certainly worthy of scholarly exploration. For now, I note these examples not only for their frightening and overt demonstrations of hostility toward reproductive justice, but also for how they are predicated on an understanding of abortion as a cultural crisis. The erosion of reproductive rights and facilities has long been a target of antiabortion activism, and violence and intimidation, paired with public defunding and legislative restrictions, have taken an undeniable toll. Comprehensive women's health care facilities are closing at record pace; in five states, only a single abortion care provider remains.[120]

The logic of homeland maternity—vested in the differential regulation, protection, and proliferation of domestic bodies—is once again present within crisis teen pregnancy narratives, producing and reproducing national identity through the bodies of certain women and families and in the broader cultural project of securing the nation and its future. Crisis in any context, but particularly in that of the homeland security state, warrants swift and decisive action.

The naming of reproductive crisis specifically taps into a web of meaning, from a young woman's experience of unintended pregnancy and the childlessness of wealthy white women, to CPC discourses of "rescue" in reference to fetal life, teenagers, and single and/or non-Christian women alike. Thus, the use of "crisis" in teen pregnancy narratives and by the CPC movement has promoted a narrow vision of motherhood, intensified the policing of young women's lives, and fueled the colonization of reproductive health clinics across the country.

Tracing these patterns is the place we begin. I now broaden my gaze to consider homeland maternity writ large and its implications for reproductive justice.

Conclusion

Just Pregnancy, Just Parenting in the Age of Homeland Maternity

Constitutional recognition of the right to abortion care in the United States has never, to date, turned on citizenship or immigration status. But in the fall of 2017, an unaccompanied minor from Central America crossed the United States–Mexico border.[1] Jane Doe—as she has been referred to in media accounts and legal proceedings—was taken into federal custody and placed in the care of the Office of Refugee Resettlement (ORR) as an undocumented minor. While in detention, she was informed that she was pregnant. Doe knew immediately that, in her own words, she "was not ready to be a parent."[2] In her country of origin, abortion remains illegal. In her family of origin, her parents beat her older sister for an unintended pregnancy so severely that the beating resulted in pregnancy loss. The seventeen-year-old pursued abortion care in the United States immediately, complying with strict Texas state laws: she successfully sought a judicial waiver for parental consent and met with the abortion care provider at least twenty-four hours in advance of the procedure. Nevertheless, ORR refused transport to her medical appointment, in direct violation of federal law. The federal agency transported Doe, instead, to a religiously affiliated crisis pregnancy center, where antiabortion staff with no medical training subjected her to an ultrasound against her will and pressured her to continue the pregnancy. The harassment continued in detention, where personnel repeatedly asked what she planned to name the baby and forced Doe to place an international phone call to her mother in order to disclose her pregnancy.

With the help of the American Civil Liberties Union and Jane's Due Process,[3] she filed a lawsuit. The Trump administration pressed back. Days and weeks passed as she edged closer to the twenty-week mark, the point at which abortion is outlawed in Texas. After a monthlong legal battle, a federal appellate court granted her constitutional right to abortion care and she terminated her pregnancy within twenty-four hours.

Jane Doe's plight captured national headlines as she struggled for just treatment under the law by a state increasingly and overtly hostile to both immigrants and reproductive self-determination. Like many stories that detail surveillance, coercion, and abuse of pregnant women in the United States, her case is not isolated—although it was quite clearly compounded by her migration status and rendered transparent as she was positioned at the mercy of the state. Many of the recent Central American refugees seeking asylum in the United States are women and children, described by the UN High Commissioner for Refugees as "women on the run"[4]—a reference to escalating levels of violence in El Salvador, Guatemala, and Honduras that threaten the lives women and children in the region. Estimates suggest that as many as 80 percent of the women making this perilous journey are raped in the process, and the vast majority of pregnant minors in ORR custody are pregnant as a result of rape.[5] In 2016, the ACLU filed a lawsuit against the federal government for granting millions of dollars to organizations tasked with providing care—including medical care—for undocumented minors because those same organizations repeatedly refused access to reproductive health care on religious grounds.[6] Reports detail how some religious shelters have evicted young women for simply inquiring about abortion. And under the Trump administration, young migrant women's health care has worsened considerably—for example, a policy revised in the spring of 2017 prohibits any federally funded shelter from facilitating access to abortion care without "direction and approval" from Scott Lloyd, an outspoken, vehement opponent of abortion rights and the current director of ORR.[7]

The case of Jane Doe is many things—it is, for one, an egregious display of state violence and abuse of power, lodged at the very heart of cultural struggles over gender, race, age, citizenship, immigration, and reproductive justice. But it also reveals the incongruities and vexations of homeland maternity. Take, for example, the dehumanizing treatment of this young woman, and others like her, as pregnant individuals are positioned against the fetuses they carry. Rendering care for pregnant minors ancillary, Lloyd directed ORR personnel to consider "the unborn child [as] a child in our care." Virtually all ORR-approved counseling centers are staunchly antiabortion pseudo-clinics.[8] During legal proceedings, government counsel refuted its capacity to provide adequate postabortion care for Doe—despite the fact that abortion during the first trimester is ten times safer than childbirth—while stating that it "would be happy to provide" Doe with prenatal care. The quality of said care remained immaterial; the state of Texas, as reproductive justice advocates were quick to note, claims one of the worst maternal mortality rates in the industrialized world.[9]

In this way, Doe's case marks the challenge of reproductive justice for many facing unintended pregnancy, and particularly minors—paltry prenatal care, laws that restrict birth control and mandate (in some cases notarized) parental consent for abortion, and cultural stigmas attached to teen pregnancy and parenting. The stunning attempt to turn to citizenship as a metric for rights and recognition under the law may anticipate additional challenges to reproductive self-determination on the horizon, even within US borders. For example, conservative members of Congress have attempted, repeatedly, to criminalize the transport of a minor across state lines to receive abortion care in a more permissive state, although these proposed legislative restrictions have yet to gain significant traction.[10] In a world where the threat of overturning *Roe v. Wade* looms large, it is not difficult to imagine the criminalization of *any* border crossing for *anyone*—regardless of age or circumstance—seeking comprehensive and compassionate reproductive health care.

And of course, Doe's treatment by the federal government is profoundly shaped by migration, documentation, and citizenship status. The attempt to deny her abortion care is rendered particularly cruel when considered alongside recent accelerated attacks on immigrant families and deportations that sever undocumented parents from their US-born children.[11] Moreover, Doe's treatment reflects assumptions of criminality that uniquely target pregnant and parenting migrant women. Despite the fact that seeking asylum at the US border is perfectly legal under federal immigration law, in response to increasing numbers of Central American women and children seeking asylum in the United States, the Department of Homeland Security adopted a strategy of "aggressive deterrence"[12] by implementing a number of draconian practices under the Obama administration—including mass detention in for-profit carceral facilities, denying bond and due process, and relying on expedited removal. While some lawsuits have successfully challenged this inhumane treatment of asylum seekers,[13] President Trump's 2017 Border Enforcement Order issued a large-scale expansion of this system, which treats all migrants as criminals and threats to the security of the United States. In March 2017, the Department of Homeland Security considered a formal policy that would separate undocumented families at the United States–Mexico border, detaining parents and children in separate carceral facilities. In a series of stunning assertions, the state defended its proposed action in the interests of national security, as a calculated "deterrent to other mothers" seeking refuge in the United States.[14] Public outcry was swift, effectively derailing a formal change in immigration policy—although then-DHS secretary John Kelly maintained that separating mothers and children would remain warranted under certain circumstances. As this book goes to press, mainstream media are reporting that the separation of children and parents at the border has indeed become routine under the Trump administration. Public outrage is, rightfully, soaring. And yet, the conversation is conspicuously bereft of gender politics as publics rally around the refrain that "families belong together." Surely, they do. And with homeland maternity as critical heuristic, we are compelled to critique not only the role of the carceral state left largely unexamined here but also the specificity of the *gendered* and *reproductive* state violence enacted in this moment.

In short, in the unfolding asylum crisis at the United States–Mexico border, motherhood has been weaponized; pregnant and parenting women have become sites where the security of the nation is imagined to be at stake. This cruel fallacy is only possible in a cultural context that regularly scapegoats racialized migrants as threats to national security, and one in which motherhood is figured as a primary vehicle for the nation. Doe's case, the plight of minors in similar circumstances, and changes in immigration policies offer clear examples of how women continue to be policed and punished under the banner of nation, and in ways that are unique to their sex, gender, race, citizenship, or immigration status—denied reproductive and maternal dignity, their children and reproductive capacities used against them in attempts to "secure" the southern US border. Recent human rights abuses of migrant mothers at the hands of the homeland security state are egregious—and they are also, importantly, *logical extensions of the treatment of pregnancy, reproduction, and motherhood in US security culture writ large*. Homeland maternity, here, is rendered transparent in its overt, acute, and most vicious manifestation.

Most of the sites in this study are less obvious. They signal, but do not overtly evidence, the persistent surveillance and policing of motherhood and reproduction in homeland security culture; they are less visibly demonstrative of egregious human rights violations under the banner of the homeland security state. The sites in this study were selected, in part, because of their subtle but insidious qualities—they illustrate the everyday contexts that undergird alignments between motherhood and nation and fuel the (discursive and material) conditions necessary to police motherhood and reproduction in the ways that we currently do. Put another way, most of the cases noted in this book focus on quotidian processes of surveillance—processes that function to normalize severe treatment of pregnant and parenting people under particular circumstances. The treatment of Jane Doe is a stunning demonstration of attempts by the state to curtail the constitutional rights of a minor based on pregnancy and migration status, but the point of this book is that this does not emerge from nowhere. It is authorized, naturalized, and made palatable by all of the myriad other forms of reproductive injustice that are lodged in the very words we speak, in the narratives we regularly weave around reproduction, motherhood, race, nation, migration, citizenship, sexuality, and family formation in the modern state.

Indeed, alignments between motherhood and nation are no less salient now than in the past. The intimate entanglements of motherhood and nation are rooted in the early formation of the US republic and extend through the antebellum period, postwar containment culture, and into the early twenty-first century. The responsibilities and requirements of motherhood have changed over time, shifting in their differential quality to interpolate women according to dominant hierarchies of reproductive stratification and mythic notions of maternal worth.[15] Homeland maternity is distinguished from earlier alignments of motherhood and nation by its rootedness in postfeminist culture, its reliance on neoliberal forms of governmentality, and its indebtedness to post-9/11 US culture that traffics in discourses of security, risk, emergency, and crisis. And yet, its fundamental animating assumption—that white, heteronuclear domesticity remains central to the flourishing of the nation, that reproduction and mothering outside of these contexts are constituted as a public threat—remains stubbornly intact. Contemplating the recent history of homeland maternity remains critical, then, to struggles on behalf of maternal and reproductive justice. Offered in the spirit of provocation, I elaborate here on the stakes and significance of this study. I hope that these remarks might usefully inform ongoing critical scholarship and advocacy efforts.

To begin, I offer three points of summation. *First, homeland maternity mobilizes discourses that mask reproductive stratification and injustice.* The grammar of homeland security purportedly knows no allegiance. It functions in the technical sphere of argumentation, jettisoning critiques of partisanship or bias through the ethos of expertise.[16] But as evidenced in the cases of Nadya Suleman and Tamara Loertscher, the rhetorical deployment of risk is differentially dispersed. While risk is often asserted with the presumption of neutrality, it is written differently on the bodies of women presumed to mother well versus those presumed to mother poorly—which we might also understand as a distinction drawn between those imagined to parent *in* or *against* the interests of the nation.[17] Similarly, as explored in the chapters on emergency contraception and teen pregnancy media, rhetorics of crisis and emergency are regularly deployed in public discourse to name *particular* reproductive bodies—those already rendered vulnerable within the homeland security state—as a kind of cultural exigence, as troubled, potentially pathological, and in need of intervention. And finally, rhetorics of security have been articulated in two distinct directions—in attempts to justify the separation of asylum-seeking mothers and children at the southern US border, but also used to propel the possibility of motherhood itself, a strategy largely aimed at women of means (see chapter one). From the opt-out revolution to the marketing of egg freezing technologies, the logic of security frames elite white women's motherhood—present or future—as a pinnacle achievement, and as such, vital to safeguard by any means necessary.

This differential valuation of motherhood in homeland security culture is of profound consequence. For those presumed incompetent, a culture of homeland maternity drives troubling trends that include rising rates of incarceration, involuntary commitment, and coerced reproductive decision making. Consider the treatment of Purvi Patel by the State of Indiana under then-governor Mike Pence's leadership. In 2013, Patel was arrested after seeking emergency medical care for what she maintained was a miscarriage. Law enforcement first questioned Patel in the hospital as she awoke from sedation. Pause to consider those circumstances for a moment. Patel had just lost a significant amount of blood. Her medical care necessitated anesthesia. She did not have a lawyer present; she was never read her Miranda rights.[18] There was no trace of an abortifacient in Patel's body, no scientific evidence that the fetus was born alive, and yet a jury convicted Patel of two contradictory felonies: child neglect and feticide.[19] She was the first woman in the United States to be sentenced for this nonsensical combination of crimes, facing twenty years in prison before the decision was overturned in 2016 by the Indiana Court of Appeals. The treatment of Patel as a criminal for seeking medical treatment after pregnancy loss—whether by miscarriage or self-induced abortion, which we will likely never know—is unconscionable. This treatment could, in theory, extend to women of means as well, but states are far more likely to target marginalized pregnant and parenting peoples for criminalization and punishment.[20] In addition to this brutal treatment, a culture of homeland maternity severely restricts the reproductive options available to those most vulnerable—whether limiting timely access to postcoital contraceptives or forcing the closure of clinics that offer a full range of compassionate, professional, and nonjudgmental health care services to patients regardless of their ability to pay.

Women of means are differently subject to the dictates of homeland maternity. Elite women who do not have children are assailed with pronatalist cultural pressures—diminished as selfish, neurotic, or naive—as those who parent are subject to the demands of intensive mothering with little structural support. And yet, elite mothers' struggles are more likely to garner publicity and sympathy, while the indignities and hardships suffered by working-class and indigent mothers fail to register within public discussions of work and family. Moreover, the differential impact of homeland maternity is rendered acutely insidious by its invisibility—an invisibility made possible through the presumed objectivity of related rhetorics of risk, security, and so on. In this way, challenging the rhetorics of homeland maternity—rhetorics that rely on themes of security, risk, emergency, and crisis—is central to the project of reproductive justice.

Second, homeland maternity intensifies the surveillance and policing of women's lives. Increased surveillance is inarguably a central feature of all lives in homeland security culture. Still, homeland maternity provides a guiding set of cultural assumptions and beliefs that fuels the surveillance of the lives of women of reproductive age specifically. Consider that crisis pregnancy centers (CPCs) have begun using mobile technologies in novel ways to target "abortion-minded women" with their advertising.[21] With the use of mobile geo-framing, a common mode of directing ads to users in specific geographical locations, CPCs track women visiting abortion clinics and tailor their advertising to appear on these women's mobile devices. As women sit in the waiting room of a comprehensive reproductive health clinic, CPCs are now able to direct them to biased and even false information regarding pregnancy, abortion, and reproductive health as they scroll through a Facebook feed or open an app that integrates location information. Put another way, in addition to harassing women on the sidewalks, anti-choice activists can now follow women into the interior of the clinic itself, targeting them with misleading information and anti-choice sentiments. It is a trend made possible by a symphony of forces that include technological innovation and piecemeal legal safeguards on privacy and data collection, but that also includes a culture shaped by homeland maternity, one in which pregnant and parenting individuals are increasingly subject to scrutiny, judgment, discipline, and even violence in homeland security culture.

As we have seen, specific iterations of this trend fracture significantly along lines of class, race, sexuality, immigration, and family formation, but it is nonetheless a trend remarkably consistent across a range of discourses and practices—for example, in the amplified requirements of intensive mothering or in public figurations of fetal risk that inspire state actions against pregnant individuals. Importantly, these trends are not exclusive to those already pregnant and parenting but include increased surveillance and policing of women of reproductive age in general. Women—particularly those who are wealthy, white, cisgender, and straight—who do not have children are often presumed incomplete; this is evidenced in mainstream depictions of white women pursuing adoption, such as Vanessa Loring of *Juno* or Shelby Cochran of *Glee*. Or, as discussed in chapter 2, infertility panics in the wake of the great recession spurred collective hand-wringing over the rise of cosmopolitan millennials' "child-free lifestyles" and fueled the rigorous marketing of egg freezing technologies to twenty- and thirtysomething professional women living in major urban centers in the United States. And as pronatalist sentiments were aimed at professional and elite women, the reproductive and maternal lives of teenagers became sites for the expression of cultural anxieties of another ilk—those connected to presumptions of "transgressive" sexuality, or that which fell outside of heteronuclear family formation, as clearly evidenced in the EC debates and crisis teen pregnancy narratives.

As women face growing surveillance in their reproductive lives, they are caught in a deep double bind of powerlessness and responsibility. They are faced, at once, with diminishing reproductive options and increasing personal liability for their decision making. Take, for example, Jennie McCormack, a young, white, single mother of three in Idaho charged with a felony in 2011 for terminating her pregnancy. The structural forces informing McCormack's circumstances were substantial—her sole income amounted to between $200 and $250 each month, and the nearest abortion clinic was located in another state 138 miles from her home and, due to mandatory delay laws, would have required multiple visits and cost between $400 and $2,000.[22] Already parenting three children on her own, McCormack obtained a medication abortion online and terminated her pregnancy. She confided in a friend, whose sister reported McCormack to state authorities, and McCormack was arrested in her home and charged with an "unlawful abortion" under an Idaho statute that predated *Roe v. Wade*.[23] Her story demonstrates how structural conditions render women virtually choiceless, and yet, simultaneously, accountable for their actions. McCormack was caught in a web of structural hostility to reproductive rights—geographic inaccessibility to women's health services, laws that force women to postpone health care procedures to their own detriment, and a woefully inadequate social safety net that forces mothers and children into abject poverty. In seeking a medication abortion, McCormack simply did what she could for the well-being of her family and herself, and, because she did so, was subject to state punishment. While the Ninth Circuit Court ruled in McCormack's favor in 2015, her plight is echoed in similar cases. Indeed, state actions against women like McCormack and Patel signal a new trend in the use of "feticide" legislation to punish women for inducing a miscarriage or simply for pregnancy loss of any kind.

Notably, the intensification of surveillance does not reside exclusively in more overt or egregious acts of discrimination or violence, but also persists in everyday conversations about reproduction and mothering in an age of homeland maternity. Consider, for example, the impossible standards to which mothers are held, deeply inflected by binary gender norms that celebrate fathers for negligible contributions to domestic labor but that simultaneously censure mothers for minute failings in the fulfillment of housework or childcare. This trend is exhibited elsewhere in the persistent (and even public) criticism of pregnant women's behaviors—from exercise and diet to the regulation of caffeine consumption, from varied critiques of "too much" or "too little" applied to everything from weight gain to work habits.[24] This form of criticism has seeped into the censure of "prepregnant" women's behaviors, as in fertility awareness marketing and the preconception services aimed at young cosmopolitan women.[25] Or, in another example, a February 2016 CDC warning to all women of reproductive age clearly embodied this troubling trend, advising them to abstain from alcohol consumption if not actively using contraception: "Alcohol can permanently harm a developing baby before a woman knows she is pregnant. . . . The risk is real. Why take the chance?"[26] While new research does, indeed, suggest that fetal alcohol spectrum disorders (FASDs) are underdiagnosed and of concern, it is worth noting that public warnings to date have been aimed at women's individual behaviors exclusively, and with far less consideration of other factors that inform FASDs—access to prenatal care and nutrition, levels of stress, genetic factors, and the influence of male partners.[27] Significantly, these trends are not easily challenged with mainstream frameworks for reproductive choice and rights. As all women of reproductive age are increasingly interpellated by homeland maternity regardless of maternal status or intent, the possibility of reproductive justice demands new modes of thinking and engagement.

This brings me to a third observation: *homeland maternity points to the significant work that remains undone in securing reproductive dignity and justice.* I refer here not simply to the more overt forms of reproductive injustice regularly challenged by feminist advocates—from anti-choice legislation to sterilization abuse in prisons and environmental toxins geographically concentrated in low-income communities and communities of color—but also to the discursive conditions that render those material effects possible. In other words, one fundamental premise of this book is that the ways in which we publicly narrate motherhood and reproduction matter profoundly to all women's lives—regardless of their desire or ability to birth or parent children—and it also matters, albeit differently, to those who carry and parent children outside of the gender binary. Indeed, for trans and nonbinary parents, a gender-conformist culture seeps into the lived experience of creating family, from access to culturally competent reproductive health and birthing care to daily negotiations of claiming parental identity against the grain of narrow and exclusive gendered norms. Challenging these injustices is in no small part shaped by our collective capacity to tell different—more capacious and inclusive—stories about parenting, family, and belonging. Put another way, the *communicative conditions* of reproductive justice are indeed central to our ability to assert this form of justice as a lived material and political reality.

I draw on reproductive justice as an established critical framework (see introduction) to consider a set of questions regarding its possibilities and requirements within the context of homeland maternity.[28] Reproductive justice is inextricably bound to a broad range of social justice struggles that include wealth disparities, the prison-industrial complex, environmental injustice, and inequities grounded in race, class, gender, nationality, immigration status, citizenship, age, ability and disability, and sexuality. Reproductive justice affirms the right of every person to decide whether, when, and with whom to create intimacy and family. It supports the full and unique expression of gender and sexuality as a critical dimension of human dignity.[29] It includes challenging current systems of foster care and adoption that target the children of poor families and families of color, as well as affirming access to knowledge of one's social, familial, and biological origins, and the right to information regarding one's body, health, and ancestry.[30] And, as a critical informant to each of the aforementioned tenets, reproductive justice necessitates access to the social, political, medical, and economic resources that enable health and prosperity for oneself, one's family, and one's community.[31] In other words, we cannot simply refer to reproductive justice as a set of freedoms tied to individual decision making, although the concept is certainly inclusive of that. It demands transformation of the social conditions that craft the architecture of institutionalized inequities. It is not solely about protecting or defending freedoms, but is also about actively supporting an expansion of rights and dignities for vulnerable and historically disenfranchised communities.

In an age of homeland maternity specifically, the project of reproductive justice demands that we interrogate the cultural logics and, relatedly, the discursive conditions under which reproductive injustices occur. It would include, for example, critical interrogations of the cultural designation of "deserving" or "fit" mothers, explorations of how sexuality and reproduction are discursively constrained through policy debates, and calling into question the force of race, class, and disability in the practice and politics of genetic testing, assessments of risk, and assisted fertility. In tracing rhetorics of security, risk, emergency, and crisis as they intersect with reproductive and maternal politics, we are better able to understand how cultural understandings of "legitimate" motherhood both shape and are shaped by homeland security culture and its attendant forms of discipline and governance.

Moreover, homeland maternity clarifies some of the circumstances under which reproductive injustices have been veiled by salient discourses of homeland security culture. To be sure, some instances of injustice have registered prominently in public arenas, with feminist communities rallying in response—for example, the reprehensible tactics of antiabortion crisis pregnancy centers, as well as state actions against pregnant women, have garnered sympathetic media coverage and significant advocacy efforts. But homeland maternity also calls our attention to the relative degree of silence surrounding other forms of injustice. The case of Nadya Suleman, for instance, generated significant public anger and demonstrative racism and misogyny, but very little critical questioning from feminist or reproductive justice advocates. Making a feminist perspective more available in Suleman's case not only affords us the opportunity to reconsider biased attitudes related to maternal legitimacy and belonging, but also pushes us to question current regulatory regimes and cultural beliefs that govern the use of reproductive technologies. For instance, we might question the extent to which we should place restrictions on the use of assisted reproductive technologies, or how we might initiate ART industry and health care reform to promote fair and just access. In another example, the persistent framing of teen mothers as inescapably in crisis curtails our capacity to question the circumstances under which this may or may not be the case. Is it possible to recast teen pregnancy, as some scholars have claimed, as an adaptive response to poverty and lack of employment or educational opportunity? If so, how might this shift the ways in which dominant cultural discourses narrate teen pregnancy and motherhood? How might we simultaneously equip young people with the information they need to make empowered decisions about their reproductive health and sexuality, while also expanding the notion of empowerment to include an integrated sense of wellness, including opportunities for education, decent employment, and freedom from violence and environmental harm? These dimensions of homeland maternity are perhaps less visible than more flagrant actions against women, but they are intimately bound together in the contemporary landscape of reproductive politics. Homeland maternity is, in this way, the broader cultural terrain in which specific attacks on pregnant and parenting individuals' lives and dignity are made possible; its interrogation offers us a framework to understand these attacks and reimagine the questions we might ask in the spirit of reproductive justice.

What, then, are the subtle forms of negotiation or more active modes of resistance that we might craft in response to homeland maternity? The following possibilities, discrete but overlapping in various ways, warrant our critical attention. I sketch them here not in their totality, but in the spirit of inviting ongoing, creative, critical exploration.

First, co-optation affords a rich set of rhetorical possibilities for challenging homeland maternity. If we understand co-optation in this context as an appropriation of the strategically valuable dimensions of motherhood, then a number of considerations arise. A rich body of scholarship traces how activists and movements exploit the cultural currency of motherhood in order to advance political struggle, despite its obvious shortcomings and problematics.[32] At its best, Sara Hayden writes that "maternity is the grounding for an alternative vision of society in which the social welfare of citizens is privileged."[33] The examples are plentiful and diverse—including struggles for suffrage, temperance, labor laws, welfare rights, civil rights, peace, gun control, and challenges to oppressive regimes.[34] Environmental justice activists have successfully leveraged maternal identities to challenge toxic waste distribution and the proliferation of nuclear power plants, Cindy Sheehan's public performances of "matriotism" challenged the legitimacy of the US invasion of Iraq, Black Lives Matter activist mothers have organized against racist violence and police brutality under the moniker Mothers of the Movement, cisgender mothers have drawn on the status of mothering to defend the rights and dignity of their trans children, and lesbians and queer-identified peoples have claimed motherhood in defense of state-recognized LGBTQ family formation.[35] In short, claiming "mother" as a strategic political identity borrows on the ethos of mothering, and thus imbues a political struggle with moral weight and urgency as it compels social change.

It is worthy of note, however, that the use of "mother" as a strategic political identity is differentially available to women; it remains far more pervasive (perhaps even more effective) when linked to, but not centered on, public struggles over reproductive and maternal politics. Put another way, the cultural cachet of motherhood travels well, but it seems to do very little when the site of struggle is, in fact, reproduction and motherhood itself. Women can and do organize under the "mother" moniker when it comes to challenging environmental injustice, drunk driving, gun control, nuclear proliferation, war, racism, and police brutality—and, to be clear, these issues are central to reproductive justice as a vision of a world free from coercion or violence regarding family formation and the capacity to parent in dignity and wellness. Still, and significantly, motherhood is far less frequently mobilized within these contexts to offer explicit attention to reproductive violence and oppression. Even MomsRising, which claims a space "where moms and people who love them go to change our world" and is dedicated specifically to "building a more family-friendly America,"[36] ignores the centrality of reproductive politics to obtaining justice for mothers and families. While MomsRising's organizational platform includes a range of issues central to the wellness of families, mothers, and children, the organization remains silent on matters of reproductive health and rights, even as threats to said rights continue to rise at astonishing speed. This omission suggests that the utility of motherhood, while leveraged effectively on behalf of other political causes, is less easily or readily mobilized on behalf of maternal health and wellness.

There are, of course, a few examples of attempts to leverage maternal identity on behalf of reproductive rights. As Lindal Buchanan details in her study of maternal appeals, Margaret Sanger drew on the cultural capital of white, wealthy, married motherhood to garner mainstream acceptance for contraception—a far cry from the staunchly feminist free love and emancipation arguments that Sanger favored in the early 1910s.[37] Sanger's appeals paired with the popularity of eugenics and scientific racism in the early twentieth century, aligning motherhood and contraceptive rights at great cost.[38] Twenty-first-century examples of maternal appeals, however, are more likely to reflect an ethic of reproductive justice. At the 2004 March for Women's Lives in Washington, DC, which drew over one million people to the National Mall under the banner of reproductive justice, individuals with pro-choice slogans written across their pregnant bellies and parents pushing children in strollers declared reproductive justice critical to motherhood; their actions suggest the largely untapped utility of similar strategies on a larger scale.[39] Some community-based reproductive justice organizations like the Brooklyn Young Mothers Collective place reproductive justice and motherhood at the heart of their platform and organizational identity, but this is less common in organizations that are national in scope and addressing a mainstream audience under the moniker of "mother." In short, motherhood has functioned powerfully in a variety of political contexts, in part because reproductive justice includes an attentiveness to all of the dimensions that make women's lives whole, but its use in contexts explicitly connected to reproductive health and dignity is alarmingly absent, save those that have leveraged the power of elite motherhood to forward the rights of some at the expense of many.

What, then, might it take or look like to co-opt and foreground motherhood in the service of reproductive justice? As the above examples might suggest, it seems far easier to *assume*, rather than to actually *affirm*, the value of motherhood, and it is far more common to draw on this assumption in order to validate allied political struggles and movements. It seems a complicated endeavor indeed to simultaneously claim the status of motherhood while illuminating the unique ways in which women's reproductive lives are subject to scrutiny, coercion, and violence. To do so, publicly and effectively, would encourage a deep and collectively felt sense of cognitive dissonance. But it might also provide a necessary corrective—what we might label in Burkean terms as "perspective by incongruity"—as an articulation of opposites in order to invite new ways of seeing the world.[40] A number of communication scholars have traced the use of perspective by incongruity in feminist activist contexts from the Guerrilla Girls to radical second-wave abortion speak-outs,[41] for in its capacity to highlight inequities and inconsistencies, perspective by incongruity functions as a powerful strategy of rhetorical invention. Affording the capacity to rethink and reinvent dominant symbolic codes, perspective by incongruity might lend itself well to challenging contemporary reproductive and maternal politics. Homeland maternity invites us to imagine the possibility of leveraging the status of motherhood to affirm and support substantively reproductive justice and dignity.

Co-optation is perhaps even more complicated than this. In addition to scholars who astutely explore how maternal appeals might be used to render reproductive rights palatable to broader publics,[42] I believe that taking co-optation seriously demands that we recognize how this may entail the use of motherhood to undo its own purchase. In other words, the mobilization of motherhood on behalf of reproductive justice insists, first and foremost, on recognizing the *human* rights of those who carry, birth, and/or parent children, as well as those who do not. I admit I find it curious that reproductive rights and justice seem to be the locus where maternal appeals are most silenced. It is, I would argue, the ultimate wresting away of motherhood from mythic norms toward radical ends—an insistence of the right of pregnant and parenting people to be *persons*; their right to freely determine when, whether, and with whom they might embark on that journey. Put another way, maternal appeals for reproductive justice insist on inverting the naturalness or essentialism of motherhood; they turn the equation on its head—insisting on personhood as a precursor to motherhood and perhaps even creating a space for gender expansiveness and creativity in "mothering" and/or parenting. What radical notions indeed.

A second mode of engagement worthy of our consideration is subversion, by which I mean the disruption or erosion of dominant codes of reproductivity and motherhood in order to challenge those codes and expand the range of possibilities available for the expression of sexuality and family formation. A few examples come to mind. For one, how might we amplify or otherwise productively engage instances in which motherhood—as compulsory, as always already virtuous, as the pinnacle experience of white women's lives—is productively queried or otherwise complicated by mobilizing discourses beyond normative heteronuclear reproductivity? While "childfree" or "childless" identities have proven to be sites of contention, due in part to the powerful logic of homeland maternity and its pronatalist proclivities, they have also been more explicitly claimed and embraced in the latter 2010s.[43] Crafting a life without children remains a vexed task for women in particular, in no small part because it demands a significant rethinking of womanhood itself—a disentangling of "woman" and "mother" that confronts longstanding cultural beliefs. Even so, resisting or refusing motherhood does not necessarily avoid women's interpellation by hegemonic familialism. For example, as Hayden notes in her study of "auntrepreneurialism," cultural discourses aimed at "savvy aunties" simultaneously disrupt and fuel intensive mothering. They challenge the belief that all women mother, and yet, they work to cast meaningful relationships with children as central to *all* women's lives, including those who do not birth or parent children.[44] But despite these difficulties, challenging compulsory motherhood stands to contribute significantly to the overall goal of reproductive justice, insofar as it could invite a re-valuation of *both* motherhood-parenting and the individual lives of those who shoulder this work in general. Put another way, challenging compulsory motherhood is decidedly not about devaluing motherhood, but rather it is fundamentally concerned with rendering its quotidian labors visible. As such, it stands to value the labor of caregiving and nurturance *more* in terms of structural support while, simultaneously, resisting attempts to fashion it requisite of femininity.

In addition to challenging pronatalist sentiments, subverting homeland maternity would also include resisting ideologies of perfectionism, intensive mothering, and competitive mothering that often position elite "working" mothers against "stay-at-home" mothers. A growing body of research provides examples of how women have actively contested dominant ideologies surrounding motherhood.[45] Andrea O'Reilly's prolific scholarship on mothering—which includes several books as well as the founding of a journal and research institute devoted to mothering studies—theorizes feminist mothering as an individual creative practice, an intentionally crafted "outlaw" mothering designed to parent against the institution of motherhood.[46] Extending beyond individualized practices of mothering, scholars such as Tasha Dubriwny, Lori Kido Lopez, and Valerie Palmer-Mehta and Sherianne Shuler have examined the potential of mommy blogging and social media as platforms for collective resistance to motherhood as a narrowly defined and limiting cultural institution—their utility in building community, disrupting totalizing assumptions about "good" and "bad" motherhood, and resisting the standards of perfection to which mothers are relentlessly held.[47]

Subverting homeland maternity not only entails resistance of pronatalism or the ideology of intensive mothering, but must include a critical undoing and transformation of racist, heteronuclear, classist assumptions regarding family formation and the figuration of particular maternal bodies as a threat to the nation, as risky, in crisis, or otherwise in need of intervention. Scholarship to expand here includes that which specifies how, in the words of Susana Martínez Guillem and Lisa A. Flores, "maternal transgressions rely upon assumptions of an ideal that, in its naturalness and its perfection, is grounded in Whiteness and patriarchy in ways that link transgression to race."[48] It includes that which challenges the circumstances under which some mothers are figured as cultural "outsiders," as threats to US identity and futurity through racialization and nativist logics.[49] It demands increased attention to how immigration law governs, in the words of Eithne Luibhéid, "peripheral sexualities" and the reproductive lives of racialized immigrant women in order "to produce particular visions of the U.S. nation and citizenry."[50]

Thus, feminists might build on the essential work initiated by Valerie Palmer-Mehta, Sara Hayden and Heather Hundley, and Alexis Pauline Gumbs, China Martens, and Mai'a Williams, which traces resistance to the conflation of motherhood, whiteness, and wealth in popular culture.[51] For example, in her essay on the activist work of Staceyann Chin, Palmer-Mehta notes the radical potentiality of queering and claiming motherhood in Chin's guest columns for *Huffington Post*, which intimately describe Chin's "journey to motherhood as a single, immigrant lesbian" and pose "critical questions regarding how we rhetorically fashion what is considered 'legitimate' motherhood, who counts as family, and what constitutes home, providing an important challenge to deeply entrenched but understudied Western domestic rhetorics."[52] In another example, Thomas Beatie has publicly claimed a fatherhood inclusive of pregnancy and childbirth. In so doing, he continues to challenge dominant cultural scripts for family formation as well as the legal architecture that sutures binary notions of sex and gender to reproductivity.[53] In activist locales, we can witness the wresting of motherhood away from dominant logics in teen mothers' collectives such as the Brooklyn Young Mothers Collectives and in similarly aligned teen mothers' support services like Iowa City–based United Action for Youth.[54] Similar investments are evident in the Boston-based Prison Birth Project, the legal advocacy of National Advocates for Pregnant Women, the online community building of trans and nonbinary birthing parents, and the expansion of care services provided by radical doulas and midwives.[55] In each of these examples, scholars, activists, and everyday parents work to transform the way we conceptualize family, many with an explicit commitment to respecting the dignity of those historically diminished, pathologized, and disenfranchised by and within dominant discourses.

Finally, subverting homeland maternity compels us to consider everyday practices that, beyond queering motherhood, invite alternate modes of crafting kin. The possibilities of productively queering kin are made visible in families composed beyond and outside of heteronuclearity. These include blended families, adoptive families, foster families, chosen families, families of surrogate origin, families with single parents, multigenerational families, and LGBTQ families, to name a few. And indeed, non-heteronuclear family formation is not new, nor is its guiding impulse necessarily predicated on radical visions of social justice, but rather it is born of survival and resistance to myriad forms of oppression and violence. African American communities, for example, have long embraced intergenerational and "other mothering," in part as an adaptive response to white supremacy and its violent destruction of black families and communities, from slavery to foster care, mass incarceration, and police brutality.[56] The concept of "chosen family" continues to animate LGBTQ forms of belonging, affirmation, and love in the absence of family-of-origin support, which is often compounded by social stigma, ostracization, and legal and cultural barriers to familial recognition.[57] In short, family formation evidences the intimate entanglement of agency and constraints as well as the creative, world making art of making do in an imperfect and sometimes cruel world. Still, for all of the ways in which we might actively reimagine family *against* homeland maternity and hegemonic familialism, powerful ideological forces shape, even determine, how we are able to create it. Cultural pressures compound structural impediments to queering kin, as heteronuclearity becomes the template for state legitimacy and recognition. In short, the work of queering kin is challenging at best. It demands deep consideration of the forces that shape normative family formation and the active, ongoing navigation of matters as intensely personal as they are unavoidably political.

In this way, subverting homeland maternity (and its correlative, hegemonic familialism)[58] requires ongoing, difficult labor in its requisite grappling with systems of disenfranchisement and ongoing legacies of racism, colonization, and institutionalized poverty. People strive in this direction nonetheless. Narrating his journey in creating family, Don Romesburg writes that he "advocate[s] for 'queer transracial family' not as a descriptive synonym for 'gay interracial adoptive family' but as a particular form of 'differential becoming' that can effect a blended open vision for belonging attentive to complex power relations."[59] For Romesburg, this process necessarily includes navigating painful and deeply unjust terrain in the formal adoption of his foster daughter, as well as in the informal integration of her family of origin as a regular fixture in their lives and family. As Romesburg rightly states, "we cannot love our way out of the psychic and structural preconditions of loss and disorientation upon which we build a family, so we develop tools to live through them."[60] This mode of queer family formation is not simply a demand for legal and cultural recognition of a gay adoptive interracial family, but rather is one committed to confronting and living with the legacies of violence that brought them together, actively challenging notions of "family" as bounded by a two-parent household or created in a vacuum. The spirit of queering kin is evidenced in other spaces, as well—in the building of donor sibling registries to connect individuals across time and space who share a genetic history, the uptick in women pursuing motherhood without a partner but with extended networks of support, in trans and nonbinary parents who challenge gendered conceptualizations of pregnancy and parenting, the integration of extended family or voluntary kin as long-term fixtures in day-to-day life, and in families of adoptive or surrogate origin that maintain active and open ties to donors, birth parents, families, and/or communities. In the daily work of creating family, messy and imperfect but rich with possibilities nonetheless, we hold the promise of transforming the way we imagine family and, in so doing, broadening the possibilities for imagining the nation as well.

Thus, in search of an alternative vision to ground reproductive and maternal justice alongside our collective commitments to one another more broadly, I wish to invest in the radical possibilities of rhetorical (re)invention to harness and adapt the potentialities of motherhood, family, and citizenship.[61] Quotidian practices in historical and contemporary contexts suggest that this is, indeed, possible—that communities can and do remake what it means to be a family, to parent or mentor meaningfully young people in our communities, to craft a relationship to nation, to challenge and to reinvent that relationship, to leverage its power on behalf of more radical politics.[62] I draw inspiration from a rich tradition in rhetorical studies that emphasizes the generative, inventive, and reparative dimensions of criticism to tether critique to the possibilities of a just world.[63] If family is indeed the central metaphor for the nation,[64] a capacious reimagining of family might thus inspire more ethical, just, and cooperative models for structuring public relationships and animating collective life. It follows, then, that we might rearticulate the relationship between motherhood and nation in new and expansive ways. In lieu of rendering reproduction and motherhood serviceable to the nation, for example, we might rearticulate alignments in ways that make the nation more readily responsive to longstanding forms of injustice that disproportionately impact mothers, parents, and families. And as we imagine new alignments in the spirit of reproductive justice, we might also invent novel forms of attachment and belonging that exceed our current conceptualizations of family as the metaphor for collective life.

To ground this abstraction in the recent history of US culture and collective life, what might be different if we wrested motherhood, parenting, and reproduction away from homeland security logics? Away from fear, intimidation, risk, and neoliberal responsibility? What would happen if we imagined reproduction and parenting not as central to security on the home front, but as core questions residing at the heart of individual and community-based struggles to create whole and meaningful lives? How might we advocate for *just pregnancy and parenting*—at once an investment in challenging the everyday surveillance and judgment of those pregnant and/or parenting, as well as an affirmation of reproductive justice and dignity? Relatedly, how might we undo the cultural lauding of some mothers at the expense of others, the powerful discourses of risk or crisis that differentially discipline and constrain reproductive decision making, the demands of intensive mothering, pronatalist culture, and compulsory motherhood? How might we claim maternal, parental, and reproductive dignity as an inviolable human right? While full answers to these questions exceed the parameters of my current project, I raise them as the central provocations of *Homeland Maternity*.

These concluding remarks are aimed less at declaration than generation, with a desire to suggest how critical feminist and rhetorical perspectives might encourage a productive rethinking of the terrain of dilemmas signaled by homeland maternity. For homeland maternity shows no sign of abating. From US immigration policy to CPCs' geotargeting of "abortion-minded" women and increasing state actions against women in the name of fetal risk, the reigning logics of homeland security have achieved a stunning salience and velocity in shaping the politics of reproduction and motherhood in contemporary US culture. Understanding these twenty-first-century alignments between motherhood and nation thus reorients our interrogation of systems in need of challenge and transformation.

Homeland maternity has a deep and expansive footprint. The possibilities of reproductive justice rely on our capacity to dream other ways of relating into existence.

Notes

Introduction: Homeland Maternity, the New Reproductive Regime

1. James D. Peterson, *Tamara M. Loertscher v. Eloise Anderson, Brad D. Schimel, and Taylor County*, no. 14-cv-870-jdp (United States District Court for the Western District of Wisconsin, April 28, 2017). This detailed court document provides the foundation for my brief sketch of Loertscher's case, corroborated by journalists and legal advocates (additional citations below).

2. "Unborn Child Protection Act, Wis. Stat." (1997).

3. National Advocates for Pregnant Women, "Federal Court Declares Wisconsin 'Unborn Child Protection' Law Unconstitutional: Law Permitting Forced Treatment and Detention of Pregnant Women Is Struck down, Effective Immediately," *National Advocates for Pregnant Women* (blog), May 1, 2017, http://advocatesforpregnantwomen.org/blog/2017/05/federal_court_declares_wiscons.php; Janet Reitman, "Abortion Rights at Risk: The GOP's War on Women Rages On," *Rolling Stone*, www.rollingstone.com/politics/news/abortion-rights-at-risk-the-gop-opens-a-new-front-in-the-war-on-women-20150422.

4. Jessica Mason Pieklo, "Pregnant Wisconsin Woman Jailed under State's 'Personhood'-Like Law," *Rewire*, December 12, 2014, https://rewire.news.

5. Andrew Chung, "Supreme Court Lifts Block on Wisconsin 'Cocaine Mom' Law during Appeal," Reuters, July 10, 2017, www.reuters.com; Caroline Modarressy-Tehrani, "'Cocaine Mom Law' That Locks up Pregnant Women Might Be Done in Wisconsin," Vice News, May 28, 2017, https://news.vice.com; David Wahlberg, "Judge Who Blocked 'Cocaine Mom' Law Partially Lifts Ruling as State Appeals," *Wisconsin State Journal*, May 5, 2017, http://host.madison.com.

6. National Women's Law Center and Law Students for Reproductive Justice, "Fact Sheet: If You Really Care about Criminal Justice, You Should Care about Reproductive Justice!," National Women's Law Center, October 3, 2014, https://nwlc.org.

7. Lynn Paltrow and Jeanne Flavin, "Arrests of and Forced Interventions on Pregnant Women in the United States (1973–2005): The Implications for Women's Legal Status and Public Health," *Journal of Health Politics, Policy and Law* 38, no. 2 (2013): 299–343. More research is needed on this trend. The numbers are difficult to estimate because of the dearth of comprehensive records or data tracking this phenomenon. Paltrow and Flavin's 2013 report studied 413 cases from 1973 to 2005, a number they noted was underestimated. As of 2016, Paltrow and Flavin have documented over four hundred additional cases since 2005.

8. Chung, "Supreme Court Lifts Block."

9. Juliette Kayyem, *Security Mom: An Unclassified Guide to Protecting Our Homeland and Your Home* (New York: Simon and Schuster, 2016), 6, 10, 8.

10. "Description of *Security Mom: An Unclassified Guide to Protecting Our Homeland and Your Home*," Amazon, accessed May 17, 2016, www.amazon.com/Security-Mom-Unclassified-Protecting-Homeland/dp/1476733740.

11. A body of scholarship is dedicated to interrogating homeland security logics at a range of cultural sites. See, for example, Barbara A. Biesecker, "Homeland Security [Special Section]," *Communication and Critical/Cultural Studies* 4, no. 2 (2007): 204–31; James Hay and Mark Andrejevic, eds., "Homeland Insecurities," special issue, *Cultural Studies* 20, nos. 4–5 (2006).

12. Linda K. Kerber, *Women of the Republic: Intellect and Ideology in Revolutionary America* (Chapel Hill: University of North Carolina Press, 1980); Elaine Tyler May, *Homeward Bound: American Families during the Cold War Era*, 20th ann. ed. (New York: Basic Books, 2008); Dorothy Roberts, *Killing the Black Body: Race, Reproduction, and the Meaning of Liberty* (New York: Pantheon Books, 1997); Andrea Smith, *Conquest: Sexual Violence and American Indian Genocide* (Boston: South End, 2005); Rickie Solinger, *Pregnancy and Power: A Short History of Reproductive Politics in America* (New York: New York University Press, 2005).

13. My attention in this project is to dominant discourses within US culture, to how motherhood and reproduction are imagined to participate in nation building. It is worth noting, however, that the alignment of motherhood and nation is evidenced not just in dominant cultural discourses, but also within counterpublic enclaves as well. Scholars have documented these trends, for example, as an assertion of class status or in movements for ethnic sovereignty, independence, and/or nationalism. Many women have resisted these pressures to reproduce "for the revolution," so to speak. Thus, histories of motherhood and nation within counterpublic enclaves converge with republican motherhood in some significant ways, and underscore the consistency with which women's reproductive capacities have been imagined and marshaled toward the future of the "nation." Attention to dominant discourses reveals, however, consistent distinctions that fracture along lines of race, class, sexuality, immigration,

and marital status. This consistency signals the importance of motherhood and reproduction in racializing the nation and maintaining long-standing power structures in domestic and global settings. It is toward illuminating the latter that this project is primarily committed.

14. Natalie Fixmer-Oraiz, "Speaking of Solidarity: Surrogacy and the Rhetorics of Reproductive (in)Justice," *Frontiers: A Journal of Women's Studies* 34, no. 3 (2013): 126–64.

15. Angela McRobbie, *The Aftermath of Feminism: Gender, Culture and Social Change* (Thousand Oaks, CA: Sage, 2009).

16. Solinger, *Pregnancy and Power*, 4.

17. Kerber, *Women of the Republic*, 283.

18. Barbara Welter, "The Cult of True Womanhood: 1820–1860," *American Quarterly* 18, no. 2 (1966): 151–74.

19. Roberts, *Killing the Black Body*; A. Smith, *Conquest*; Solinger, *Pregnancy and Power*.

20. Solinger, *Pregnancy and Power*.

21. Ibid., 29.

22. Roberts, *Killing the Black Body*.

23. bell hooks, *Yearning: Race, Gender, and Cultural Politics* (Boston: South End, 1990); Roberts, *Killing the Black Body*; Solinger, *Pregnancy and Power*.

24. A. Smith, *Conquest*, 15–16.

25. Ibid., 36.

26. Ibid., 37.

27. A. Smith, *Conquest*.

28. Jessica Enoch, "Survival Stories: Feminist Historiographic Approaches to Chicana Rhetorics of Sterilization Abuse," *Rhetoric Society Quarterly* 35, no. 3 (2005): 5–30; Luibhéid Eithne, *Entry Denied: Controlling Sexuality at the Border* (Minneapolis: University of Minnesota Press, 2002); Sara L. McKinnon, "Essentialism, Intersectionality, and Recognition: A Feminist Rhetorical Approach to the Audience," in *Standing in the Intersection: Feminist Voices, Feminist Practices in Communication Studies*, ed. Karma R. Chávez and Cindy L. Griffin (Albany: State University of New York Press, 2012), 189–210.

29. Luibhéid, *Entry Denied*.

30. Ibid., 7.

31. Luibhéid, *Entry Denied*.

32. Ibid.

33. Angela Y. Davis, *Women, Race, and Class* (New York: Vintage Books, 1983); Linda Gordon, *The Moral Property of Women: A History of Birth Control Politics in America* (Chicago: University of Illinois Press, 2007).

34. A. Davis, *Women, Race, and Class*, 215.

35. Ibid.; Gordon, *Moral Property*.

36. May, *Homeward Bound*.

37. Patricia Hill Collins, *Black Feminist Thought: Knowledge, Consciousness, and the Politics of Empowerment*, 2nd ed. (New York: Routledge, 2000); Premilla Nadasen, *Welfare Warriors: The Welfare Rights Movement in the United States* (New York: Routledge, 2005).

38. Collins, *Black Feminist Thought*; Enoch, "Survival Stories."

39. Roberts, *Killing the Black Body*; A. Smith, *Conquest*.

40. Roberts, *Killing the Black Body*.

41. Ibid.

42. May, *Homeward Bound*, 130.

43. Jeremiah Favara, "A Maternal Heart: Angelina Jolie, Choices of Maternity, and Hegemonic Femininty in *People* Magazine," *Feminist Media Studies* 15, no. 4 (2015): 626–42; Raka Shome, *Diana and Beyond: White Femininity, National Identity, and Contemporary Media Culture* (Urbana: University of Illinois Press, 2014).

44. Betty Friedan, *The Feminine Mystique* (New York: Norton, 1963).

45. Susan J. Douglas and Meredith W. Michaels, *The Mommy Myth: The Idealization of Motherhood and How It Has Undermined All Women* (New York: Free Press, 2004), 104.

46. D. Lynn O'Brien Hallstein, "Public Choices, Private Control: How Mediated Mom Labels Work Rhetorically to Dismantle the Politics of Choice and White Second Wave Feminist Successes," in *Contemplating Maternity in an Era of Choice: Explorations into Discourses of Reproduction*, ed. Sara Hayden and D. Lynn O'Brien Hallstein (Lanham, MD: Lexington Books, 2010), 7.

47. Judith Warner, *Perfect Madness: Motherhood in the Age of Anxiety* (New York: Riverhead Books, 2005), 56–57.

48. McRobbie, *Aftermath of Feminism*.

49. For more on postfeminism, see Susan J. Douglas, *Enlightened Sexism: The Seductive Message That Feminism's Work Is Done* (New York: Times Books, 2010); Bonnie J. Dow, *Prime-Time Feminism: Television, Media Culture, and the Women's Movement since 1970* (Philadelphia: University of Pennsylvania Press, 1996); Rosalind Gill, "Postfeminist Media Culture: Elements of a Sensibility," *European Journal of Cultural Studies* 10, no. 2 (2007): 147–66, doi:10.1177/1367549407075898; Rosalind Gill, "Post-Postfeminism? New Feminist Visibilities in Postfeminist Times," *Feminist Media Studies* 16, no. 4 (July 3, 2016): 610–30, doi:10.1080/14680777.2016.1193293; McRobbie, *Aftermath of Feminism*; Yvonne Tasker and Diane Negra, eds., *Interrogating Post-Feminism: Gender and the Politics of Popular Culture* (Durham, NC: Duke University Press, 2007).

50. Linda Steiner and Carolyn Bronstein, "When Tiger Mothers Transgress: Amy Chua, Dara-Lynn Weiss and the Cultural Imperative of Intensive Mothering," in *Mediated Moms: Contemporary Challenges to the Motherhood Myth*, ed. Heather L. Hundley and Sara E. Hayden (New York: Peter Lang Publishing, 2015), 247–74; Julie A. Wilson and Emily Chivers Yochim, *Mothering through Precarity: Women's Work and Digital Media* (Durham, NC: Duke University Press, 2017).

51. Stephanie Coontz, *The Way We Never Were: American Families and the Nostalgia Trap* (New York: Basic Books, 1992).

52. Julie Wilson and Yochim, *Mothering through Precarity*.

53. Joan Wolf, *Is Breast Best? Taking on the Breastfeeding Experts and the New High Stakes of Motherhood* (New York: New York University Press, 2011), 76.

54. Miranda Waggoner, *The Zero Trimester: Pre-Pregnancy Care and the Politics of Reproductive Risk* (Berkeley: University of California Press, 2017).

55. Shome, *Diana and Beyond*, 59.

56. Christine Hauser, "Florida Woman Whose 'Stand Your Ground' Defense Was Rejected Is Released," *New York Times*, February 7, 2017, sec. U.S., www.nytimes.com; Paltrow and Flavin, "Arrests of and Forced Interventions."

57. Paltrow and Flavin, "Arrests of and Forced Interventions."

58. Benedict Anderson, *Imagined Communities: Reflections on the Origin and Spread of Nationalism* (London: Verso, 1983).

59. Kelly Gates, "The Globalization of Homeland Security," in *Routledge Handbook of Surveillance Studies*, ed. Kristie Ball, Kevin Haggerty, and David Lyon (New York: Routledge, 2012), 292–300; James Hay and Mark Andrejevic, "Toward an Analytic of Governmental Experiments in These Times: Homeland Security as the New Social Security," *Cultural Studies* 20, nos. 4–5 (2006): 331–48.

60. Nicholas De Genova, "The Production of Culprits: From Deportability to Detainability in the Aftermath of 'Homeland Security,'" *Citizenship Studies* 11, no. 5 (November 2007): 421–48, https://doi.org/10.1080/13621020701605735; Gates, "The Globalization of Homeland Security"; Sarah Jaffe, "The Militarization of Everything," *Bitch* 17, no. 73 (2017): 36–42.

61. Gates, "Globalization of Homeland Security."

62. Mark B. Salter, "Conclusion: Risk and Imagination in the War on Terror," in *Risk and the War on Terror*, ed. Louise Amoore and Marieke de Goede (New York: Routledge, 2008), 243.

63. Salter, quoted in Marieke de Goede, "Beyond Risk: Premediation and the Post-9/11 Security Imagination," *Security Dialogue* 39, nos. 2–3 (April 2008): 155, https://doi.org/10.1177/0967010608088773.

64. Richard Grusin, "Premediation," *Criticism* 46, no. 1 (2004): 29.

65. Goede, "Beyond Risk"; Salter, "Conclusion."

66. Ulrich Beck, *World at Risk*, trans. Ciaran Cronin (Malden, MA: Polity, 2009).

67. Ulrich Beck, "Living in the World Risk Society," *Economy and Society* 35, no. 3 (2006): 329–45, 332.

68. Beck, *World at Risk*, 188.

69. Claudia Aradau and Rens Van Munster, "Taming the Future: The Dispositif of Risk in the War on Terror," in *Risk and the War on Terror*, ed. Louise Amoore and Marieke de Goede (New York: Routledge, 2008), 23–40.

70. Andrea Smith, "Not-Seeing: State Surveillance, Settler Colonialism, and Gender Violence," in *Feminist Surveillance Studies*, ed. Rachel E. Dubrofsky and Shoshana Amielle Magnet (Durham, NC: Duke University Press, 2015), 21.

71. ASIS International and Institute of Finance and Management, "The United States Security Industry: Size and Scope, Insights, Trends, and Data," 2013; Hay and Andrejevic, "Homeland Insecurities."

72. Joshua Reeves, "If You See Something, Say Something: Lateral Surveillance and the Uses of Responsibility," *Surveillance and Society* 10, nos. 3–4 (2012): 235–48.

73. Michel Foucault, *Security, Territory, Population: Lectures at the Collège de France, 1977–78*, trans. Graham Burchell (New York: Palgrave Macmillan, 2007); Nikolas Rose and Peter Miller, *Governing the Present* (Cambridge, UK: Polity, 2008).

74. N. Rose and P. Miller, *Governing the Present*, 82.

75. Ibid., 54.

76. Hay and Andrejevic, "Toward an Analytic," 343.

77. Mark Andrejevic, "Interactive (In)Security: The Participatory Promise of Ready .Gov," *Cultural Studies* 20, nos. 4–5 (2006): 441–58 ; Rachel Hall, *The Transparent Traveler: The Performance and Culture of Airport Security* (Durham, NC: Duke University Press, 2015).

78. Hay and Andrejevic, "Toward an Analytic," 344.

79. James Hay, "Designing Homes to Be the First Line of Defense: Safe Households, Mobilization, and the New Mobile Privatization," *Cultural Studies* 20, nos. 4–5 (2006): 375.

80. Michel Foucault, *The History of Sexuality*, vol. 1, *An Introduction*, trans. Robert Hurley (New York: Vintage Books, 1990).

81. Nikolas S. Rose, *The Politics of Life Itself: Biomedicine, Power, and Subjectivity in the Twenty-First Century* (Princeton, NJ: Princeton University Press, 2007).

82. Reprogenetics refers to the integration of genetic technologies into reproductive medicine and is defined by the Hastings Center "as the field of research and application that involves the creation, use, manipulation, or storage of gametes or embryos." Erik Parens and Lori P. Knowles, "Reprogenetics and Public Policy: Reflections and Recommendations," *Hastings Center Report*, (July–August 2003): S1–S25.

83. N. Rose, *Politics of Life Itself*, 3.

84. Ibid., 254.

85. Ibid., 24.

86. For a deft exploration of disability and the failures of reproductive "choice," see Alison Piepmeier, "The Inadequacy of 'Choice': Disability and What's Wrong with Feminist Framings of Reproduction," *Feminist Studies* 39, no. 1 (2013): 159–86.

87. Dorothy Roberts, "Race, Gender, and Genetic Technologies: A New Reproductive Dystopia?" *Signs: Journal of Women in Culture and Society* 34, no. 4 (summer 2009): 783–804.

88. N. Rose, *Politics of Life Itself*; Silja Samerski, "Genetic Counseling and the Fiction of Choice: Taught Self-Determination as a New Technique of Social Engineering," *Signs: Journal of Women in Culture and Society* 34, no. 4 (summer 2009): 735–61.

89. Samerski, "Genetic Counseling," 744.

90. Tasha N. Dubriwny, *The Vulnerable Empowered Woman: Feminism, Postfeminism, and Women's Health* (New Brunswick, NJ: Rutgers University Press, 2013); Wolf, *Is Breast Best?*

91. Judith Butler, *Precarious Life: The Powers of Mourning and Violence* (New York: Verso, 2006); Nicholas De Genova, "Antiterrorism, Race, and the New Frontier: American Exceptionalism, Imperial Multiculturalism, and the Global Security State," *Identities* 17,

no. 6 (December 15, 2010): 613–40, https://doi.org/10.1080/1070289X.2010.533523; De Genova, "Production of Culprits"; Sarah Jaffe, "The Militarization of Everything," *Bitch* 17, no. 73 (2017): 36–42.

92. NYU School of Law Global Justice Clinic and Fordham Law School Center for International Law and Justice, "Suppressing Protest: Human Rights Violations in the U.S. Response to Occupy Wall Street," Protest and Assembly Rights Project (New York 2012), http://chrgj.org/wp-content/uploads/2012/10/suppressingprotest.pdf; Bruce Taylor et al., "Changes in Officer Use of Force over Time: A Descriptive Analysis of a National Survey," *Policing: An International Journal of Police Strategies and Management* 34, no. 2 (May 31, 2011): 211–32, https://doi.org/10.1108/13639511111131058; John Wihbey and Leighton Walter Kille, "Excessive or Reasonable Force by Police? Research on Law Enforcement and Racial Conflict," *Journalist's Resource* (blog), July 28, 2016, https://journalistsresource.org/studies/government/criminal-justice/police-reasonable-force-brutality-race-research-review-statistics.

93. Jaffe, "Militarization of Everything."

94. Ibid.

95. Sarah Wheaton and Ben Schreckinger, "Police Union Accuses White House of Politicizing Cop Safety," Politico, May 18, 2015, www.politico.com/story/2015/05/white-house-limiting-military-equipment-for-police-118041.

96. Various reports document extensive police brutality against black and brown communities, as well as political protestors. See, for example, NYU School of Law Global Justice Clinic and Fordham Law School Center for International Law and Justice, "Suppressing Protest"; U.S. Department of Justice, Civil Rights Division, "Investigation of the Albuquerque Police Department," April 10, 2014, https://www.justice.gov/sites/default/files/crt/legacy/2014/04/10/apd_findings_4-10-14.pdf; U.S. Department of Justice, Civil Rights Division, "Investigation of the Ferguson Police Department," March 4, 2015, http://apps.washingtonpost.com/g/documents/national/department-of-justice-report-on-the-ferguson-mo-police-department/1435/. Moreover, public trust in just policing practices has deteriorated; see Pew Research Center, "Few Say Police Forces Nationally Do Well in Treating Races Equally," Pew Research Center/*USA Today*, August 25, 2014, www.people-press.org/2014/08/25/few-say-police-forces-nationally-do-well-in-treating-races-equally/.

97. Jaffe, "Militarization of Everything."

98. For more on how the insistence on "civility" evacuates protest of its power and silences those most marginalized among us, see Nina M. Lozano-Reich and Dana L. Cloud, "The Uncivil Tongue: Invitational Rhetoric and the Problem of Inequality," *Western Journal of Communication* 73, no. 2 (2009): 220–26.

99. Butler, *Precarious Life*; De Genova, "Production of Culprits"; Gates, "Globalization of Homeland Security."

100. Butler, *Precarious Life*; Naomi Klein, *The Shock Doctrine: The Rise of Disaster Capitalism* (New York: Metropolitan Books, 2007); Setha Low and Neil Smith, eds., *The Politics of Public Space* (New York: Routledge, 2006); Don Mitchell, *The Right to the City: Social Justice and the Fight for Public Space* (New York: Guilford, 2003).

101. Annette D. Beresford, "Homeland Security as an American Ideology: Implications for U.S. Policy and Action," *Journal of Homeland Security and Emergency Management* 1, no. 3 (January 1, 2004), doi:10.2202/1547-7355.1042; Susan Faludi, *The Terror Dream: Myth and Misogyny in an Insecure America* (New York: Metropolitan Books, 2007); Isabel Fay, "The Home Front: Citizens behind the Camera," *Critical Studies in Media Communication* 33, no. 3 (May 26, 2016): 264–78, doi:10.1080/15295036.2016.1193210; Gates, "The Globalization of Homeland Security"; Jennifer Gillan, "Extreme Makeover Homeland Security Edition," in *The Great American Makeover: Television, History, Nation*, ed. Dana Heller (New York: Palgrave Macmillan, 2006), 193–209; Diane Negra, "Structural Integrity, Historical Reversion, and the Post-9/11 Chick Flick," *Feminist Media Studies* 8, no. 1 (2008): 51–68; Carol A. Stabile, "'Sweetheart, This Ain't Gender Studies': Sexism and Superheroes," *Communication and Critical/Cultural Studies* 6, no. 1 (2009): 86–92.

102. Amy Kaplan, "Homeland Insecurities: Some Reflections on Language and Space," *Radical History Review*, no. 85 (winter 2003): 82–93.

103. Ibid., 86.

104. De Genova, "Production of Culprits," 423.

105. Kaplan, "Homeland Insecurities," 87.

106. Faludi, *Terror Dream*; Gates, "Globalization of Homeland Security"; Gillan, "Extreme Makeover"; May, *Homeward Bound*.

107. Kaplan, "Homeland Insecurities."

108. Gillan, "Extreme Makeover," 196.

109. May, *Homeward Bound*, 221.

110. Ibid., 218.

111. Faludi, *Terror Dream*; May, *Homeward Bound*.

112. Faludi, *Terror Dream*; Katie Gentile, "What about the Baby? The New Cult of Domesticity and Media Images of Pregnancy," *Studies in Gender and Sexuality* 12 (2011): 38–58; Inderpal Grewal, "'Security Moms' in the Early Twentieth-Century United States: The Gender of Security in Neoliberalism," *Women's Studies Quarterly* 34, nos. 1–2 (spring/summer 2006): 25–39; Negra, "Structural Integrity"; Melody Rose and Mark O. Hatfield, "Republican Motherhood Redux?: Women as Contingent Citizens in 21st Century America," *Journal of Women, Politics, and Policy* 29, no. 1 (2008): 5–30; Stabile, "Sweetheart"; Carol A. Stabile and Carrie Rentschler, "States of Insecurity and the Gendered Politics of Fear," *NWSA Journal* 17, no. 3 (2005): vii–xxv.

113. Faludi, *Terror Dream*.

114. Ibid.; Grewal, "Security Moms."

115. Faludi, *Terror Dream*, 151.

116. Ibid.

117. Ibid., 28–29.

118. Stabile and Rentschler, "States of Insecurity," viii.

119. Alison Bailey, "Reconceiving Surrogacy: Toward a Reproductive Justice Account of Indian Surrogacy," *Hypatia* 26, no. 4 (2011): 715–41; Catalina (Kathleen) M. de Onís, "Lost in Translation: Challenging (white, Monolingual Feminism's) with Justicia Re-

productiva," *Women's Studies in Communication* 38, no. 1 (2015): 1–19; Forward Together (formerly Asian Communities for Reproductive Justice), "What Is Reproductive Justice?," Forward Together, n.d.), https://forwardtogether.org/what-is-reproductive-justice/, accessed August 14, 2018; Sara Hayden, "Revitalizing the Debate between <Life> and <Choice>: The 2004 March for Women's Lives," *Communication and Critical/Cultural Studies* 6, no. 2 (2009): 111–31; Piepmeier, "Inadequacy of 'Choice'"; Loretta Ross and Rickie Solinger, *Reproductive Justice: An Introduction* (Oakland: University of California Press, 2017); Jael Silliman et al., *Undivided Rights: Women of Color Organize for Reproductive Justice* (Cambridge, MA: South End, 2004).

120. A. Davis, *Women, Race, and Class*; the literature on this is quite extensive. See, for example, de Onís, "Lost in Translation"; Michaele L. Ferguson, "Choice Feminism and the Fear of Politics," *Perspectives on Politics* 8, no. 1 (March 2010): 247–53; Hayden, "Revitalizing the Debate"; Rickie Solinger, *Beggars and Choosers: How the Politics of Choice Shapes Adoption, Abortion, and Welfare in the United States* (New York: Hill and Wang, 2001); Roberts, *Killing the Black Body*; Loretta J. Ross, "The Color of Choice: White Supremacy and Reproductive Justice," in *The Color of Violence: The Incite! Anthology*, ed. Incite! Women of Color Against Violence (Cambridge, MA: South End Press, 2006), 53–65.

121. Loretta Ross, "Understanding Reproductive Justice," Trust Black Women, March 2011, www.trustblackwomen.org/our-work/what-is-reproductive-justice/9-what-is-reproductive-justice; Ross and Solinger, *Reproductive Justice*.

122. Ross, "Color of Choice"; Ross and Solinger, *Reproductive Justice*.

123. Loretta J. Ross, "The Movement for Reproductive Justice: Six Years Old and Growing," *Collective Voices* 4, no. 10 (2009): 8.

124. Ibid.

125. Ross and Solinger, *Reproductive Justice*.

126. Bonnie J. Dow, "Criticism and Authority in the Artistic Mode," *Western Journal of Communication* 65, no. 3 (2001): 336–48.

127. For example, Jeffrey A. Bennett and Charles E. Morris, eds., "Rhetorical Criticism's Multitudes," special issue, *Review of Communication* 16, no. 1 (January 2, 2016): 1–107; Robert L. Ivie, "Productive Criticism Then and Now," *American Communication Journal* 4, no. 3 (2001), http://ac-journal.org/journal/vol4/iss3/special/ivie.htm; Robert L. Ivie, "Productive Criticism," *Quarterly Journal of Speech* 81, no. 1 (1995): 2.

128. Raymond Williams, *The Long Revolution* (London: Chatto and Windus, 1961), 63.

129. I am indebted to Isaac West for this astute observation, e-mail correspondence, February 6, 2017.

Chapter 1. Securing Motherhood on the Home Front

1. Sylvia Ann Hewlett, *Creating a Life: Professional Women and the Quest for Children* (New York: Talk Miramax Books, 2002), 33.

2. Faludi, *Terror Dream*.

3. Sylvia Ann Hewlett, "Executive Women and the Myth of Having It All," *Har-*

vard Business Review 80, no. 4 (April 2002): 66–73, https://hbr.org/2002/04/executive-women-and-the-myth-of-having-it-all.

4. Hewlett, *Creating a Life*, 50, 35.

5. Ibid., 307–8.

6. Faludi, *Terror Dream*.

7. Hewlett specifies a range of policy changes to promote family-friendly working conditions, including flexible workloads, expansions to the Family Medical Leave Act to cover all workers and guarantee six months of paid leave, and tax code changes to disincentivize long hours and benefit companies who offer generous policies to enhance work/life balance.

8. Faludi, *Terror Dream*, 162; Negra, "Structural Integrity."

9. For more on the concept of the "pre-pregnant" body, see Miranda Waggoner, *The Zero Trimester: Pre-Pregnancy Care and the Politics of Reproductive Risk* (Oakland: University of California Press, 2017).

10. Stabile, "Sweetheart," 87; Negra, "Structural Integrity," 55.

11. Claudia Kalb, "Have Another 'Fertilitini,'" *Newsweek*, January 26, 2009.

12. Robin E. Jensen, *Infertility: Tracing the History of a Transformative Term*, RSA Series in Transdisciplinary Rhetoric (University Park: Pennsylvania State University Press, 2016); Margaret Marsh and Wanda Ronner, *The Empty Cradle: Infertility in America from Colonial Times to the Present* (Baltimore: Johns Hopkins University Press, 1996).

13. Susan Faludi, *Backlash: The Undeclared War against American Women*, 15th anniv. ed. (New York: Three Rivers, 2006); Roberts, *Killing the Black Body* (New York: Pantheon Books, 1997).

14. Guttmacher Institute, *Benefits of Contraceptive Use in the United States*, 2013, www.guttmacher.org; Nicholas D. Kristof and Sheryl WuDunn, *Half the Sky: Turning Oppression into Opportunity for Women Worldwide* (New York: Vintage Books, 2009); Marsh and Ronner, *Empty Cradle*; Rachael Rettner, "US Infertility Rates Drop Over Last 3 Decades," *Live Science*, August 14, 2013, https://www.livescience.com/38877-infertility-rates-drop-united-states.html; United Nations, "Senior UN Officials Spotlight Women's Health Rights to Accelerate Global Development," *UN News Centre*, May 30, 2013.

15. Lorraine Culley, Nicky Hudson, and Floor van Rooij, eds., *Marginalized Reproduction: Ethnicity, Infertility, and Reproductive Technologies* (London: Earthscan, 2009). The National Institutes of Health recognizes infertility as a health care disparity, noting it is under-examined as such.

16. *The Birth Dearth* and *The Bell Curve* cited in Roberts, *Killing the Black Body*; Jonathan V. Last, *What to Expect When No One's Expecting: America's Coming Demographic Disaster* (New York: Encounter Books, 2013).

17. Centers for Disease Control and Prevention, "National Survey of Family Growth" (Centers for Disease Control and Prevention, February 14, 2011).

18. See, for example, Douglas and Michaels, *Mommy Myth*; Bonnie J. Dow, "Michelle Obama, 'Mom-in-Chief': Gender, Race, and Familialism in Media Representations of the First Lady," in *The Rhetoric of Heroic Expectations: Establishing the Obama Presidency*, ed.

Justin S. Vaughn and Jennifer R. Mercieca, 235–56 (College Station: Texas A&M University Press, 2014); Faludi, *Terror Dream*; Gentile, "What about the Baby?"; Hallstein, "Public Choices"; Negra, "Structural Integrity"; M. Rose and Hatfield, "Republican Motherhood Redux"; Stabile, "Sweetheart"; Warner, *Perfect Madness*; Wolf, *Is Breast Best?*

19. Hewlett, "Executive Women."

20. Patricia Sellers, "Power: Do Women Really Want It?," *Fortune*, October 13, 2003, http://archive.fortune.com/magazines/fortune/fortune_archive/2003/10/13/350932/index.htm.

21. Negra, "Structural Integrity"; Pew Research Center, "Public Attitudes toward the War in Iraq: 2003–2008," *Pew Research Center* (blog), March 19, 2008, www.pewresearch.org/2008/03/19/public-attitudes-toward-the-war-in-iraq-20032008/; Stabile, "Sweetheart."

22. The so-called mommy wars pitted stay-at-home mothers against working mothers, individualizing and privatizing structural inequities that disproportionately burden women in balancing work and family. See, for example, Bernie D. Jones, "Introduction: Women, Work, and Motherhood in American History," in *Women Who Opt Out: The Debate over Working Mothers and Work-Family Balance*, ed. Bernie D. Jones (New York: New York University Press, 2012), 3–32; Toni Schindler Zimmerman et al., "Deconstructing the 'Mommy Wars': The Battle over the Best Mom," *Journal of Feminist Family Therapy* 20, no. 3 (2008): 203–19.

23. Lisa Belkin, "The Opt-Out Revolution," *New York Times Magazine*, October 26, 2003.

24. Christine Percheski, "Opting Out? Cohort Differences in Professional Women's Employment Rates from 1960 to 2005," *American Sociological Review* 73, no. 3 (June 2008): 497–517.

25. Authority via repetition is a key marker of a trend story. See Faludi, quoted in Bonnie J. Dow, *Watching Women's Liberation: Feminism's Pivotal Years on the Network News* (Urbana: University of Illinois Press, 2014).

26. Sellers, "Power"; Linda Tischler, "Where Are the Women?," *Fast Company*, no. 79 (February 2004): 52–60; Claudia Wallis, "The Case for Staying Home," *Time* 163, no. 12 (March 22, 2004): 50–59.

27. Stephanie Coontz, "The Myth of the Opt-Out Mom," *Christian Science Monitor*, March 30, 2006; Joan Williams, "The Opt-Out Revolution Revisited," *American Prospect*, February 19, 2007.

28. B. Jones, "Introduction"; Meredith W. Michaels, "Mothers 'Opting Out': Facts and Fiction," *Women's Studies Quarterly* 37, no. 3 & 4 (2009): 317–22; Pamela Stone and Lisa Ackerly Hernandez, "The Rhetoric and Reality of 'Opting Out,'" in *Women Who Opt Out: The Debate over Working Mothers and Work-Family Balance*, ed. Bernie D. Jones (New York: New York University Press, 2012), 33–56; Mary Douglas Vavrus, "Opting Out Moms in the News: Selling New Traditionalism in the New Millennium," *Feminist Media Studies* 7, no. 1 (2007): 47–63.

29. Heather Boushey, *Are Women Opting Out? Debunking the Myth* (Washington,

DC: Center for Economic and Policy Research, 2005), http://cepr.net/documents/publications/opt_out_2005_11_2.pdf; Faludi, *Terror Dream*; Michaels, "Mothers 'Opting Out'"; Stone and Hernandez, "Rhetoric and Reality."

30. Heather Antecol, "The Opt-Out Revolution: Recent Trends in Female Labor Supply," *Research in Labor Economics* 33 (2011): 45–83; Boushey, *Are Women Opting Out?*; Sharon R. Cohany and Emy Sok, "Trends in Labor Force Participation of Married Mothers of Infants," *Monthly Labor Review*, February 2007, 9–16; David Cotter, Paula England, and Joan Hermsen, *Moms and Jobs: Trends in Mothers' Employment and Which Mothers Stay Home* (Coral Gables, FL: Council on Contemporary Families, 2007), https://www.contemporaryfamilies.org/wp-content/uploads/2013/10/2007_Briefing_Cotter_Moms-and-jobs1.pdf; Percheski, "Opting Out?"; Stone and Hernandez, "Rhetoric and Reality."

31. Pamela Stone, *Opting Out? Why Women Really Quit Careers and Head Home* (Berkeley: University of California Press, 2008); Stone and Hernandez, "Rhetoric and Reality."

32. Stone, *Opting Out?*

33. Coontz, "Myth of the Opt-Out Mom"; Stone and Hernandez, "Rhetoric and Reality."

34. Stone and Hernandez, "Rhetoric and Reality," 43, 55.

35. Gwendolyn Mink, *Welfare's End* (Ithaca, NY: Cornell University Press, 1998); Nadasen, *Welfare Warriors*; Rickie Solinger, *Beggars and Choosers*; Stone and Hernandez, "Rhetoric and Reality."

36. Michaels, "Mothers 'Opting Out'"; Vavrus, "Opting Out Moms."

37. Michaels, "Mothers 'Opting Out'"; Stone and Hernandez, "Rhetoric and Reality"; Vavrus, "Opting Out Moms."

38. Belkin, "Opt-Out Revolution," 44.

39. Sally Sears, quoted in ibid., 47.

40. Vavrus, "Opting Out Moms," 51, 54.

41. I borrow the phrase taking "feminism into account" from Angela McRobbie, and draw on her work to integrate postfeminism into my analysis. McRobbie, *Aftermath of Feminism*.

42. Quoted in Belkin, "Opt-Out Revolution," 47, 46.

43. Quoted in Lesley Stahl, "Staying at Home," *60 Minutes*, October 10, 2004.

44. Amelia Warren Tyagi, "Why Women Have to Work," *Time* 163, no. 12 (March 22, 2004): 56.

45. Catalyst's Paulette Gerkovich, quoted in Wallis, "Case for Staying Home."

46. Louise Story, "Many Women at Elite Colleges Set Career Path to Motherhood," *New York Times*, September 20, 2005.

47. Amy Cunningham Atkinson, quoted in Stahl, "Staying at Home."

48. Stahl, "Staying at Home."

49. Sally Sears and Katherine Brokaw, quoted in Belkin, "Opt-Out Revolution."

50. Belkin, "Opt-Out Revolution."

51. Wallis, "Case for Staying Home."

52. Stahl, "Staying at Home."

53. Frelinghuysen, quoted in ibid.

54. Tarkenton, quoted in Belkin, "Opt-Out Revolution," 47.

55. Frelinghuysen, quoted in Stahl, "Staying at Home."

56. Sarah Blaffer Hrdy, quoted in Belkin, "Opt-Out Revolution," 47.

57. Ibid., 47.

58. Wallis, "Case for Staying Home."

59. Tori Hall, quoted in Stahl, "Staying at Home."

60. Pew Research Center, "Public Attitudes toward the War in Iraq: 2003–2008," *Pew Research Center* (blog), March 19, 2008, http://www.pewresearch.org/2008/03/19/public-attitudes-toward-the-war-in-iraq-20032008/.

61. Belkin, "Opt-Out Revolution," 45.

62. Ibid., 45.

63. Faludi, *Terror Dream*.

64. Judith Warner, "The Opt-Out Generation Wants Back In," *New York Times Magazine*, August 7, 2013.

65. Quoted in Peg Tyre, "Daddy's Home, and a Bit Lost," *New York Times*, January 11, 2009.

66. Rakesh Kochhar, "Employment in the Recession," *Pew Research Center's Social and Demographic Trends Project* (blog), July 6, 2011, www.pewsocialtrends.org/2011/07/06/iii-employment-in-the-recession/.

67. Mark Peters and David Wessel, "Idled Americans: More Men in Their Prime Are Out of Work and at Home," *Wall Street Journal*, February 6, 2014, sec. J.

68. D'Vera Cohn, "Divorce and the Great Recession," *Pew Research Center's Social and Demographic Trends Project* (blog), May 2, 2012, www.pewsocialtrends.org/2012/05/02/divorce-and-the-great-recession/; Drew DeSilver, "Chart of the Week: The Great Baby Recession," *Pew Research Center* (blog), July 25, 2014, www.pewresearch.org/fact-tank/2014/07/25/chart-of-the-week-the-great-baby-recession/; Richard Fry and D'Vera Cohn, "Women, Men and the New Economics of Marriage," *Pew Research Center's Social and Demographic Trends Project* (blog), January 19, 2010, www.pewsocialtrends.org/2010/01/19/women-men-and-the-new-economics-of-marriage/; Gretchen Livingston, "Growing Number of Dads Home with the Kids," *Pew Research Center's Social and Demographic Trends Project* (blog), June 5, 2014, www.pewsocialtrends.org/2014/06/05/growing-number-of-dads-home-with-the-kids/; Wendy Wang, Kim Parker, and Paul Taylor, "Breadwinner Moms," *Pew Research Center's Social and Demographic Trends Project* (blog), May 29, 2013, www.pewsocialtrends.org/2013/05/29/breadwinner-moms/.

69. Lauren Sandler and Kate Witteman, "None Is Enough," *Time* 182, no. 7 (August 12, 2013): 38. It is worth noting that long-term demographic trends are notoriously difficult to anticipate. In other words, delayed childbearing does not necessarily result in childbearing forgone. This fact seemed to register very little in public discourse.

70. Sheryl Sandberg, *Lean In: Women, Work, and the Will to Lead* (New York: Knopf, 2013).

71. Quoted in bell hooks, "Dig Deep: Beyond Lean In," Feminist Wire, October 28, 2013, http://thefeministwire.com/2013/10/17973/.

72. Susan Faludi, "Facebook Feminism, Like It or Not," *Baffler* 23 (August 2013), https://thebaffler.com/salvos/facebook-feminism-like-it-or-not; hooks, "Dig Deep."

73. For information on the primary causes of female-factor infertility, see Mauricio S. Abrao, Ludovico Muzii, and Riccardo Marana, "Anatomical Causes of Female Infertility and Their Management," *International Journal of Gynaecology and Obstetrics: The Official Organ of the International Federation of Gynaecology and Obstetrics* 123, suppl. 2 (December 2013): S18–24, https://doi.org/10.1016/j.ijgo.2013.09.008; Katherine Kaproth-Joslin and Vikram Dogra, "Imaging of Female Infertility: A Pictorial Guide to the Hysterosalpingography, Ultrasonography, and Magnetic Resonance Imaging Findings of the Congenital and Acquired Causes of Female Infertility," *Radiologic Clinics of North America* 51, no. 6 (November 2013): 967–81, https://doi.org/10.1016/j.rcl.2013.07.002; Mayo Clinic Staff, "Female Infertility: Causes," Mayo Clinic, accessed July 27, 2016, www.mayoclinic.org/diseases-conditions/female-infertility/basics/causes/con-20033618 (dead); Hans-Rudolf Tinneberg and Antonio Gasbarrini, "Infertility Today: The Management of Female Medical Causes," *International Journal of Gynaecology and Obstetrics: The Official Organ of the International Federation of Gynaecology and Obstetrics* 123, suppl. 2 (December 2013): S25–30, https://doi.org/10.1016/j.ijgo.2013.09.004.

Diet and lifestyle factors have been demonstrated to have only some impact on certain kinds of infertility, such as anovulatory infertility. For more on diet and lifestyle, see Jorge E. Chavarro, Walter C. Willett, and Patrick J. Skerrett, *The Fertility Diet: Groundbreaking Research Reveals Natural Ways to Boost Ovulation and Improve Your Chances of Getting Pregnant* (New York: McGraw-Hill, 2008); Jorge E. Chavarro, Walter C. Willett, and Patrick J. Skerrett, "Fertility & Diet: How What You Eat Affects Your Odds of Getting Pregnant," *Newsweek*, December 10, 2007; Roberta Fontana and Sara Torre, "The Deep Correlation between Energy Metabolism and Reproduction: A View on the Effects of Nutrition for Women Fertility," *Nutrients* 8, no. 2 (February 11, 2016): 87, https://doi.org/10.3390/nu8020087; Meike A. Q. Mutsaerts et al., "Randomized Trial of a Lifestyle Program in Obese Infertile Women," *New England Journal of Medicine* 374, no. 20 (May 19, 2016): 1942–53, https://doi.org/10.1056/NEJMoa1505297; David F. Yao and Jesse N. Mills, "Male Infertility: Lifestyle Factors and Holistic, Complementary, and Alternative Therapies," *Asian Journal of Andrology* 18, no. 3 (June 2016): 410–18, https://doi.org/10.4103/1008-682X.175779.

For rates of infertility according to sex, see American Society for Reproductive Medicine, "Frequently Asked Questions about Infertility," American Society for Reproductive Medicine, 2016, www.asrm.org/awards/index.aspx?id=3012. Age-related infertility is a point of contentious debate, but significant evidence exists to suggest that the decline in fertility is quite gradual for individuals in their thirties, and that conception is quite possible but may take longer. David B. Dunson, Donna D. Baird, and Bernardo Colombo, "Increased Infertility with Age in Men and Women:," *Obstetrics and Gynecology* 103, no. 1 (January 2004): 51–56, https://doi.org/10.1097/01.AOG.0000100153.24061.45; David S. Guzick, "Age and Fertility: A Social-Biologic Balance," *Fertility and Sterility* 105, no. 6 (June 2016): 1461, https://doi.org/10.1016/j.fertnstert.2016.03.021; Anne Z. Steiner and Anne Marie Z. Jukic, "Impact of Female Age and Nulligravidity on Fecundity in an Older Reproductive Age Cohort," *Fertility and Sterility* 105, no. 6 (June 2016): 1584–1588.e1, https://doi.org/10.1016/j.fertnstert.2016.02.028; Jean Twenge, "How Long Can You Wait to Have a Baby?," *Atlantic*, August 2013, www.theatlantic.com/magazine/archive/2013/07/how-long-can-you-wait-to-have-a-baby/309374/.

74. Lisa Lombardi, "Protect Your Fertility," *Shape*, September 2003.

75. Michelle Stacey, "How to Keep Your Body Baby-Ready," *Cosmopolitan*, January 2009.

76. Hillary Frey, "How to Get Pregnant Exactly When You Want To," *Glamour*, June 2010.

77. Stacey, "How to Keep Your Body Baby-Ready"; "Fire Up Fertility," *Shape*, November 2011; Stacey, "How to Keep Your Body Baby-Ready"; Christie Aschwanden, "Fertility 101," *Marie Claire*, February 2009.

78. Stacey Colino, "Are You Gambling with Your Fertility?," *Shape*, June 2012.

79. Miranda R. Waggoner, "Motherhood Preconceived: The Emergence of the Preconception Health and Health Care Initiative," *Journal of Health Politics, Policy and Law* 38, no. 2 (January 1, 2013): 345–71, https://doi.org/10.1215/03616878-1966333.

80. Aschwanden, "Fertility 101."

81. Dubriwny, *Vulnerable Empowered Woman*, 32.

82. Sawyer was reported to have sent employees to egg-freezing seminars; Inhorn wrote for CNN that she would advise her female graduate students to consider the process as a means of balancing family and an academic career. See Johanna Gohmann, "Chill Out," *Bust*, March 2013; Marcia C. Inhorn, *Women, Consider Freezing Your Eggs*, CNN, updated April 9, 2013, www.cnn.com/2013/04/09/opinion/inhorn-egg-freezing.

83. Kalb, "Have Another 'Fertilitini.'"

84. American College of Obstetricians and Gynecologists, "Oocyte Preservation. Committee Opinion No. 584," *Obstetrics and Gynecology* 123 (January 2014): 221–22; Practice Committee, "Mature Oocyte Cryopreservation."

85. American College of Obstetricians and Gynecologists, "Oocyte Preservation." Unlike freezing sperm or embryos, oocyte preservation has proven particularly challenging for researchers and practitioners—as the largest cells in the human body, eggs are largely composed of water, making them susceptible to chromosomal damage during traditional (slower) processes of cryopreservation. Early attempts at egg freezing were designated experimental due to low rates of fertilization and pregnancy success, and selectively made available to women of childbearing age who were facing severe medical prognoses that threatened fertility. However, the development of vitrification, or flash freezing, has led to greater success in oocyte preservation, similar to rates associated with the use of fresh eggs in assisted reproduction procedures.

See Practice Committee, "Mature Oocyte Cryopreservation"; Catrin E. Argyle, Joyce C. Harper, and Melanie C. Davies, "Oocyte Cryopreservation: Where Are We Now?," *Human Reproduction Update* 22, no. 4 (June 2016): 440–49, https://doi.org/10.1093/humupd/dmw007.

86. Sarah Elizabeth Richards, "Do You Know Where Your Eggs Are?," *Cosmopolitan*, June 2013.

87. Gohmann, "Chill Out," 47.

88. Ibid., 44.

89. Jennifer Bleyer, "Should You Freeze Your Eggs?," *Cosmopolitan*, January 2012.

90. Ibid.

91. Sarah Elizabeth Richards, "Why I Froze My Eggs (and You Should, Too)," *Wall Street Journal*, May 3, 2013.

92. Emma Rosenblum, "Freeze Your Eggs, Free Your Career," *Bloomberg Business Week*, April 17, 2014.

93. Bleyer, "Should You Freeze Your Eggs?"

94. Lara Naaman, "Now that Everyone's Freezing Their Eggs, Should You?," *Glamour*, April 2013.

95. Ibid.

96. Dr. Jamie Grifo, quoted in Gohmann, "Chill Out," 44.

97. Sarah Elizabeth Richards, *Motherhood, Rescheduled: The New Frontier of Egg Freezing and the Women Who Tried It* (New York: Simon and Schuster, 2013), 210.

98. Quoted in Nancy Hass, "Time to Chill? Egg Freezing Technology Offers a Chance to Extend Fertility," *Vogue*, May 2011, 264.

99. Brigitte Adams, quoted in Gohmann, "Chill Out," 47.

100. Richards, *Motherhood*, 57.

101. Ibid., 10.

102. Brigette Adams, quoted in Rosenblum, "Freeze Your Eggs."

103. Sarah Elizabeth Richards, "Freezing Your Eggs—Is This What We're All Doing Now?," *Cosmopolitan*, June 13, 2013, www.cosmopolitan.com/lifestyle/advice/a4477/fertility-fears/.

104. Richards, *Motherhood*, 243.

105. Ibid., 97.

106. Ibid., 243.

107. "What He Thinks about Your, Um, Eggs," *Glamour*, January 2014, 70.

108. Sarah Elizabeth Richards, "The Freedom of Freezing," *Marie Claire*, May 2013.

109. Sarah Elizabeth Richards, "Should You Freeze Your Eggs?," *Marie Claire*, May 2007.

110. A recent study indicates that banking eggs does not seem to impact relational or reproductive decision making, at least in the three years following the procedure, but it does confer significant psychological benefits to women in that same time frame. D. Stoop et al., "Does Oocyte Banking for Anticipated Gamete Exhaustion Influence Future Relational and Reproductive Choices? A Follow-Up of Bankers and

Non-Bankers," *Human Reproduction* (Oxford, UK) 30, no. 2 (February 2015): 338–44, doi:10.1093/humrep/deu317.

111. Rosenblum, "Freeze Your Eggs."

112. Inhorn, *Women.*

113. Richards, "Why I Froze My Eggs."

114. Ibid.

115. Rachel Lehman-Haupt, quoted in Gohmann, "Chill Out."

116. Richards, "Should You Freeze Your Eggs?"

117. Hass, "Time to Chill?," 264.

118. Rosenblum, "Freeze Your Eggs."

119. B. Adams, quoted in Gohmann, "Chill Out," 47.

120. Vanessa Grigoriadis, "Waking Up from the Pill," *New York Magazine*, December 6, 2010.

121. Hass, "Time to Chill?," 264.

122. Claudia Kalb, "Fertility and the Freezer," *Newsweek*, August 1, 2004; Jennifer Ludden, "Egg Freezing Puts the Biological Clock on Hold," *Morning Edition*, NPR, aired May 31, 2011; Kyra Phillips, "DNA on Ice: The Next Step in Women's Equality," CNN, April 20, 2015, www.cnn.com/2015/04/20/opinions/phillips-egg-freezing/; Rosenblum, "Freeze Your Eggs."

123. Rosenblum, "Freeze Your Eggs."

124. Quoted in Richards, "Freezing Your Eggs."

125. McRobbie, *Aftermath of Feminism*, 18.

126. Richards, *Motherhood*, 87.

127. Ferguson, "Choice Feminism."

128. Anne-Marie Slaughter, "Why Women Still Can't Have It All," *Atlantic*, August 2012, www.theatlantic.com/magazine/archive/2012/07/why-women-still-cant-have-it-all/309020/; Claire Suddath, "Labor Crisis: Maternity Leave Isn't Working for Working Women," *Bloomberg Businessweek*, January 19, 2015; (Obama) White House, Office of the Press Secretary, "Fact Sheet: The White House Summit on Working Families," whitehouse.gov, June 23, 2014, https://obamawhitehouse.archives.gov/the-press-office/2014/06/23/fact-sheet-white-house-summit-working-families.

129. Rene Almeling, Joanann Radien, and Sarah S. Richardson, "Egg-Freezing a Better Deal for Companies than for Women," Opinion, CNN, October 20, 2014, www.cnn.com/2014/10/20/opinion/almeling-radin-richardson-egg-freezing/; J. Maureen Henderson, "Why We Should Be Alarmed that Apple and Facebook Are Paying for Employee Egg Freezing," *Forbes*, October 15, 2014, www.forbes.com/sites/jmaureenhenderson/2014/10/15/dont-work-for-or-trust-a-company-that-pays-you-to-freeze-your-eggs/; Rebecca Mead, "Cold Comfort: Tech Jobs and Egg Freezing," *New Yorker*, October 17, 2014, www.newyorker.com/news/daily-comment/facebook-apple-egg-freezing-benefits; Sabrina Parsons, "Female Tech CEO: Egg-Freezing 'Benefit' Sends the Wrong Message to Women," *Business Insider*, October 20, 2014, www.businessinsider.com/apple-facebook-egg-freezing-benefit-is-bad-for-women-2014-10.

130. See, for example, Erin Matson, "'Freeze Your Eggs, Free Your Career' Is Insulting to Women," RH Reality Check, April 22, 2014, http://rhrealitycheck.org/article/2014/04/22/freeze-eggs-free-career-insulting-women/.

131. Facebook is a leader among tech giants in providing comprehensive workplace benefits, including paid parental leave, subsidized childcare, workout facilities, free gourmet meals, and comprehensive health care packages, to name a few. While Apple lags behind other industry leaders like Facebook and Google in this regard, it far outperforms other US companies in offering, for example, relatively generous paid parental leave, health care, and 401K benefits for part-time employees, shuttle services, and compensation for travel. See, for example, Seth Fiegerman, "Actually, Sometimes It Sucks to Work at Apple—Here's Why," *Business Insider*, June 14, 2012, www.businessinsider.com/the-biggest-complaints-employees-have-about-working-at-apple-2012-6; Seth Fiegerman, "Why Working at Apple Is a Dream Job," *Business Insider*, June 18, 2012, www.businessinsider.com/heres-what-employees-really-love-about-working-for-apple-2012-6; Mead, "Cold Comfort."

132. Fixmer-Oraiz, "(In)Conceivable"; Lori Kido Lopez, "The Radical Act of 'Mommy Blogging': Redefining Motherhood through the Blogosphere," *New Media and Society* 11, no. 5 (2009): 729–47.

133. Lisa Miller, "The Retro Wife: Feminists Who Say They're Having It All—by Choosing to Stay Home," *New York Magazine*, March 17, 2013.

Chapter 2. Risky Reproduction and the Politics of Octomom

1. Judith Daar, "Federalizing Embryo Transfers: Taming the Wild West of Reproductive Medicine?," *Columbia Journal of Gender and Law* 23, no. 2 (2012): 257–325; Camille M. Davidson, "Octomom and Multi-Fetal Pregnancies: Why Federal Legislation Should Require Insurers to Cover in Vitro Fertilization," *William & Mary Journal of Women and the Law* 17 (2010): 135–86; Deborah L. Forman, "When 'Bad' Mothers Make Worse Law: A Critique of Legislative Limits on Embryo Transfer," *University of Pennsylvania Journal of Law and Social Change* 14 (2010): 273–312; Theresa Glennon, "Choosing One: Resolving the Epidemic of Multiples in Assisted Reproduction," *Villanova Law Review* 55 (2010): 147–203; Michele Goodwin, "A Few Thoughts on Assisted Reproductive Technology," *Law and Inequality: A Journal of Theory and Practice* 27 (2009): 465–79; Kimberly D. Krawiec, "Why We Should Ignore the 'Octomom,'" *Northwestern University Law Review* 104 (2009): 120–31; Radhika Rao, "How (Not) to Regulate ARTs: Lessons from Octomom," *Albany Law Journal of Science and Technology* 21, no. 2 (2011): 313–21; Stephanie N. Sivinski, "Putting Too Many (Fertilized) Eggs in One Basket: Methods of Reducing Multifetal Pregnancies in the United States," *Texas Law Review* 88, no. 4 (March 2010): 897–916; Kayte K. Spector-Bagdady, "Artificial Parentage: Screening Parents for Assisted Reproductive Technologies," *Michigan State University Journal of Medicine and Law* 14 (2010): 457–76.

2. Pew Research Center, "Public Attitudes."

3. Pew Research Center, "Psychology of Bad Times Fueling Consumer Cutbacks: Job Worries Mount, 73% Spending Less on Holidays," Pew Research Center for the People and the Press (press release), December 12, 2008, http://assets.pewresearch.org/wp-content/uploads/sites/5/legacy-pdf/475.pdf.

4. Mark Greif, "Octomom, One Year Later," *N+1*, no. 9 (2010): 128.

5. I conducted searches for US newspaper reports in LexisNexis using the search terms "Nadya Suleman" and "octuplets" between January 1, 2009 and July 1, 2011. Additionally, I tracked coverage in mainstream periodicals such as *Time* and *People*, reviewed transcripts from news broadcasts and talk shows, including *Oprah*, the *The View*, and *Dr. Phil*, and tended to online forums for each show.

6. Strict compliance with ASRM guidelines is approximated at less than 20 percent. See Sivinski, "Putting Too Many (Fertilized) Eggs"; ASRM guidelines state: "These guidelines have been developed to assist physicians with clinical decisions regarding the care of their patients. They are not intended to be a protocol to be applied in all situations, and cannot substitute for the individual judgment of the treating physicians based on their knowledge of their patients and specific circumstances." American Society for Reproductive Medicine, "Practice Committee Guidelines," 2011, http://www.asrm.org/Guidelines/.

7. See the sources cited in note 1.

8. C. Davidson, "Octomom," 139.

9. Rao, "How (Not) to Regulate ARTs."

10. Forman, "When 'Bad' Mothers," 303.

11. Dana-Ain Davis, "The Politics of Reproduction: The Troubling Case of Nadya Suleman and Assisted Reproductive Technology," *Transforming Anthropology* 17, no. 2 (2009): 105–16.

12. I use the term *sym/pathetic* to signal both the cultural sympathy that infertility often elicits when suffered by privileged white women, but also the ways in which privileged women without children are often diminished, pitied, or viewed as incomplete within dominant cultural discourses.

13. Nadya Suleman, "Her Side of the Story," interview by Ann Curry, *Dateline News*, NBC, February 10, 2009.

14. Ibid.

15. Nadya Suleman, "Octuplets' Mom Talks with Dr. Phil," interview by Phil McGraw, *Dr. Phil*, February 25, 2009.

16. Suleman, quoted in "Octuplets' Mom: 'All I Ever Wanted,'" CNN, February 6, 2009, http://articles.cnn.com/2009-02-06/us/octuplets.mom_1_octuplets-birth-nadya-suleman-octuplets-mom?_s=PM:US.

17. For additional scholarship on the discursive politics of epidemics, see Jeffrey A. Bennett, "Troubled Interventions: Public Policy, Vectors of Disease, and the Rhetoric of Diabetes Management," *Journal of Medical Humanities* 34, no. 1 (March 2013): 15–32, https://doi.org/10.1007/s10912-012-9198-0.

18. Jensen, *Infertility*, 6.

19. The National Institute of Health recognizes infertility as a health care disparity, noting it is under-examined as such; see Culley, Hudson, and van Rooij, *Marginalized Reproduction*.

20. This survey has been compiled a total of seven times since 1973 by the National Center for Health Statistics, Centers for Disease Control and Prevention, "National Survey of Family Growth."

21. Jeff Gottlieb and Sam Quinones, "The Eighth Baby Was a Surprise," *Los Angeles Times*, January 27, 2009.

22. "California Woman Gives Birth to Rare Octuplets," CBSNews, January 26, 2009, www.cbsnews.com/news/calif-woman-gives-birth-to-rare-octuplets/; Raquel Maria Dillon, "Octuplets Born in California Doing 'Very Well,'" Associated Press, January 27, 2009.

23. Michael Inbar, "First U.S. Octuplets Offer Advice to New Parents of Eight: Now Ten Years Old, Seven Surviving Chukwu Octuplets Are Healthy, 'Beautiful,'" Today, January 28, 2009, http://today.msnbc.msn.com/id/28891400/.

24. Jill Smolowe et al., "A Mom's Controversial Choice," *People*, February 16, 2009; Bonnie Rochman, "Octuplets Fallout: Should Fertility Doctors Set Limits?," *Time*, February 2, 2009; Alison Motluk, "When Eight Is Seven Too Many," *New Scientist* 201, no. 2695 (2009): 24; Kay Hymowitz, "Where in the World Is Octodad?," *Wall Street Journal*, February 20, 2009.

25. Patricia Hill Collins, *Black Sexual Politics: African Americans, Gender, and the New Racism* (New York: Routledge, 2005); Nadasen, *Welfare Warriors*.

26. Solinger, *Beggars and Choosers*.

27. For example, Ginia Bellafante, "In Documentary, an Obsessed 'Octomom,'" *New York Times*, August 20, 2009; Katherine Thomson, "Does Nadya Suleman Think She's Angelina Jolie?," *HuffPost Entertainment*, February 10, 2009; "Being Angelina Not an Easy Role," *Chicago Tribune*, February 12, 2009.

28. Alison Stateman, "The Octuplets' Mom Speaks, and the Questions Grow," *Time*, February 7, 2009.

29. Dr. Jeff Gardere, quoted in Suleman, "Her Side."

30. Jeanne Flavin, *Our Bodies, Our Crimes: The Policing of Women's Reproduction in America* (New York: New York University Press, 2009); Paltrow and Flavin, "Arrests of and Forced Interventions."

31. D. Davis, "Politics of Reproduction"; Greif, "Octomom."

32. "Octuplets' Family Filed for Bankruptcy," CBSNews, January 30, 2009, https://www.cbsnews.com/news/octuplets-family-filed-for-bankruptcy/.

33. The terms used to describe individuals and communities originating from the "Middle East" are contested. My use of Southwest Asian and North African (SWANA) follows scholars who advocate this term for its inclusivity and refusal of Eurocentricity, "as an alternative [to Arab, Muslim, or Middle Eastern] that includes non-Arab minorities, transcends patriarchal and homophobic nationalism, and opens up possibilities for alliance building between people from Arab nations and other nations

in the region, such as Iran, who share a similar history in the context of US imperialism and war in the region." Nadine Christine Naber, "Introduction: Arab Americans and US Racial Formations," in *Race and Arab Americans before and after 9/11: From Invisible Citizens to Visible Subjects*, edited by Amaney Jamal and Nadine Naber, 1–45 (Syracuse, NY: Syracuse University Press, 2008), 8.

The term "Southwest Asian" seems particularly appropriate in Suleman's case. Suleman is the daughter of an Iraqi immigrant who claims Assyrian ethnicity, rendering both "Arab" and "Muslim" inaccurate. "Middle Eastern" is, as many scholars note, Eurocentric in its orientation. SWANA can encompass the ethnic diversity of the region while simultaneously signaling shared histories and—particularly in the context of this project—post-9/11 experiences of racialization, marginalization, and violence within the United States.

34. Arab American Institute, "AAI Issue Brief: Hate Crimes," Arab American Institute, http://www.aaiusa.org/aai_issue_brief_hate_crimes, accessed August 2, 2018; Amaney A. Jamal and Nadine Christine Naber, eds., *Race and Arab Americans before and after 9/11: From Invisible Citizens to Visible Subjects* (Syracuse, NY: Syracuse University Press, 2008).

35. Jane Velez-Mitchell, "Issues with Jane Velez-Mitchell," HLN, November 24, 2009.

36. See "Suz Orman's Intervention with 'Octomom' Nadya Suleman," *Oprah Show*, January 14, 2011; Nadya Suleman, "A Conversation with Nadya Suleman," interview by Oprah Winfrey, *Oprah Show*, April 20, 2010; Suleman, "Octuplets' Mom."

37. Velez-Mitchell, "Issues."

38. David Finnigan, "First Peek at Octo-Cuties—Report Reveals Serial Mom Was Already on Food Stamps," *New York Post*, February 10, 2009.

39. Natalie Cisneros, "'Alien' Sexuality: Race, Maternity, and Citizenship," *Hypatia* 28, no. 2 (2013): 290–306.

40. "Octomom vs. Illegal Aliens," *Topix: Immigration Reform Form*, February 16, 2009, www.topix.com.

41. Pew Research Center, "Black-White Conflict Isn't Society's Largest," *Pew Research Center's Social and Demographic Trends Project* (blog), September 24, 2009, www.pewsocialtrends.org/2009/09/24/black-white-conflict-isnt-societys-largest/.

42. Whoopi Goldberg, quoted in Liz Brown, "Octomom Nadya Suleman's 'The View' Appearance Evokes Criticism, Anger," *View Examiner*, February 25, 2009.

43. Tina Moore, "Octuplet Grandma's Shame: Daughter Has 14 Kids, No Husband," *New York Daily News*, January 31, 2009.

44. Jill Smolowe et al., "The Challenge of Her Life," *People*, February 23, 2009.

45. Russell, quoted in Velez-Mitchell, "Issues."

46. Mike Celizic, "First Look: Octuplet Mom Shows Off Babies," Today.com, February 10, 2009, www.today.com/id/29086126/ns/today-parenting_and_family/t/first-look-octuplet-mom-shows-babies/.

47. See, for example, Douglas and Michaels, *Mommy Myth*; Dubriwny, *Vulnerable*

Empowered Woman; Heather L. Hundley and Sara E. Hayden, eds., *Mediated Moms: Contemporary Challenges to the Motherhood Myth* (New York: Peter Lang, 2016); Hallstein, "Public Choices"; Wolf, *Is Breast Best?*

48. Smolowe et al., "Challenge."

49. Carolyn R. Miller, "The Presumptions of Expertise: The Role of Ethos in Risk Analysis," *Configurations* 11 (2004): 185.

50. Stephanie Saul, "Birth of Octuplets Puts Focus on Fertility Clinics," *New York Times*, February 11, 2009.

51. Ashley Surdin, "Octuplet Mother Also Gives Birth to Ethical Debate," *Washington Post*, February 4, 2009.

52. Smolowe et al., "Mom's Controversial Choice," 80.

53. Dr. Robert Stillman, quoted in Susan Donaldson James, "Octomom Lesson: More Couples Pressure Doctors," *ABC News*, October 25, 2010.

54. The rhetoric of health is a growing area of interest in the field of communication studies. See, for example, Jeffrey A. Bennett, *Banning Queer Blood: Rhetorics of Citizenship, Contagion, and Resistance* (Tuscaloosa: University of Alabama Press, 2009); Bennett, "Troubled Interventions"; Lisa Keranen, "Concocting Viral Apocalypse: Catastrophic Risk and the Production of Bio(in)security," *Western Journal of Communication* 75, no. 5 (2011): 451–72; J. Blake Scott, *Risky Rhetoric: AIDS and the Cultural Practices of HIV Testing* (Carbondale: Southern Illinois University Press, 2003); Robin E. Jensen, "An Ecological Turn in Rhetoric of Health Scholarship: Attending to the Historical Flow and Percolation of Ideas, Assumptions, and Arguments," *Communication Quarterly* 63, no. 5 (October 20, 2015): 522–26, doi:10.1080/01463373.2015.1103600; Jensen, *Infertility*.

For more on the vexed relationship between disability and reproductive politics, see Piepmeier, "Inadequacy of 'Choice.'"

55. Smolowe et al., "Mom's Controversial Choice."

56. James, "Octomom Lesson."

57. James, "Octomom Lesson."

58. Karen Grigsby Bates, "Octuplets Make 14 for Mom, Stirring Debate," *All Things Considered*, NPR, January 30, 2009.

59. Guttmacher Institute, "The Number of States Considered Hostile to Abortion Skyrocketed between 2000 and 2014," Guttmacher Institute, November 12, 2015, https://www.guttmacher.org/infographic/2015/number-states-considered-hostile-abortion-skyrocketed-between-2000-and-2014; Piepmeier, "Inadequacy of 'Choice.'"

60. David Perry, "Anti-Choice Legislators Try to Force Wedge between Reproductive, Disability Rights Activists," Rewire, January 16, 2015, https://rewire.news/article/2015/01/16/anti-choice-legislators-try-force-wedge-reproductive-disability-rights-activists/; Piepmeier, "Inadequacy of 'Choice.'"

61. For example, Celeste Condit, *Decoding Abortion Rhetoric: Communicating Social Change* (Urbana: University of Illinois Press, 1990); Lynn M. Morgan and Meredith W. Michaels, eds., *Fetal Subjects, Feminist Positions* (Philadelphia: University of Pennsylvania

Press, 1999); Rosalind Pollack Petchesky, "Fetal Images: The Power of Visual Culture in the Politics of Reproduction," *Feminist Studies* 13, no. 2 (1987): 263–92; Samerski, "Genetic Counseling"; Scott, *Risky Rhetoric*; Nathan Stormer, "Embodying Normal Miracles," *Quarterly Journal of Speech* 83, no. 2 (5): 172.

62. Piepmeier, "Inadequacy of 'Choice'"; Samerski, "Genetic Counseling."

63. Samerski, "Genetic Counseling," 744.

64. High-order multiples are defined as triplets or more.

65. James, "Octomom Lesson," 24.

66. Motluk, "When Eight."

67. Wolf, *Is Breast Best?*, xv.

68. "Fertility Ethics," *Los Angeles Times*, February 3, 2009, http://articles.latimes.com/2009/feb/03/opinion/ed-octuplet3.

69. "Mothers Gone Wild," *Maclean's*, February 23, 2009.

70. Arthur Caplan quoted in Stateman, "Octuplets' Mom."

71. Arthur Caplan, "Ethics and Octuplets: Society Is Responsible," *Philadelphia Inquirer*, February 6, 2009.

72. Sean Tipton quoted in James, "Octomom Lesson"; Rita Rubin, "A Singular Approach to IVF," *USA Today*, March 4, 2009.

73. Greif, "Octomom."

74. Hymowitz, "Where in the World."

75. Scott, *Risky Rhetoric*, 87.

76. N. Rose, *Politics of Life Itself*, 3, 143. See also Dubriwny, *Vulnerable Empowered Woman*; Davi Johnson Thornton, "Race, Risk, and Pathology in Psychiatric Culture: Disease Awareness Campaigns as Governmental Rhetoric," *Critical Studies in Media Communication* 27, no. 4 (2010): 311–35; Wolf, *Is Breast Best?*

77. Grifo, quoted in Summer Johnson McGee, "Don't Blame Momma," *Bioethics.Net* (blog), February 6, 2009, http://www.bioethics.net/2009/02/dont-blame-momma.

78. Current regulations refuse issues of ethics or access and the rate of compliance with ASRM guidelines is approximately 20 percent. Other countries have opted for nationally uniform and enforceable protocols that determine, for example, under what circumstances parents might select or avoid genetic characteristics (e.g., gender, birth defects, disabilities, or donor tissue matches), or in the affirmation (or refusal) of marginalized patients, like single women or LGBTQ families. See Connie Cho, "Regulating Assisted Reproductive Technology," *Yale Journal of Medicine and Law* 7, no. 1 (2010): 40–41.

79. In Georgia, the bill was quickly criticized for its retooled definition of an embryo as a "biological human being who is not the property of any person or entity." But the Missouri bill avoided abortion politics altogether, sticking strictly to the enforcement of ASRM guidelines, so the grounds for its refusal are less clear. Michelle N. Meyer, "States' Regulation of Assisted Reproductive Technologies: What Does the U.S. Constitution Allow?," Nelson A. Rockefeller Institute of Government, Harvard Public Law Working Paper, July 1, 2009, 13. See also James, "Octomom Lesson."

80. For more on gender, race, and monstrosity, see Bernadette Marie Calafell, *Monstrosity, Performance, and Race in Contemporary Culture* (New York: Peter Lang, 2015).

81. At the time of the Suleman birth, *Jon & Kate Plus Eight* was in its fourth season and the highest rated show on TLC. See Raina Kelley, "Octomom Hypocrisy," *Newsweek*, March 3, 2009, www.newsweek.com/2009/03/02/octomom-hypocrisy.print.html; Susan Stewart, "Big Brood Spawns Big Ratings," *New York Times*, February 15, 2009.

82. "Arkansas Woman Has 15th Child," *NBC News*, May 25, 2004, www.nbcnews.com/id/5060048/#.UZz2t5WRCos.

83. D. Davis, "Politics of Reproduction"; Gordon, *Moral Property*; Roberts, *Killing the Black Body*; Solinger, *Pregnancy and Power*.

84. Samerski, "Genetic Counseling."

85. Amie Newman, "Iowa 'Feticide' Law Could Be Used to Target Mothers," *Huffington Post* (blog), April 18, 2010, www.huffingtonpost.com/amie-newman/iowa-feticide-law-could-b_b_463153.html.

86. Erik Eckholm, "Case Explores Rights of Fetus versus Mother," *New York Times*, October 23, 2013.

87. Manny Fernandez and Erik Eckholm, "Pregnant, and Forced to Stay on Life Support," *New York Times*, January 7, 2014, sec. U.S., www.nytimes.com.

88. Anna Halkidis, "Bei Bei Shuai Case Exposes Pregnancy-Suicide Risk," Women's eNews, August 3, 2013, http://womensenews.org/2013/08/bei-bei-shuai-case-exposes-pregnancy-suicide-risk/; Anemona Hartocollis, "Mother Accuses Doctors of Forcing a C-Section and Files Suit," *New York Times*, May 16, 2014, www.nytimes.com; Katha Pollitt, "Protect Pregnant Women: Free Bei Bei Shuai," *Nation*, March 7, 2012, www.thenation.com/article/protect-pregnant-women-free-bei-bei-shuai/.

89. Catherine Pearson, "Montana County Has Plan for Moms-to-Be Who Drink or Do Drugs: Jail 'Em," AOL.com, January 27, 2018, https://www.aol.com/article/news/2018/01/27/montana-county-has-plan-for-moms-to-be-who-drink-or-do-drugs-jail-em/23345328/.

90. Flavin, *Our Bodies*; Nicole Knight, "Report: Criminalizing Pregnancy a 'Noose around Your Neck,'" Rewire, May 23, 2017, https://rewire.news/article/2017/05/23/report-criminalizing-pregnancy-noose-around-neck/; Paltrow and Flavin, "Arrests of and Forced Interventions."

91. U.S. Centers for Disease Control and Prevention, "More than 3 Million US Women at Risk for Alcohol-Exposed Pregnancy," CDC Newsroom, February 2, 2016, www.cdc.gov/media/releases/2016/p0202-alcohol-exposed-pregnancy.html.

92. Judith Graham, "This Chicago Doctor Stumbled on a Hidden Epidemic of Fetal Brain Damage," *PBS NewsHour*, May 21, 2016, www.pbs.org/newshour/rundown/this-chicago-doctor-stumbled-on-a-hidden-epidemic-of-fetal-brain-damage/.

93. Dubriwny, *Vulnerable Empowered Woman*, 66.

94. RESOLVE: The National Infertility Association, "Infertility Coverage By State" (RESOLVE: The National Infertility Association, 2018).

95. Daar, "Federalizing Embryo Transfers."

96. Piepmeier, "Inadequacy of 'Choice,'" 166.

97. Ibid.; Dorothy Roberts, "Race, Gender, and Genetic Technologies: A New Reproductive Dystopia?," *Signs: Journal of Women in Culture and Society* 34, no. 4 (summer 2009): 783–804; Samerski, "Genetic Counseling."

98. Perry, "Anti-Choice Legislators."

99. Piepmeier, "Inadequacy of 'Choice.'"

100. Bailey, "Reconceiving Surrogacy"; de Onís, "Lost in Translation"; Hayden, "Revitalizing the Debate"; Ross, "Movement for Reproductive Justice."

101. Katherine Ellison and Nina Martin, "Nearly Dying in Childbirth: Why Preventable Complications Are Growing in U.S.," NPR, December 22, 2017, https://www.npr.org/2017/12/22/572298802/nearly-dying-in-childbirth-why-preventable-complications-are-growing-in-u-s.

102. Ibid.; Nina Martin and Renee Montagne, "Focus on Infants during Childbirth Leaves U.S. Moms in Danger," *Morning Edition*, NPR, March 12, 2017, https://www.npr.org/2017/05/12/527806002/focus-on-infants-during-childbirth-leaves-u-s-moms-in-danger.

103. U.S. Centers for Disease Control and Prevention, "Pregnancy Mortality Surveillance System," Centers for Disease Control and Prevention, November 9, 2017, https://www.cdc.gov/reproductivehealth/maternalinfanthealth/pmss.html.

104. Nina Martin and Renee Montagne, "Black Mothers Keep Dying After Giving Birth," *All Things Considered*, NPR, December 7, 2017, https://www.npr.org/2017/12/07/568948782/black-mothers-keep-dying-after-giving-birth-shalon-irvings-story-explains-why.

105. Paltrow and Flavin, "Arrests of and Forced Interventions."

106. Midwives Alliance, "New Studies Confirm Safety of Home Birth With Midwives in the U.S.," Midwives Alliance of North America, January 30, 2014, http://mana.org/blog/home-birth-safety-outcomes. See also Melissa Cheyney et al., "Outcomes of Care for 16,924 Planned Home Births in the United States: The Midwives Alliance of North America Statistics Project, 2004 to 2009," *Journal of Midwifery and Women's Health* 59, no. 1 (January 2014): 17–27, https://doi.org/10.1111/jmwh.12172.

107. Elizabeth G. Raymond and David A. Grimes, "The Comparative Safety of Legal Induced Abortion and Childbirth in the United States," *Obstetrics and Gynecology* 119, no. 2, part 1 (February 2012): 215–19, https://doi.org/10.1097/AOG.0b013e31823fe923.

Chapter 3. Post-Prevention? Conceptualizing Emergency Contraception

1. Suz Redfearn, "Preparing for a Mistake: For Emergency Birth Control, Plan Ahead," *Washington Post*, May 21, 2002, sec. Health.

2. Heather Munro Prescott, *The Morning After: A History of Emergency Contraception in the United States*, Critical Issues in Health and Medicine (New Brunswick, NJ: Rutgers University Press, 2011), 118.

3. Andrew Feenberg, *Critical Theory of Technology* (New York: Oxford University Press, 1991), 14.

4. See, for example, Andrew Feenberg, "Democratic Rationalization: Technology, Power, and Freedom," in *Philosophy of Technology: The Technological Condition*, ed. Robert C. Scharff and Val Dusek, 652–65 (Malden, MA: Blackwell, 2003); Feenberg, *Critical Theory*; Valerie Hartouni, *Cultural Conceptions: On Reproductive Technologies and the Remaking of Life* (Minneapolis: University of Minnesota Press, 1997); Carolyn Marvin, *When Old Technologies Were New: Thinking about Communications in the Late Nineteenth Century* (New York: Oxford University Press, 1988); Lynn Spigel, *Welcome to the Dreamhouse: Popular Media and Postwar Suburbs* (Durham, NC: Duke University Press, 2001).

5. For this chapter, I studied all articles having to do with EC published in prominent newspapers and periodicals with national circulation, including the *New York Times*, *Washington Post*, *New York Times Magazine*, *Time*, and *Newsweek*, between January 1, 1997, and December 31, 2006. These ten years are particularly significant for the EC debates because 1997 marks the original approval of EC for prescription sale in the United States; 2006 marks Plan B's final approval by the FDA to go "behind the counter" for those eighteen and older. While not all articles are included in the direct quotations provided in this study, each readily informs my analysis of these discourses and contributes to my overall argument.

6. A thorough history of the politics of EC exceeds the parameters of this book but is documented elsewhere. See Prescott, *Morning After*.

7. The FDA does not intervene in the practice of medicine but rather regulates which medications are available for sale in the United States and how they are to be distributed (over-the-counter, or by prescription only). An off-label use of a drug, then, refers to "use for an indication, dosage form, dose regimen, population or other use parameter not mentioned in the approved labeling." See Judith A. Johnson and Vanessa K. Burrows, *Emergency Contraception: Plan B*, CRS Report for Congress RL33728 (Washington, DC: Congressional Research Service: Report for Congress, 2007).

8. Johnson and Burrows, "Emergency Contraception"; Prescott, *Morning After*.

9. Johnson and Burrows, "Emergency Contraception."

10. As historian Heather Munro Prescott explains, EC awareness remained low into the early twenty-first century, despite the promotional efforts of various health care organizations: "A 1997 survey indicated that only 11 percent of women of reproductive age had heard of emergency contraception. Even providers who knew about emergency contraception were not consistent about getting the word out to their patients: only 10 percent of those surveyed in 1997 indicated that they routinely counseled patients about this contraceptive option" (93). Moreover, Title X clinics were prohibited from prescribing contraceptives off-label, thus barring low-income women from accessing EC altogether. Prescott, *Morning After*.

11. Prescott, *Morning After*.

12. Johnson and Burrows, "Emergency Contraception."

13. Prescott, *Morning After*.

14. David Grimes, quoted in Redfearn, "Preparing for a Mistake."

15. Prescott, *Morning After*.

16. Kathleen Adams and Bruce Crumley, "Health Report," *Time*, March 10, 1997.

17. Sandra G. Boodman, "The 'Morning-After' Kit; New Emergency Contraceptive Gives Women a Second Chance to Prevent Pregnancy," *Washington Post*, September 22, 1998, final ed., sec. Health; Adam Rogers, "Options beyond the Pill," *Newsweek*, spring/summer special ed., 1999.

18. Prescott, *Morning After*.

19. Mifepristone is approved by the FDA to terminate a pregnancy within the first seventy days of gestation. While entirely distinct from EC in its synthetic composition and use, mifepristone is also (perhaps obviously) used after unprotected sex and was approved for sale in the United States in September 2000, just over a year after Plan B. Confusion of these medications in mediated and public forums abounds.

20. Rogers, "Options."

21. Russell Shorto, "Contra-Contraception," *New York Times Magazine*, May 7, 2006.

22. Laurie Goodstein, "Falwell: Blame Abortionists, Feminists and Gays," World News, *Guardian*, September 19, 2001, US ed., www.theguardian.com/world/2001/sep/19/september11.usa9.

23. Faludi, *Terror Dream*, 27.

24. Elizabeth Nash et al., "Laws Affecting Reproductive Health and Rights: 2014 State Policy Review," Guttmacher Institute, January 5, 2015, www.guttmacher.org/statecenter/updates/2014/statetrends42014.html.

25. Guttmacher Institute, *Facts on Induced Abortion in the United States* (New York: Guttmacher Institute, March 2016), accessed March 23, 2016.

26. Ibid.

27. Ellen Goodman, "A Workable Plan for Fewer Abortions," *Washington Post*, February 29, 2004, sec. Editorial B07.

28. Laura Sessions Stepp, "With Birth Control, Plan B Is Topic A," *Washington Post*, February 10, 2004, sec. Style C01.

29. Quoted in Monica Davey and Pam Belluck, "Pharmacies Balk on After-Sex Pill and Widen Fight," *New York Times*, April 19, 2005.

30. Kate Zernike, "Use of Morning-After Pill Rising and It May Go over the Counter," *New York Times*, May 19, 2003, sec. A1.

31. Lisa Rein and Craig Timberg, "Emergency Birth Control Approved; Bill Calls for Access without Prescription," *Washington Post*, February 21, 2001, sec. A.

32. David Bjerklie, Alice Park, and Sora Song, "A to Z Guide," *Time*, January 19, 2004.

33. Quoted in Gina Kolata, "A Contraceptive Clears a Hurdle to Wider Access," *New York Times*, December 17, 2003.

34. See, for example, Jennifer Baumgardner, "Would You Pledge Your Virginity to Your Father?," *Glamour*, January 1, 2007, www.glamour.com; Monica J. Casper and Laura M. Carpenter, "Sex, Drugs, and Politics: The HPV Vaccine for Cervical Cancer," *Sociology of Health and Illness* 30, no. 6 (September 2008): 886–99, https://doi

.org/10.1111/j.1467-9566.2008.01100.x; M. Gigi Durham, *The Lolita Effect: The Media Sexualization of Young Girls and What We Can Do about It* (Overlook, 2008); Breanne Fahs, "Daddy's Little Girls: On the Perils of Chastity Clubs, Purity Balls, and Ritualized Abstinence," *Frontiers: A Journal of Women's Studies* 31, no. 3 (2010): 116–42; Christine J. Gardner, *Making Chastity Sexy: The Rhetoric of Evangelical Abstinence Campaigns* (Berkeley: University of California Press, 2001); Casey Ryan Kelly, *Abstinence Cinema: Virginity and the Rhetoric of Sexual Purity in Contemporary Film* (New Brunswick, NJ: Rutgers University Press, 2016); Casey Ryan Kelly and Kristen E. Hoerl, "Shaved or Saved? Disciplining Women's Bodies," *Women's Studies in Communication* 38, no. 2 (April 3, 2015): 141–45, https://doi.org/10.1080/07491409.2015.1027088; Jessica Valenti, *The Purity Myth: How America's Obsession with Virginity Is Hurting Young Women* (Berkeley, CA: Seal Press, 2009).

35. While sex education has proven a recurrent site of struggle for over a century, the 1981 Adolescent Family Life Act initiated abstinence-only curricula in the United States, granting federal funding to "chastity education" developed by conservative religious organizations. Early curricula were censured for violation of the separation of church and state; abstinence-only education was nevertheless renewed through the 1996 Personal Responsibility and Work Opportunity Reconciliation Act. This legislation dismantled state assistance for impoverished families and increased regulation of marginalized women's childbearing and parenting, but it also set the stage for the transformation of sex education in public schools by requiring abstinence-only curricula in exchange for federal funding.

36. SIECUS: Sexuality Information and Education Council of the United States, "A History of Federal Funding for Abstinence-Only-Until-Marriage Programs" (SIECUS: Sexuality Information and Education Council of the United States), accessed April 13, 2016, www.siecus.org/index.cfm?fuseaction=page.viewpage&pageid=1340&nodeid=1.

37. Henry Waxman, "The Content of Federally Funded Abstinence-Only Education Programs" (Washington, DC: U.S. House of Representatives Committee on Government Reform—Minority Staff Special Investigations Division, 2004).

38. Casey Ryan Kelly, "'True' Love Waits: The Construction of Facts in Abstinence-until-Marriage Discourse," in *Disturbing Argument: Selected Works from the 18th NCA/AFA Alta Conference on Argumentation*, ed. Catherine H. Palczewski (New York: Routledge, 2015), 376–81; SIECUS: Sexuality Information and Education Council of the United States, "A History"; Waxman, "Content."

39. Robin E. Jensen, *Dirty Words: The Rhetoric of Public Sex Education, 1870–1924* (Champaign: University of Illinois Press, 2010).

40. Jon Knowles, *Issue Brief: Sex Education in the United States* (New York: Katharine Dexter McCormick Library and the Education Division of Planned Parenthood Federation of America, 2012), https://www.plannedparenthood.org/files/3713/9611/7930/Sex_Ed_in_the_US.pdf.

41. SIECUS: Sexuality Information and Education Council of the U.S., "President's FY 2017 Budget Applauded by the Sexuality Information and Education Council of the U.S.

(SIECUS)," February 9, 2016, www.siecus.org/index.cfm?fuseaction=Feature.show Feature&featureid=2437&pageid=611.

42. See, for example, Durham, *Lolita Effect*; Gardner, *Making Chastity Sexy*; C. Kelly, *Abstinence Cinema*; C. Kelly, "'True' Love."

43. C. Kelly, *Abstinence Cinema*; C. Kelly and Hoerl, "Shaved or Saved?"; Hortense Smith, "Abstinence, the 'Sexy' Way," Jezebel, August 9, 2009, http://jezebel.com/5333434/abstinence-the-sexy-way; Lisa Wade, "Sexing Up Abstinence—Sociological Images," August 8, 2009, http://thesocietypages.org/socimages/2009/08/08/sexing-up-abstinence/.

44. C. Kelly and Hoerl, "Shaved or Saved?"; H. Smith, "Abstinence"; Wade, "Sexing Up Abstinence."

45. C. Kelly and Hoerl, "Shaved or Saved?," 142.

46. Durham, *Lolita Effect*.

47. Gardner, *Making Chastity Sexy*.

48. Ibid., 28.

49. Jimmie Manning, "Exploring Family Discourses about Purity Pledges: Connecting Relationships and Popular Culture," *Qualitative Research Reports in Communication* 15, no. 1 (January 2014): 92–99, https://doi.org/10.1080/17459435.2014.955597.

50. Baumgardner, "Would You Pledge Your Virginity."

51. Ibid.; Jimmie Manning, "Paradoxes of (Im)Purity: Affirming Heteronormativity and Queering Heterosexuality in Family Discourses of Purity Pledges," *Women's Studies in Communication* 38, no. 1 (January 2, 2015): 99–117, https://doi.org/10.1080/07491409.2014.954687.

52. Valenti, *Purity Myth*.

53. Fahs, "Daddy's Little Girls"; C. Kelly, "'True' Love"; Manning, "Paradoxes"; Valenti, *Purity Myth*.

54. Quoted in Lisa L. Wynn, "United States: Activism, Sexual Archetypes, and the Politicization of Science," in *Emergency Contraception: The Story of a Global Reproductive Health Technology*, ed. Angelina Marguerite Foster and Lisa L. Wynn (New York: Palgrave Macmillan, 2012), 50.

55. Prescott, *Morning After*.

56. Casper and Carpenter, "Sex, Drugs, and Politics."

57. Gina Kolata, "Debate on Selling Morning-After Pill over the Counter," *New York Times*, December 12, 2003.

58. Stepp, "With Birth Control."

59. Marc Kaufman, "FDA Delays Decision on Plan B Contraceptive," *Washington Post*, August 27, 2005.

60. Sarah Projansky, "Mass Magazine Cover Girls: Some Reflections on Postfeminist Girls and Postfeminism's Daughters," in *Interrogating Postfeminism: Gender and the Politics of Popular Culture*, ed. Yvonne Tasker and Diane Negra, 4–72 (Durham, NC: Duke University Press, 2007).

61. Emily Vasquez and Kate Hammer, "Easier Access to Plan B Pill Evokes Praise, and Concern," *New York Times*, August 2006.

62. Stepp, "With Birth Control."

63. "A Public Health Victory," Opinion, *New York Times*, December 18, 2003, sec. A42.

64. Zernike, "Use of Morning-After Pill."

65. Stepp, "With Birth Control."

66. Abigail Trafford, "Second Opinion," *Washington Post*, May 15, 2001.

67. Marc Kaufman, "Compromise May Restrict 'Morning-After' Pill," *Washington Post*, April 8, 2004, sec. A.

68. Kolata, "Contraceptive."

69. Sarah Lyall, "Britain Allows Over-the-Counter Sales of Morning-After Pill," *New York Times*, January 15, 2001, sec. A4.

70. Gardiner Harris, "U.S. Again Delays Decision on Sale of Next-Day Pill," *New York Times*, August 27, 2005.

71. Goodman, "Workable Plan."

72. Karen Judd Lewis, quoted in Marc Kaufman, "FDA Plan B Sales Rejected against Advice; Official Denies that Politics Blocked Contraceptive's Over-the-Counter Status," *Washington Post*, May 8, 2004, sec. A.

73. Gardiner Harris, "Official Quits on Pill Delay at the F.D.A.," *New York Times*, September 1, 2005.

74. U.S. Food and Drug Administration, "Postmarket Drug Safety Information for Patients and Providers—Plan B: Questions and Answers—August 24, 2006; Updated December 14, 2006," WebContent, August 24, 2006, https://www.fda.gov/Drugs/DrugSafety/PostmarketDrugSafetyInformationforPatientsandProviders/ucm109783.htm.

75. Quoted in Susan F. Wood, "Inappropriate Obstructions to Access: The FDA's Handling of Plan B," *American Medical Association Journal of Ethics* 16, no. 4 (April 2014): 295–301.

76. Megan L. Kavanaugh, Sanithia L. Williams, and E. Bimla Schwarz, "Emergency Contraception Use and Counseling after Changes in United States Prescription Status," *Fertility and Sterility* 95, no. 8 (June 2011): 2578–81, https://doi.org/10.1016/j.fertnstert.2011.03.011.

77. Anna Glasier, "Emergency Contraception: Clinical Outcomes," *Contraception* 87, no. 3 (March 2013): 309–13, https://doi.org/10.1016/j.contraception.2012.08.027; Jennifer L. Meyer, Melanie A. Gold, and Catherine L. Haggerty, "Advance Provision of Emergency Contraception among Adolescent and Young Adult Women: A Systematic Review of Literature," *Journal of Pediatric and Adolescent Gynecology* 24, no. 1 (February 2011): 2–9, https://doi.org/10.1016/j.jpag.2010.06.002; Maria I. Rodriguez et al., "Advance Supply of Emergency Contraception: A Systematic Review," *Contraception* 87, no. 5 (May 2013): 590–601, https://doi.org/10.1016/j.contraception.2012.09.011.

78. Sally Rafie et al., "Assessment of Family Planning Services at Community Pharmacies in San Diego, California," *Pharmacy* 1, no. 2 (October 11, 2013): 153–59, https://doi.org/10.3390/pharmacy1020153; Tracey A. Wilkinson et al., "Access to Emergency Contraception for Adolescents," *JAMA* 307, no. 4 (January 25, 2012), https://doi.org/10.1001/jama.2011.1949; Tracey A. Wilkinson et al., "Evaluating Com-

munity Pharmacy Responses about Levonorgestrel Emergency Contraception by Mystery Caller Characteristics," *Journal of Adolescent Health*, February 2018, https://doi.org/10.1016/j.jadohealth.2017.11.303; Tracey A. Wilkinson et al., "'I'll See What I Can Do': What Adolescents Experience When Requesting Emergency Contraception," *Journal of Adolescent Health* 54, no. 1 (January 2014): 14–19, https://doi.org/10.1016/j.jadohealth.2013.10.002; Tracey. A. Wilkinson et al., "Pharmacy Communication to Adolescents and Their Physicians Regarding Access to Emergency Contraception," *Pediatrics* 129, no. 4 (April 1, 2012): 624–29, https://doi.org/10.1542/peds.2011-3760.

79. Olivia Sampson et al., "Barriers to Adolescents' Getting Emergency Contraception through Pharmacy Access in California: Differences by Language and Region," *Perspectives on Sexual and Reproductive Health* 41, no. 2 (June 2009): 110–18, https://doi.org/10.1363/4111009.

80. National Women's Law Center, "Emergency Contraception Coverage under Family Planning §1115 Waivers" (Washington, DC: National Women's Law Center, December 2007); Office of Population Research at Princeton University, "Get Emergency Contraception Now," Emergency Contraception Website, August 14, 2017, http://ec.princeton.edu/locator/concerned-about-cost.html#Medicaid.

81. Wilkinson et al., "Access."

82. Native American Women's Health Education Resource Center, "Lack of Access to Emergency Contraception Continues," 2014, www.nativeshop.org/m/news-110/783-the-lack-of-access-to-emergency-contraception-continues.html.

83. Native American Community Board, "Indian Health Service and Tribal Health Center Plan B Accessibility Survey," 2017, www.nativeshop.org/images/pdf/2017-05-Plan-B-IHS-and-Tribal-Health-Center-final-report-2.pdf.

84. American Society for Emergency Contraception, "Inching towards Progress: ASEC's 2015 Pharmacy Access Study" (American Society for Emergency Contraception, December 2015), http://americansocietyforec.org/uploads/3/4/5/6/34568220/asec_2015_ec_access_report_1.pdf.

85. Ibid., 1.

86. Christian Fiala and Joyce H. Arthur, "'Dishonourable Disobedience'—Why Refusal to Treat in Reproductive Healthcare Is Not Conscientious Objection," *Woman—Psychosomatic Gynaecology and Obstetrics* 1 (December 2014): 2, https://doi.org/10.1016/j.woman.2014.03.001.

87. Guttmacher Institute, "State Policies in Brief: Refusing to Provide Health Services" (New York: Guttmacher Institute, March 2016), 1.

88. As of 2016, eleven states allow pharmacists and pharmacies to refuse to dispense EC, while a total of five states require either a pharmacist or a pharmacy to fill valid prescriptions for EC. Guttmacher Institute, "State Policies in Brief: Emergency Contraception" (New York: Guttmacher Institute, March 2016).

89. National Women's Law Center, "Pharmacy Refusals 101," *National Women's Law Center: Expanding the Possibilities* (blog), August 4, 2015, http://nwlc.org/resources/pharmacy-refusals-101/.

90. Ibid.

91. Claire E. Eades, Jill S. Ferguson, and Ronan E. O'Carroll, "Public Health in Community Pharmacy: A Systematic Review of Pharmacist and Consumer Views," *BMC Public Health* 11, no. 1 (2011): 582; Sampson et al., "Barriers"; Wilkinson et al. "'I'll See What I Can Do.'"

92. In one study, only 55 percent of U.S. pharmacists indicated an interest in providing EC to patients; in another study, 25 percent of pharmacists were opposed, citing concerns about potential "overuse" and related increases in sexually transmitted infections. See Eades, Ferguson, and O'Carroll, "Public Health"; Ryan E. Lawrence et al., "Obstetrician-Gynecologist Physicians' Beliefs about Emergency Contraception: A National Survey," *Contraception* 82, no. 4 (October 2010): 324–30.

93. National Women's Law Center, "Pharmacy Refusals 101."

94. Casper and Carpenter, "Sex, Drugs, and Politics," 887.

Chapter 4. Crisis Pregnancy and the Colonization of the Clinic

1. "MTV's Premiere of 'Teen Mom' Marks the Highest-Rated New Series Launch in Over a Year," *TV by the Numbers* (blog), December 9, 2009, http://tvbythenumbers.zap2it.com/network-press-releases/mtvs-premiere-of-teen-mom-marks-the-highest-rated-new-series-launch-in-over-a-year/.

2. Laurie Ouellette, *Lifestyle TV* (New York: Routledge, 2016), 80.

3. John Seery, "The Juno Effect," blog, *Huffington Post*, January 22, 2008, www.huffingtonpost.com/john-seery/the-juno-effect_b_82582.html.

4. Kristen Hoerl and Casey Ryan Kelly, "The Post-Nuclear Family and the Depoliticization of Unplanned Pregnancy in *Knocked Up*, *Juno*, and *Waitress*," *Communication and Critical/Cultural Studies* 7, no. 4 (2010): 360–80; Pamela Thoma, "Buying Up Baby: Modern Feminine Subjectivity, Assertions of 'Choice,' and the Repudiation of Reproductive Justice in Postfeminist Unwanted Pregnancy Films," *Feminist Media Studies* 9, no. 4 (2009): 409–25.

5. An exposé in *Time* on the startling incidence of teen pregnancy in a small town north of Boston hit the newsstand in the summer of 2008, coinciding with the birth of Jamie Lynn Spears's baby, and stoked a media firestorm. Kathleen Kingsbury, "Pregnancy Boom at Gloucester High," *Time*, June 18, 2008, http://content.time.com/time/magazine/article/0,9171,1816486,00.html.

6. Popular teen clothing line Forever 21 faced much public criticism for its release of a maternity line in July 2010. The line was quietly retired a few years later. See Kate Abbott, "Forever 21 Launches Maternity Line—Is It Targeted at Teens?," *Time*, July 21, 2010, http://newsfeed.time.com/2010/07/21/forever-21-launches-maternity-line-for-teens/.

7. Jennifer Stevens Aubrey, Elizabeth Behm-Morawitz, and Kyungbo Kim, "Understanding the Effects of MTV's *16 and Pregnant* on Adolescent Girls' Beliefs, Attitudes, and Behavioral Intentions toward Teen Pregnancy," *Journal of Health Communication* 19, no. 10 (October 3, 2014): 1145–60, https://doi.org/10.1080/10810730.2013.872721;

James Dinh, "MTV's '16 and Pregnant' Credited for Decline in Teen Pregnancy Rates," MTV News, December 12, 2010, www.mtv.com/news/1654818/mtvs-16-and-pregnant-credited-for-decline-in-teen-pregnancy-rates/; Lauren Dolgen, "Why I Created MTV's '16 and Pregnant,'" May 5, 2011, www.cnn.com/2011/SHOWBIZ/TV/05/04/teen.mom.dolgen/index.html; Patrik Jonsson, "A Force behind the Lower Teen Birthrate: MTV's '16 and Pregnant,'" *Christian Science Monitor*, December 21, 2010, www.csmonitor.com/USA/Society/2010/1221/A-force-behind-the-lower-teen-birthrate-MTV-s-16-and-Pregnant; Annie Lowrey, "MTV's '16 and Pregnant,' Derided by Some, May Resonate as a Cautionary Tale," *New York Times*, January 13, 2014; Jennifer Trudeau, "The Role of New Media on Teen Sexual Behaviors and Fertility Outcomes—the Case of *16 and Pregnant*," *Southern Economic Journal*, March 17, 2015, https://doi.org/10.1002/soej.12034; Jacque Wilson, "Study: '16 and Pregnant,' 'Teen Mom' Led to Fewer Teen Births—CNN.Com," CNN, January 13, 2014, www.cnn.com/2014/01/13/health/16-pregnant-teens-childbirth/index.html; Paul J. Wright, Ashley K. Randall, and Analisa Arroyo, "Father–Daughter Communication about Sex Moderates the Association between Exposure to MTV's *16 and Pregnant/Teen Mom* and Female Students' Pregnancy-Risk Behavior," *Sexuality and Culture* 17, no. 1 (March 2013): 50–66, https://doi.org/10.1007/s12119-012-9137-2.

8. Much of the scholarship concerned with film does not focus on teen pregnancy, but rather offers insight into crisis pregnancy narratives more broadly as postfeminist texts that work to commodify maternity, depoliticize reproduction, and "valorize pregnancy and motherhood as women's imperatives" (Hoerl and Kelly, "Post-Nuclear Family," 360).

Scholarship that attends exclusively to crisis teen pregnancy is focused largely on the popular genre of reality programming, which, despite its name, is heavily curated, edited, and staged. Both *16 and Pregnant* and *Teen Mom* have garnered a wealth of critical attention in the blogosphere, academic journals, and in an edited volume as well. See Carolyn M. Cunningham, "Sixteen and Not Pregnant: Teen-Created YouTube Parody Videos and Sexual Risk-Taking in the United States," *Journal of Children and Media* 8, no. 1 (January 2, 2014): 53–68, doi:10.1080/17482798.2014.863479; Clare Daniel, "'Taming the Media Monster': Teen Pregnancy and the Neoliberal Safety (Inter)net," *Signs: Journal of Women in Culture and Society* 39, no. 4 (2014): 973–98; Letizia Guglielmo and Kimberly Wallace Stewart, "*16 and Pregnant* and the 'Unvarnished' Truth about Teen Pregnancy," in *MTV and Teen Pregnancy: Critical Essays on "16 and Pregnant" and "Teen Mom,"* ed. Letizia Guglielmo (Lanham, MD: Scarecrow, 2013), 19–34; Nicholas D. Kristof, "TV Lowers Birthrate (Seriously)," *New York Times*, March 20, 2014, sec. A; Aubrey, Behm-Morawitz, and Kim, "Understanding the Effects"; Jessica Valenti, "Why No Abortions on MTV's '16 and Pregnant'?," February 10, 2010, accessed July 24, 2015. In this chapter, I extend both bodies of literature by investigating texts across genres in order to provide insight into dominant figurations of teen pregnancy and motherhood in entertainment media (and public discourse writ large).

9. Ruby C. Tapia, "Impregnating Images: Visions of Race, Sex, and Citizenship in

California's Teen Pregnancy Prevention Campaigns," *Feminist Media Studies* 5, no. 1 (2005): 10.

10. My analysis of *Glee* is limited to its first season, which features crisis teen pregnancy prominently in its unfolding narrative. In the case of reality programming, rather than provide superficial analysis of several seasons, I limit my study of *16 and Pregnant* and *Teen Mom* to their first, record-breaking seasons, and, for the purposes of continuity, tend specifically to the four teens that bridge the series.

11. Solinger, *Beggars and Choosers*. Linda Gordon, *Pitied but Not Entitled: Single Mothers and the History of Welfare, 1890–1935* (Cambridge: Harvard University Press, 1994).

12. Ann Fessler, *The Girls Who Went Away: The Hidden History of Women Who Surrendered Children for Adoption in the Decades before 'Roe v. Wade'* (New York: Penguin, 2006), 183.

13. Heather Brook Adams, "Rhetorics of Unwed Motherhood and Shame," *Women's Studies in Communication* 40, no. 1 (January 2, 2017): 91–110, https://doi.org/10.1080/07491409.2016.1247401.

14. Fessler, *Girls*, 154, 8.

15. Precise statistics on adoption have been, and continue to be, scarce and incomplete. The federal government tracked data between 1945 and 1975, but the methods excluded informal adoptions and obscured significant trends in adoption. Federal data do not distinguish between relative and stranger adoption, independent and agency adoptions, infant and older child adoptions, and a range of other significant issues. Thus, while exact figures prior to 1945 are difficult to locate, available data suggest that adoption in the United States peaked at 175,000 in the year 1970. At present, states continue to collect information on the adoption of children through public foster care; data on adoptions outside of the system after 1975 are available only through private organizations.

16. Available studies of domestic adoption in the 1970s trace a precipitous decline in the number of white infants available for adoption; simultaneously, increasing numbers of single women were giving birth. Reports note that the steep decline in the number of infants available for adoption had less to do with legal abortion than with increasing numbers of single women keeping their children. See Solinger, *Beggars and Choosers*.

17. Solinger, *Beggars and Choosers*, 23.

18. Stephanie J. Ventura, Brady E. Hamilton, and T. J. Mathews, "National and State Patterns of Teen Births in the United States, 1940–2013," *National Vital Statistics Reports* 63, no. 4 (2014): 1–34.

19. Ibid.

20. Laura Briggs, *Somebody's Children: The Politics of Transracial and Transnational Adoption* (Durham NC: Duke University Press, 2012); Solinger, *Beggars and Choosers*.

21. Notably, most teen mothers are not legal minors, but rather eighteen or nineteen years old at the birth of their babies.

22. Clare Daniel, "Teen Sex, an Equal Opportunity Menace: Multicultural Politics in 16 and Pregnant," in Guglielmo, *MTV and Teen Pregnancy*, 80.

23. U.S. Department of Health and Human Services, "Voluntary Relinquishment for Adoption" (Washington, DC, 2005).

24. Briggs, *Somebody's Children*.

25. See Briggs, *Somebody's Children*; Catherine Ceniza Choy, *Global Families: A History of Asian International Adoption in America* (New York: New York University Press, 2013); Jeremiah Favara, "A Maternal Heart: Angelina Jolie, Choices of Maternity, and Hegemonic Femininty in People Magazine," *Feminist Media Studies*, 2015; E. J. Graff, "The Lie We Love," *Foreign Policy*, November/December 2008, 58–66. A. Smith, *Conquest*; Solinger, *Pregnancy and Power*.

26. Briggs, *Somebody's Children*; Graff, "Lie We Love."

27. The literature here is extensive, but a few examples illustrate this sobering point. First, in countries such as Liberia, Ukraine, and Vietnam, some orphanages function as temporary boarding schools for families struggling with poverty or illness, or just during harvest season in farming communities. Investigations have revealed instances in which illiterate birth mothers or families sign away their children under false pretenses, or where children are disappeared when their families return for them. In another example, at the height of US adoptions of Guatemalan children in 2007, Guatemalan mothers were assaulted in the streets by armed men, and their infants kidnapped to be sold for baby finder fees that far exceeded the nation's per capita GDP. And corruption and fraud are prominent within the agencies themselves. Well-known US adoption agent Lauryn Galindo was indicted in 2004 for arranging adoptions of Cambodian children who were not orphans, paying poor women and families to give their babies to US couples. See Arthur Brice, "Guatemalan Army Stole Children for Adoption, Report Says," International CNN, April 4, 2012, www.cnn.com/2009/WORLD/americas/09/12/guatemala.child.abduction/index.html; Mary Ellen Fieweger, "Stolen Children and International Adoptions," *Child Welfare* 70, no. 2 (1991): 285–91; Graff, "Lie We Love"; Schuster Institute for Investigative Journalism, "Adoption: Cambodia," February 22, 2011, www.brandeis.edu/investigate/gender/adoption/cambodia.html; Schuster Institute for Investigative Journalism, "The Baby Business: Policy Proposals for Fairer Practice," *Fraud and Corruption in International Adoptions* (Waltham, MA: Schuster Institute for Investigative Journalism), April 5, 2012; David M. Smolin, "Child Laundering: How the Intercountry Adoption System Legitimizes and Incentivizes the Practices of Buying, Trafficking, Kidnapping, and Stealing Children," *Wayne Law Review* 52, no. 1 (2006): 113–200.

28. Laura Briggs, *Somebody's Children: The Politics of Transracial and Transnational Adoption* (Durham, NC: Duke University Press, 2012); Choy, *Global Families: A History of Asian International Adoption in America*; A. Smith, *Conquest*; Solinger, *Beggars and Choosers*.

29. U.S. Department of State, "Intercountry Adoption: FY 2017 Annual Report on Intercountry Adoption" (Washington, DC: Bureau of Consular Affairs, 2018).

30. U.S. Department of State, "Adoption Statistics: Adoptions by Year," (2018), https://travel.state.gov/content/travel/en/Intercountry-Adoption/adopt_ref/adoption-statistics.html.

31. Rachel Lorenzo, "Young Women United Releases New Report, 'Dismantling Teen Pregnancy Prevention' for Immediate Release," June 1, 2016, www.youngwomenunited.org/press-advisories-and-releases/ (dead), accessed August 8, 2016.

32. Daniel, "Taming the Media Monster," 979.

33. Roberts, *Killing the Black Body*, 119.

34. Kathryn Edin and Maria Kefalas, *Promises I Can Keep: Why Poor Women Put Motherhood before Marriage* (Berkeley: University of California Press, 2005).

35. Micaela Cadena, Raquel Z. Rivera, Tannia Esparza, and Denicia Cadena, *Dismantling Teen Pregnancy Prevention* (Albuquerque, NM: Young Women United, 2016), www.youngwomenunited.org/wp-content/uploads/2016/05/ywu-dismantlingtpp-may2016-digital.pdf.

36. Lorenzo, "Young Women United."

37. Joanna D. Brown et al., "Longitudinal Study of Depressive Symptoms and Social Support in Adolescent Mothers," *Maternal and Child Health Journal* 16, no. 4 (May 2012): 894–901, https://doi.org/10.1007/s10995-011-0814-9; Nicole L. Letourneau, Miriam J. Stewart, and Alison K. Barnfather, "Adolescent Mothers: Support Needs, Resources, and Support-Education Interventions," *Journal of Adolescent Health* 35, no. 6 (December 2004): 509–25, https://doi.org/10.1016/j.jadohealth.2004.01.007; M. Cynthia Logsdon et al., "Social Support in Pregnant and Parenting Adolescents: Research, Critique, and Recommendations," *Journal of Child and Adolescent Psychiatric Nursing* 15, no. 2 (2002): 75–83; Elyse D'nn Lovell, "College Students Who Are Parents Need Equitable Services for Retention," *Journal of College Student Retention: Research, Theory and Practice* 16, no. 2 (January 1, 2014): 187–202, https://doi.org/10.2190/CS.16.2.b; Mikki Meadows-Oliver et al., "Sources of Stress and Support and Maternal Resources of Homeless Teenage Mothers," *Journal of Child and Adolescent Psychiatric Nursing* 20, no. 2 (2007): 116–25; Stefanie Mollborn, "Making the Best of a Bad Situation: Material Resources and Teenage Parenthood," *Journal of Marriage and Family* 69 (2007): 92–104; C. O'Brien Cherry et al., "Building a 'Better Life': The Transformative Effects of Adolescent Pregnancy and Parenting," *Sage Open* 5, no. 1 (February 11, 2015), https://doi.org/10.1177/2158244015571638; Mitchell Schmidt, "Organization Marks 25 Years of Teen Parent Program," *Cedar Rapids Gazette*, September 20, 2015, www.thegazette.com/subject/news/business/organization-marks-45-years-of-teen-parent-program-20150920; L. SmithBattle, "'I Wanna Have a Good Future': Teen Mothers' Rise in Educational Aspirations, Competing Demands, and Limited School Support," *Youth and Society* 38, no. 3 (March 1, 2007): 348–71, https://doi.org/10.1177/0044118X06287962.

38. SmithBattle, "I Wanna Have a Good Future."

39. See, for example, Fahs, "Daddy's Little Girls"; Gardner, *Making Chastity Sexy*.

40. Heather D. Boonstra, "Advocates Call for a New Approach after the Era of Abstinence-Only Sex Education," *Guttmacher Policy Review* 12, no. 1 (2009): 6–11; Jensen, *Dirty Words*.

41. Guttmacher Institute, "Minors' Rights as Parents," Guttmacher Institute, July 1, 2017, https://www.guttmacher.org/state-policy/explore/minors-rights-parents; Guttmacher Institute, "Parental Involvement in Minors' Abortions," Guttmacher Institute: State Laws and Policies, July 1, 2017, https://www.guttmacher.org/state-policy/explore/parental-involvement-minors-abortions.

42. Heather D. Boonstra, "Meeting the Sexual and Reproductive Health Needs of Adolescents in School-Based Health Centers," *Guttmacher Policy Review* 18, no. 1 (2015): 21–26; Amy Adele Hasinoff, *Sexting Panic: Rethinking Criminalization, Privacy, and Consent* (Urbana: University of Illinois Press, 2015).

43. Sady Doyle, *Trainwreck: The Women We Love to Hate, Mock, and Fear . . . and Why* (Brooklyn, NY: Melville House, 2016), 204.

44. Laurie Ouellette and James Hay, *Better Living through Reality TV: Television and Post-Welfare Citizenship* (Malden, MA: Blackwell, 2008).

45. Mark Andrejevic, "'Securitainment' in the Post-9/11 Era," *Continuum: Journal of Media and Cultural Studies* 25, no. 2 (2011): 165–75. See also Rachel E. Dubrofsky, "Surveillance on Reality Television and Facebook: From Authenticity to Flowing Data," *Communication Theory* 12 (2011): 111–29; Ouellette and Hay, *Better Living*.

46. IMDb: The Internet Movie Database, "Awards for *Juno*," accessed April 26, 2010.

47. IMDb: The Internet Movie Database, "Awards for *Glee*," accessed February 21, 2011.

48. Shirley Halperin, "The Business of *Glee*," *Hollywood Reporter*, February 2, 2011.

49. Rob Sheffield, "*Glee*'s Unstoppable Roll," *Rolling Stone*, November 25, 2010; Michael O'Connell, "TV Ratings: 'Glee' Exits Stage Left," Hollywood Reporter, March 21, 2015, www.hollywoodreporter.com/live-feed/tv-ratings-glee-exits-stage-783509.

50. Kathryn Kost, Stanley Henshaw, and Liz Carlin, *U.S. Teenage Pregnancies, Births and Abortions: National and State Trends and Trends by Race and Ethnicity* (N.p.: Guttmacher Institute, January 2010); Ventura, Hamilton, and Mathews, "National and State Patterns."

51. Dolgen, "Why I Created MTV's '16 and Pregnant.'"

52. A report released in December 2010 by the National Campaign to Prevent Teen and Unplanned Pregnancy specifically cites the show in its findings: "Among those teens who have watched MTV's 16 and Pregnant, 82% think the show helps teens better understand the challenges of teen pregnancy and parenthood and how to avoid it." Bill Albert, "With One Voice 2010: America's Adults and Teens Sound Off about Teen Pregnancy" (Washington, DC: National Campaign to Prevent Teen and Unplanned Pregnancy, 2010), 6. Additional research both refutes and supports this claim. See note 5.

53. Ginia Bellefante, "Real Life Is Like 'Juno,' Except Maybe the Dialogue," *New York Times*, June 11, 2009; Tom Shales, "*16 & Pregnant* Deftly Plumbs the Parent Trap," *Washington Post*, June 11, 2009; and Michael Essany, "*16 and Pregnant* Returns to MTV with Life after Labor Reunion and Dramatic Stories for Season 2," *Entertainment Examiner*, July 24, 2010.

54. "MTV's Premiere of 'Teen Mom'"; "Season Finale for MTV's 'Teen Mom' Scores

Series High 3.6 Million Viewers," *TV by the Numbers* (blog), January 27, 2010, http://tvbythenumbers.zap2it.com/ratings/season-finale-for-mtvs-teen-mom-scores-series-high-3-6-million-viewers/.

55. Stephanie Goldberg, "The 'Teen Mom' Phenomenon," CNN, September 10, 2010, www.cnn.com/2010/SHOWBIZ/TV/09/10/teen.mom.mtv/index.html.

56. See, for example, Mark Andrejevic, "The Kinder, Gentler Gaze of Big Brother: Reality TV in the Era of Digital Capitalism," *New Media and Society* 4, no. 2 (2002): 251–70; Andrejevic, "Securitainment"; Ron Becker, "'Help Is on the Way!': *Supernanny, Nanny 911,* and the Neoliberal Politics of the Family," in *The Great American Makeover: Television, History, Nation*, ed. Dana Heller (New York: Palgrave Macmillan, 2006), 175–92; Rachel E. Dubrofsky, "Therapeutics of the Self: Surveillance in the Service of the Therapeutic," *Television and New Media* 8 (2007): 263–84; Dubrofsky, "Surveillance"; Gillan, "Extreme Makeover"; Ouellette and Hay, *Better Living*.

57. Ouellette, *Lifestyle TV*, 90.

58. Letizia Guglielmo, ed., *MTV and Teen Pregnancy: Critical Essays on "16 and Pregnant" and "Teen Mom"* (Lanham, MD: Scarecrow, 2013), viii.

59. Hoerl and Kelly, "Post-Nuclear Family"; Thoma, "Buying Up Baby"; Valenti, "Why No Abortions."

60. Hoerl and Kelly, "Post-Nuclear Family," 336.

61. *Glee*, season 1, episode 2, "Showmance," directed by Ryan Murphy, aired September 23, 2009, on Fox.

62. *Glee*, season 1, episode 4, "Preggers," directed by Brad Falchuk, aired September 23, 2009, on Fox.

63. Krystie Lee Yandoli, "Why 'Obvious Child' Is the Abortion Movie We All Need," Bustle, December 26, 3013, www.bustle.com/articles/11370-why-obvious-child-is-the-abortion-movie-we-all-need; Valenti, "Why No Abortions."

64. Subsequent seasons of *16 and Pregnant* have responded to feminist criticism regarding the absence of abortion. While none of the teens featured in subsequent seasons chose abortion, the creators sponsored a special episode to discuss "difficult choices." The episode aired at 11:30 p.m. and, according to reports, MTV did not seek advertising for the program. Irin Carmon, "MTV's Abortion Special Didn't Disappoint," *Jezebel*, December 29, 2010, https://jezebel.com/5720450/mtvs-abortion-special-didnt-disappoint.

65. Ouellette, *Lifestyle TV*.

66. Other scholars have noted the way "teen" and "mother" are figured as discursively opposed positions in reality programming. See May Friedman, "'100% Preventable': Teen Motherhood, Morality, and the Myth of Choice," in Guglielmo, *MTV and Teen Pregnancy*, 68.

67. *16 and Pregnant*, season 1, episode 1, "Maci," produced by Morgan J. Freeman, aired June 11, 2009, on MTV. *Teen Mom*, season 1, episode 3, "Fallout," produced by Morgan J. Freeman, aired December 22, 2009, on MTV.

68. *16 and Pregnant*, season 1, episode 1, "Maci," produced by Morgan J. Freeman, aired June 11, 2009 on MTV.

69. *Teen Mom*, season 1, episode 3, "Fallout," produced by Morgan J. Freeman, aired December 22, 2009, on MTV.

70. *Teen Mom*, season 1, episode 7, "Baby Steps," produced by Morgan J. Freeman, aired January 19, 2010, on MTV.

71. An estranged ex-boyfriend, he died in a car accident during Farrah's pregnancy and is seldom mentioned in the first season of either *16 and Pregnant* or *Teen Mom*.

72. *Teen Mom*, season 1, episode 5, "A Little Help," produced by Morgan J. Freeman, aired January 4, 2010, on MTV.

73. *Teen Mom*, season 1, episode 3, "Fallout," produced by Morgan J. Freeman, aired December 22, 2009, on MTV.

74. Gareth Palmer, "On Our Best Behaviour," *FlowTV* 5 (December 15, 2006), http://flowtv.org/2006/12/on-our-best-behaviour/.

75. Guglielmo, *MTV and Teen Pregnancy*.

76. Ouellette, *Lifestyle TV*.

77. *Teen Mom*, season 1, episode 9, "Finale Special: Check Up with Dr. Drew," produced by Morgan J. Freeman, aired February 1, 2010, on MTV.

78. See Emily, "Interview: Farrah Abraham Talks Sophia, Misconceptions, Her New Restaurant and That Christian Parenting Book," Starcasm, June 3, 2014, http://starcasm.net/archives/274344.

79. For data on the teen birth rate according to race/ethnicity, see National Campaign to Prevent Teen and Unplanned Pregnancy, "National Data," https://powertodecide.org/what-we-do/information/national-state-data/national. For discussions regarding the use of Latina/o, Latin@, and Latinx, see Catalina (Kathleen) M. de Onís, "What's in an 'X'?: An Exchange about the Politics of 'Latinx,'" *Chiricú Journal: Latina/o Literatures, Arts, and Cultures* 1, no. 2 (2017): 78–91.

80. Rachel Alicia Griffin, "*Pushing* into *Precious*: Black Women, Media Representation, and the Glare of the White Supremacist Capitalist Patriarchal Gaze," *Critical Studies in Media Communication* 31, no. 3 (May 27, 2014): 182–97, https://doi.org/10.1080/15295036.2013.849354; Mia Mask, "The Precarious Politics of *Precious*: A Close Reading of a Cinematic Text," *Black Camera* 4, no. 1 (winter 2012): 96–116.

81. *16 and Pregnant*, season 1, episode 6, "Catelynn," produced by Morgan J. Freeman, aired July 16, 2009, on MTV.

82. Lynn Cinnamon, "MTV's *16 and Pregnant*—Catelynn Lowell," Starcasm.net, July 17, 2009, http://starcasm.net/archives/8416.

83. *16 and Pregnant*, season 1, episode 6, "Catelynn," produced by Morgan J. Freeman, aired July 16, 2009, on MTV.

84. Ibid.

85. The relationship between the biological and adoptive parents has been taxed in its own ways. For example, in a much later season of *Teen Mom*, adoptive parents

Brandon and Teresa asked that Catelynn and Tyler stop discussing their daughter Carly on the show and social media, or risk their ability to visit with Carly.

86. *16 and Pregnant*, season 1, episode 6, "Catelynn," produced by Morgan J. Freeman, aired July 16, 2009, on MTV.

87. *Glee*, season 1, episode 4, "Preggers," directed by Brad Falchuk, aired September 23, 2009, on Fox.

88. *Glee*, season 1, episode 20, "Theatricality," directed by Brad Falchuk, aired May 25, 2010, on Fox.

89. There are two kinds of surrogacy—traditional and gestational. In traditional surrogacy, the surrogate uses her own egg and is thus considered a biological (genetic and gestational) parent. In gestational surrogacy, the surrogate is impregnated through IVF using another woman's egg; thus, a gestational surrogate does not have a genetic link to the child she bears.

90. Jason Reitman, dir., *Juno* (Fox Searchlight Pictures, 2007).

91. Ibid.

92. *Glee*, season 1, episode 20, "Theatricality," directed by Brad Falchuk, aired May 25, 2010, on Fox.

93. *Glee*, season 1, episode 22, "Journey to Regionals," directed by Brad Falchuk, aired June 8, 2010, on Fox.

94. Kelly E. Happe, *The Material Gene: Gender, Race, and Heredity after the Human Genome Project* (New York: New York University Press, 2013); N. Rose, *Politics of Life Itself*.

95. Kimberly Kelly, "In the Name of the Mother: Renegotiating Conservative Women's Authority in the Crisis Pregnancy Center Movement," *Signs* 38, no. 1 (September 2012): 203–30, https://doi.org/10.1086/665807.

96. Caitlin Bancroft, "What I Learned Undercover at a Crisis Pregnancy Center," Huffington Post, blog, August 15, 2013, www.huffingtonpost.com/caitlin-bancroft/crisis-pregnancy-center_b_3763196.html; K. Kelly, "In the Name of the Mother"; Meaghan Winter, "'Save the Mother, Save the Baby': An Inside Look at a Pregnancy Center Conference," *Cosmopolitan*, April 6, 2015, www.cosmopolitan.com/politics/a38642/heartbeat-international-conference-crisis-pregnancy-centers-abortion/.

97. Akiba Solomon, "The Missionary Movement to 'Save' Black Babies," Colorlines, May 2, 2013, www.colorlines.com/articles/missionary-movement-save-black-babies.

98. Margot Schein and NARAL Pro-Choice North Carolina, Listserv e-mail, "The Truth about CPCs: Targeting Vulnerable Communities," July 18, 2017.

99. Ibid.

100. For example, the national umbrella organizations for individual CPCs banned graphic imagery of fetuses, implemented standardized counseling trainings, and expanded direct services. The medical information distributed at CPCs remains inaccurate, however. Kathryn E. Gilbert, "Commercial Speech in Crisis: Crisis Pregnancy Center Regulations and Definitions of Commercial Speech," *Michigan Law Review* 111, no. 4 (2013): 591–616; K. Kelly, "In the Name of the Mother."

101. Amy G. Bryant and Erika E. Levi, "Abortion Misinformation from Crisis Preg-

nancy Centers in North Carolina," *Contraception* 86, no. 6 (December 2012): 752–56, https://doi.org/10.1016/j.contraception.2012.06.001; Gilbert, "Commercial Speech"; Jennifer Ludden, "States Fund Pregnancy Centers That Discourage Abortion," NPR .org, March 9, 2015, www.npr.org/sections/health-shots/2015/03/09/391877614 /states-fund-pregnancy-centers-that-discourage-abortion; Henry Waxman, "False and Misleading Health Information Provided by Federally Funded Pregnancy Resource Centers" (Washington, DC: U.S. House of Representatives Committee on Government Reform—Minority Staff Special Investigations Division, 2006); Joanne D. Rosen, "The Public Health Risks of Crisis Pregnancy Centers," *Perspectives on Sexual and Reproductive Health* 44, no. 3 (2012): 201–5; Winter, "Save the Mother."

102. NARAL estimates that, as of 2015, CPCs have received a total of 60 million federal dollars. The examples on a state level are numerous: 11 states have "Choose Life" license plates that provide revenue for CPCs, 20 states include CPCs in service referrals, and "at least 23 states have laws supporting CPCs." As of 2005, the State of Texas has directed millions of state dollars from comprehensive family planning providers to crisis pregnancy centers, which remain free of oversight and are not bound by confidentially agreements. In another example, the Minnesota state budget makes $2.4 million available to CPCs annually; 87 percent of these CPCs were found to provide false or inaccurate medical information to women. See Lisa McIntire, *Crisis Pregnancy Centers Lie: The Insidious Threat to Reproductive Freedom* (NARAL Pro-Choice America, 2015), www.prochoiceamerica.org/assets/download-files/cpc-report-2015 .pdf. See also Ludden, "States Fund Pregnancy Centers."

103. Guttmacher Institute, "Fact Sheet: Induced Abortion in the United States," Guttmacher Institute, January 2017, https://www.guttmacher.org/fact-sheet/induced-abortion-united-states; K. Kelly, "In the Name of the Mother"; McIntire, "Crisis Pregnancy Centers."

104. See Johanna Schoen, *Abortion after Roe* (Chapel Hill: University of North Carolina Press, 2015).

105. Willie Parker, *Life's Work: A Moral Argument for Choice* (New York: Atria Books, 2017).

106. Jamilah King, "NYC Anti-Abortion Ad Is Coming Down—but the Real Battle's Just Begun," Text, Colorlines, February 24, 2011, www.colorlines.com/articles /nyc-anti-abortion-ad-coming-down-real-battles-just-begun; Trust Black Women Partnership, "Our Story," Trust Black Women, www.trustblackwomen.org/about -trust-black-women/our-story, accessed July 17, 2017.

107. Akiba Solomon, "9 Reasons to Hate Anti-Abortion Billboards That Target Black Women," Text, Colorlines, February 25, 2011, www.colorlines.com/articles /9-reasons-hate-anti-abortion-billboards-target-black-women.

108. King, "NYC Anti-Abortion Ad"; Thembisa S. Mshaka, "Commentary: Why ThatsAbortion.Com Billboard Is an Ad *Fail*," *Thembisa S. Mshaka* (blog), February 24, 2011, https://thembisamshaka.com/2011/02/24/commentary-why-thatsabortion -com-billboard-is-an-ad-fail/; Parker, *Life's Work*; Solomon, "9 Reasons."

109. Parker, *Life's Work*.

110. Solomon, "9 Reasons."

111. Parker, *Life's Work*.

112. Ellison and Martin, "Nearly Dying in Childbirth"; Martin and Montagne, "Black Mothers."

113. Quoted in Winter, "Save the Mother."

114. Guttmacher Institute, "Last Five Years Account for More than One-Quarter of All Abortion Restrictions Enacted since Roe," Guttmacher.org, January 13, 2016, www.guttmacher.org/media/inthenews/2016/01/13/index.html.

115. A Fund Inc. (Kentucky) et al., "Letter to Congress," July 27, 2015, www.apha.org/~/media/files/pdf/advocacy/letters/2015/150727_plannedparenthood.ashx.

116. Jennifer J. Frost, "Response to Inquiry Concerning Geographic Service Availability from Planned Parenthood Health Center" (New York: Guttmacher Institute, August 14, 2015), www.guttmacher.org/pubs/guttmacher-cbo-memo-2015.pdf; Planned Parenthood Action Fund, "The Cost of Defunding Planned Parenthood," September 9, 2015, https://istandwithpp.org/facts/cost-defunding-planned-parenthood/.

117. Ludden, "States Fund Pregnancy Centers"; Liz Szabo and Laura Ungar, "Family Planning Budgets in Crisis before Planned Parenthood Controversy," *USA Today*, July 31, 2015, www.usatoday.com/story/news/2015/07/30/family-planning-budgets-crisis-before-planned-parenthood-controversy/30861853/.

118. Leadership Conference on Civil and Human Rights, et al., letter to Congress, "Stand Up for Women's Access to Healthcare Services: Oppose All Efforts to Defund Planned Parenthood," July 31, 2015, https://lulac.org/advocacy/PPFADefunding Letter7-31.pdf.

119. National Abortion Federation, "NAF Violence and Disruption Statistics," 2015, http://prochoice.org/education-and-advocacy/violence/violence-statistics-and-history/.

120. At this writing, the most recent data available are from 2014 (the Guttmacher Institute gathers data every three years). As Rachel Jones confirmed in personal correspondence to the author, 2017 data should be released in 2019 (e-mail to author, July 17, 2017). Rachel K. Jones and Jenna Jerman, "Abortion Incidence and Service Availability in the United States, 2014," *Perspectives on Sexual and Reproductive Health* 49, no. 1 (March 1, 2017): 17–27, https://doi.org/10.1363/psrh.12015.

Conclusion: Just Pregnancy, Just Parenting in the Age of Homeland Maternity

1. Jane Doe's name and country of origin are unspecified here and in public and legal discourses due to her status as a minor.

2. American Civil Liberties Union, "After a Month of Obstruction by the Trump Administration, Jane Doe Gets Her Abortion," American Civil Liberties Union, October 25, 2017, https://www.aclu.org/news/after-month-obstruction-trump-administration-jane-doe-gets-her-abortion.

3. Jane's Due Process "ensur[es] legal representation for pregnant minors in Texas" (https://janesdueprocess.org/).

4. Quoted in Nina Rabin and Roxana Bacon, "Women on the Run," *Ms.* 27, no. 2 (summer 2017): 21.

5. Tina Vasquez, "Immigrant Minor Held 'Hostage' in Texas Because She Wants Abortion Care," Rewire, October 11, 2017, https://rewire.news/article/2017/10/11/immigrant-minor-held-hostage-texas-wants-abortion-care/.

6. Tina Vasquez, "'Anti-Choice Fanaticism' in the U.S. Immigration System: The Real Reason Jane Doe's Abortion Request Is Being Denied," Rewire, October 16, 2017, https://rewire.news/article/2017/10/16/anti-choice-fanaticism-u-s-immigration-system-real-reason-jane-abortion-request-denied/.

7. Ibid.

8. Quoted in Tina Vasquez, "Teenage Immigrant Forced by Government to Remain Pregnant," Rewire, October 20, 2017, https://rewire.news/article/2017/10/20/teenage-immigrant-forced-remain-pregnant/. T. Vasquez, "Teenage Immigrant."

9. United Health Foundation, "America's Health Rankings: Maternal Mortality," America's Health Rankings, 2018, https://www.americashealthrankings.org/explore/2018-health-of-women-and-children-report/measure/maternal_mortality/state/ALL; T. Vasquez, "Teenage Immigrant."

10. Center for Reproductive Rights, "House Committee Rejects Bare Minimum Exceptions to Dangerous Bill Restricting Abortion Access for Teens," Center for Reproductive Rights, March 28, 2012, https://www.reproductiverights.org/press-room/house-committee-rejects-bare-minimum-exceptions-to-dangerous-bill-restricting-abortion-ac; Cristina Marcos, "Bill Would Ban Abortions across State Lines," Text, Hill, February 9, 2015, http://thehill.com/blogs/floor-action/house/232155-bill-would-ban-abortions-across-state-lines; Brian Naylor, "Senate Limits Interstate Abortions for Minors," *Morning Edition*, NPR, July 26, 2006, https://www.npr.org/templates/story/story.php?storyId=5582615; Jen Quraishi, "New Act Prohibits Minors Traveling for Abortions," *Mother Jones* (blog), June 22, 2011, https://www.motherjones.com/politics/2011/06/new-act-prohibits-minors-traveling-abortions/.

11. Layidua Salazar, "Activist's Detainment Reminds Us Immigration Is a Reproductive Justice Issue," Rewire, March 12, 2108, https://rewire.news/article/2018/03/12/activists-detainment-reminds-us-immigration-reproductive-justice-issue/.

12. Quoted in American Civil Liberties Union, "ACLU Sues Obama Administration for Detaining Asylum Seekers as Intimidation Tactic," American Civil Liberties Union, December 16, 2014, https://www.aclu.org/news/aclu-sues-obama-administration-detaining-asylum-seekers-intimidation-tactic.

13. A federal judge in *RILR v. Johnson* ruled in favor of asylum seekers in 2015, capping at twenty the number of days that US Immigration and Customs Enforcement (ICE) can detain asylum seekers. Despite this, reports of women and children languishing in detention centers for a year or longer persist. American Civil Liberties Union, "*RILR v. Johnson*," *American Civil Liberties Union*, July 31, 2015, https://www.aclu.org/cases/rilr-v

-johnson?redirect=immigrants-rights/rilr-v-johnson; Valeria Fernández, "Moms Go on a Hunger Strike to Get Themselves and Their Kids out of Immigration Detention," Public Radio International, August 25, 2016, https://www.pri.org/stories/2016-08-25/madres-berks-are-hunger-strike-get-their-kids-out-immigration-detention.

14. Quoted in Rabin and Bacon, "Women on the Run," 21.

15. For more on stratified reproduction, see Shellee Colen, "'With Respect and Feelings': Voices of West Indian Child Care Workers in New York City," in *All American Women: Lines That Divide, Ties That Bind*, ed. Johnnetta Cole (New York: Free Press, 1986), 46–70; Faye D. Ginsburg and Rayna Rapp, eds., *Conceiving the New World Order: The Global Politics of Reproduction* (Berkeley: University of California Press, 1995).

16. See G. Thomas Goodnight, "The Personal, Technical, and Public Spheres of Argument: A Speculative Inquiry into the Art of Public Deliberation," *Journal of the American Forensic Association* 18 (1982): 214–27; Carolyn R. Miller, "Risk, Controversy, and Rhetoric: Response to Goodnight," *Argumentation and Advocacy* 42 (2005): 34–37.

17. Roberts, *Killing the Black Body*; Shome, *Diana and Beyond*; Solinger, *Pregnancy and Power*.

18. Amy Gastelum, "Purvi Patel Faces 20 Years in Prison for Feticide and Child Neglect," Public Radio International, March 31, 2015, https://www.pri.org/stories/2015-03-30/purvi-patel-faces-20-years-prison-feticide-and-child-neglect; Jessica Glenza, "Purvi Patel Case: Legal Experts Warn on Reproductive Rights in Indiana," *Guardian*, April 2, 2015, sec. US news, www.theguardian.com/us-news/2015/apr/02/purvi-patel-case-alter-reproductive-rights-indiana.

19. Emily Bazelon, "Purvi Patel Could Be Just the Beginning," *New York Times Magazine*, April 1, 2015, www.nytimes.com; Kelli Stopczynski, "Lawyer Wants Woman's Feticide Charge Dropped, Some Evidence Excluded," WSBT, November 20, 2014, wsbt.com/news/local/lawyer-wants-womans-feticide-charge-dropped-some-evidence-excluded.

20. Paltrow and Flavin, "Arrests of and Forced Interventions."

21. Sharona Coutts, "Anti-Choice Groups Use Smartphone Surveillance to Target 'Abortion-Minded Women' during Clinic Visits," Rewire, May 25, 2016, https://rewire.news/article/2016/05/25/anti-choice-groups-deploy-smartphone-surveillance-target-abortion-minded-women-clinic-visits/.

22. Brief Amici Curiae Supporting Petitioners, *Whole Woman's Health v. Cole*, No. 15-274 (Supreme Court of the United States 2016).

23. Jessica Robinson, "Idaho Woman Arrested for Abortion Is Uneasy Case for Both Sides," NPR, April 9, 2012, www.npr.org/templates/story/story.php?storyId=150312812.

24. Lynn O'Brien Hallstein, *Bikini-Ready Moms: Celebrity Profiles, Motherhood, and the Body* (Albany: State University of New York Press, 2015).

25. Waggoner, *Zero Trimester*.

26. CDC Principal deputy director Anne Schuchat, quoted in U.S. Centers for Disease Control and Prevention, "More than 3 Million."

27. Graham, "This Chicago Doctor."

28. For an excellent primer on reproductive justice, see Ross and Solinger, *Reproductive Justice*.

29. See Forward Together, "What Is Reproductive Justice?"; Ross, "Movement for Reproductive Justice"; SPARK Reproductive Justice Now, "Guiding Principles and Central Voices," accessed October 28, 2011, http://sparkrj.org/content/about/guiding principlesandcentralvoices; Young Women United, "Why We Do YWU: Young Women United's Vision of Purpose," accessed October 20, 2011, www.youngwomenunited .org/whoweare/whywedoywu.html.

30. Dorothy Roberts, *Shattered Bonds: The Color of Child Welfare* (New York: Basic Civitas Books, 2003); Solinger, *Beggars and Choosers*. See Jane Jeong Trenka et al., "Transnational and Transracial Adoption: The Right of Poor Women of Color to Keep and Raise Their Children," in *Reproductive Justice Briefing Book: A Primer on Reproductive Justice and Social Change*, ed. SisterSong Women of Color Reproductive Health Collective (n.p.: n.p., 2007), 56.

31. See Forward Together, "A New Vision for Advancing Our Movement for Reproductive Health, Reproductive Rights and Reproductive Justice" (Oakland: Asian Communities for Reproductive Justice, 2005), https://forwardtogether.org/tools /a-new-vision/; Sistas on the Rise, "Sistas on the Rise Herstory," accessed October 20, 2011, http://sistasontherise.com/About%20Us.shtml.

32. For an impressive summary of these efforts, see Sara Hayden, "Family Metaphors and the Nation: Promoting a Politics of Care through the Million Mom March," *Quarterly Journal of Speech* 89, no. 3 (January 2003): 196–215, doi:10.1080/0033563032 000125313. These forms of co-optation are in many ways similar to Gayatri Spivak's concept of strategic essentialism. Given the controversy surrounding this term, however, and its tendency to be misconstrued as essentializing, I offer co-optation for its rhetoricity—its foregrounding of contingency and malleability of identity categories, and its availability to adaptation in specific locales and contexts. See Gayatri Spivak, *The Spivak Reader: Selected Works of Gayatri Spivak*, ed. Donna Landry and MacLean (New York: Routledge, 1996).

33. Hayden, "Family Metaphors," 197.

34. Lindal Buchanan, *Rhetorics of Motherhood*, Studies in Rhetorics and Feminisms (Carbondale: Southern Illinois University Press, 2013); Valeria Fabj, "Motherhood as Political Voice: The Rhetoric of the Mothers of Plaza de Mayo," *Communication Studies* 44, no. 1 (March 1993): 1–18, https://doi.org/10.1080/10510979309368379; Lillian Faderman, *To Believe in Women: What Lesbians Have Done for America—A History* (Boston: Houghton Mifflin, 1999); Hayden, "Family Metaphors"; Mari Boor Tonn, "Militant Motherhood: Labor's Mary Harris 'Mother' Jones," *Quarterly Journal of Speech* 82 (1996): 1–21; Isaac West, "Performing Resistance in/from the Kitchen: The Practice of Maternal Pacifist Politics and la WISP's Cookbooks," *Women's Studies in Communication* 30, no. 3 (fall 2007).

35. Janis L. Edwards and Amanda Leigh Brozana, "Gendering Anti-War Rhetoric:

Cindy Sheehan's Symbolic Motherhood," *Journal of the Northwest Communication Association* 37 (2008): 78–102; Laura Knudson, "Cindy Sheehan and the Rhetoric of Motherhood: A Textual Analysis," *Peace and Change* 34, no. 2 (April 2009): 164–83; Valerie Palmer-Mehta, "Subversive Maternities: Staceyann Chin's Contemplative Voice," *QED: A Journal in GLBTQ Worldmaking* 3, no. 1 (2016): 34–60; Jennifer A. Peeples and Kevin M. DeLuca, "The Truth of the Matter: Motherhood, Community and Environmental Justice," *Women's Studies in Communication* 29, no. 1 (2006): 59–87, https://doi.org/10.1080/07491409.2006.10757628; Kenrya Rankin, "Black Lives Matter Partners with Reproductive Justice Groups to Fight for Black Women," Text, Colorlines, February 9, 2016, https://www.colorlines.com/articles/black-lives-matter-partners-reproductive-justice-groups-fight-black-women; Don Romesburg, "Where She Comes From: Locating Queer Transracial Adoption," *QED: A Journal in GLBTQ Worldmaking* 1, no. 3 (2014): 1–29. Christopher Scott Thomas, "The Mothers of East Los Angeles: (Other) Mothering for Environmental Justice." *Southern Communication* (2018): 1–17.

36. "MomsRising," MomsRising.org, accessed June 3, 2016, www.momsrising.org/.

37. Buchanan, *Rhetorics*. See also Roberts, *Killing the Black Body*.

38. Buchanan, *Rhetorics*.

39. I am indebted to Julia T. Wood for this insight, who reminded me of our encounters with these activists while reading a draft of this conclusion (June 2016).

40. Kenneth Burke, *Permanence and Change: An Anatomy of Purpose*, 3rd ed. (Berkeley: University of California Press, 1984).

41. See, for example, Anne Teresa Demo, "The Guerrilla Girls' Comic Politics of Subversion," *Women's Studies in Communication* 23, no. 2 (2000): 133–56; Bonnie J. Dow, "AIDS, Perspective by Incongruity, and Gay Identity in Larry Kramer's '1,112 and Counting,'" *Communication Studies* 45 (1994): 225–40; Tasha N. Dubriwny, "Consciousness-Raising as Collective Rhetoric: The Articulation of Experience in the Redstockings' Abortion Speak-Out of 1969," *Quarterly Journal of Speech* 91, no. 4 (11): 395–422.

42. Buchanan, *Rhetorics*; Hayden, "Family Metaphors."

43. Sandra Davidson and Anita Rao, *She and Her: Thank You, More Please*, aired May 7, 2016, https://www.acast.com/sheher/episode19-thankyou-moreplease?autoplay; Last, *What to Expect When No One's Expecting*; Charity Nebbe, "Talk of Iowa on Iowa Public Radio," *Childless by Choice*, March 4, 2016, http://iowapublicradio.org/post/childless-choice#stream/0; Sandler and Witteman, "None Is Enough"; Jessica Valenti, *Why Have Kids?: A New Mom Explores the Truth about Parenting and Happiness* (Boston: New Harvest, 2012).

44. Sara Hayden, "Constituting Savvy Aunties: From Childless Women to Child-Focused Consumers," *Women's Studies in Communication* 34, no. 1 (May 5, 2011): 1–19, https://doi.org/10.1080/07491409.2011.566531.

45. See, for example, Dubriwny, *Vulnerable Empowered Woman*; Hundley and Hayden, *Mediated Moms*; Lopez, "Radical Act"; Palmer-Mehta, "Subversive Maternities."

46. Andrea O'Reilly, ed., *Feminist Mothering* (Albany: State University of New York

Press, 2008); Andrea O'Reilly, *Maternal Theory: Essential Readings* (Toronto: Demeter, 2007).

47. Tasha N. Dubriwny, "Mommy Blogs and the Disruptive Possibilities of Transgressive Drinking," in Hundley and Hayden, *Mediated Moms*, 203–20; Lopez, "Radical Act"; Valerie Palmer-Mehta and Sherianne Shuler, "'Devil Mamas' of Social Media: Resistant Maternal Discourses in Sanctimommy," in Hundley and Hayden, *Mediated Moms*, 221–46.

48. Susana Martínez Guillem and Lisa A. Flores, "Maternal Transgressions, Racial Regressions: How Whiteness Mediates the (Worst) White Moms," in Hundley and Hayden, *Mediated Moms*, 79.

49. Luibhéid, *Entry Denied*.

50. Ibid., xi. See also Eithne Luibhéid, *Pregnant on Arrival: Making the Illegal Immigrant* (Minneapolis: University of Minnesota Press, 2013).

51. Palmer-Mehta, "Subversive Maternities"; Hundley and Hayden, *Mediated Moms*; Alexis Pauline Gumbs, China Martens, and Mai'a Williams, eds., *Revolutionary Mothering: Love on the Front Lines* (Oakland, CA: PM Press, 2016).

52. Palmer-Mehta, "Subversive Maternities," 35.

53. Thomas Beatie's story has been thoughtfully explored by scholars from different disciplines. See Paisley Currah, "Expecting Bodies: The Pregnant Man and Transgender Exclusion from the Employment Non-Discrimination Act," *Women's Studies Quarterly* 36, nos. 3–4 (fall–winter 2008): 330–36; Jamie Landau, "Reproducing and Transgressing Masculinity: A Rhetorical Analysis of Women Interacting with Digital Photographs of Thomas Beatie," *Women's Studies in Communication* 35, no. 2 (2012): 178–203; Laura Nixon, "The Right to (Trans) Parent: A Reproductive Justice Approach to Reproductive Rights, Fertility, and Family-Building Issues Facing Transgender People," *William & Mary Journal of Women and the Law* 20 (2013): 73–103; Damien W. Riggs, "What Makes a Man? Thomas Beatie, Embodiment, and 'Mundane Transphobia,'" *Feminism and Psychology* 24, no. 2 (2014): 157–71. Although Beatie's story meets some of the qualifications for inclusion in this study (i.e., a controversy centered on reproduction that garnered significant attention in dominant discourse), the rationalities and rhetorics of homeland security culture were conspicuously absent. Unlike other cases featured in this book, dominant discourses treated Beatie's story seriously for its challenging of reproductive normativities while also simultaneously trafficking in carnivalesque voyeurism. Perhaps Beatie was thus rendered too anomalous to "threaten" the nation in the ways that other cases studied in this book were imagined to do.

54. Schmidt, "Organization Marks 25 Years."

55. Monica R. Basile, "Reproductive Justice and Childbirth Reform: Doulas as Agents of Social Change" (University of Iowa, 2012), http://ir.uiowa.edu/etd/2819; Paltrow and Flavin, "Arrests of and Forced Interventions"; Prison Birth Project, "About," Prison Birth Project, accessed July 19, 2016, http://theprisonbirthproject.org/about/.

56. Collins, *Black Feminist Thought*.

57. See, for example, D. O. Braithwaite et al., "Constructing Family: A Typology of Voluntary Kin," *Journal of Social and Personal Relationships* 27, no. 3 (May 1, 2010): 388–407, https://doi.org/10.1177/0265407510361615.

58. Dow, "Michelle Obama."

59. Romesburg, "Where She Comes From," 3.

60. Ibid., 7.

61. Imagining a more radical undoing has its merits, of course, as in scholarship that advocates for an embrace of a queer, unintelligible futurity that is adamantly untethered to redemptive reproductive futurity, or that which critiques citizenship itself for its constellation of problematics and concerns. See, for example, Amy L. Brandzel, *Against Citizenship: The Violence of the Normative* (Urbana: University of Illinois Press, 2016); Lee Edelman, *No Future: Queer Theory and the Death Drive* (Durham, NC: Duke University Press, 2004).

62. See, for example, Palmer-Mehta, "Subversive Maternities"; Piepmeier, "Inadequacy of 'Choice'"; Romesburg, "Where She Comes From"; Isaac West, *Transforming Citizenships: Transgender Articulations of the Law* (New York: New York University Press, 2014).

63. This is a rich tradition in rhetorical studies. In addition to the feminist rhetorical scholars that I cite throughout this book, this critical impulse is illustrated in various areas of the discipline. See, for example, Bennett and Morris, "Rhetorical Criticism's Multitudes"; J. Robert Cox, "Argument and Environmental Advocacy," *Controversia: An International Journal of Debate and Democratic Renewal* 1 (fall 2002): 82–85; J. Robert Cox, "Nature's 'Crisis Disciplines': Does Environmental Communication Have an Ethical Duty?," *Environmental Communication* 1, no. 1 (May 2007): 5–20, https://doi.org/10.1080/17524030701333948; Ivie, "Productive Criticism"; Ivie, "Productive Criticism Then and Now"; Phaedra C. Pezzullo, *Toxic Tourism: Rhetorics of Pollution, Travel, and Environmental Justice* (Tuscaloosa: University of Alabama Press, 2007); West, *Transforming Citizenships*.

64. See, for example, Dow, "Michelle Obama"; Hayden, "Family Metaphors"; George Lakoff, *Moral Politics: How Liberals and Conservatives Think*, 2nd ed. (Chicago: University of Chicago Press, 2002).

Bibliography

Abbott, Kate. "Forever 21 Launches Maternity Line—Is It Targeted at Teens?" *Time*, July 21, 2010. http://newsfeed.time.com/2010/07/21/forever-21-launches-maternity-line-for-teens/.

Abrao, Mauricio S., Ludovico Muzii, and Riccardo Marana. "Anatomical Causes of Female Infertility and Their Management." *International Journal of Gynaecology and Obstetrics: The Official Organ of the International Federation of Gynaecology and Obstetrics* 123, suppl. 2 (December 2013): S18–24. https://doi.org/10.1016/j.ijgo.2013.09.008.

Adams, Heather Brook. "Rhetorics of Unwed Motherhood and Shame." *Women's Studies in Communication* 40, no. 1 (January 2, 2017): 91–110. https://doi.org/10.1080/07491409.2016.1247401.

Adams, Kathleen, and Bruce Crumley. "Health Report." *Time*, March 10, 1997.

A Fund Inc. (Kentucky), Abortion Care Network, Access Matters, Access Reproductive Care-Southeast ACCESS Women's Health Justice (California) Advocates for Youth, Alabama Reproductive Rights Advocates, American Association of University Women (AAUW), American Civil Liberties Union, et al. "Letter to Congress." July 27, 2015. www.apha.org/~/media/files/pdf/advocacy/letters/2015/150727_plannedparenthood.ashx.

Albert, Bill. "With One Voice 2010: America's Adults and Teens Sound Off about Teen Pregnancy." Washington, DC: National Campaign to Prevent Teen and Unplanned Pregnancy, 2010.

Almeling, Rene, Joanann Radien, and Sarah S. Richardson. "Egg-Freezing a Better Deal for Companies than for Women." Opinion, CNN, October 20, 2014. www.cnn.com/2014/10/20/opinion/almeling-radin-richardson-egg-freezing/.

American Civil Liberties Union. "ACLU Sues Obama Administration for Detaining Asylum Seekers as Intimidation Tactic." American Civil Liberties Union, December 16, 2014. https://www.aclu.org/news/aclu-sues-obama-administration-detaining-asylum-seekers-intimidation-tactic.

———. "After a Month of Obstruction by the Trump Administration, Jane Doe Gets Her Abortion." American Civil Liberties Union, October 25, 2017. https://www.aclu.org/news/after-month-obstruction-trump-administration-jane-doe-gets-her-abortion.

———."*RILR v. Johnson*." American Civil Liberties Union, July 31, 2015. https://www.aclu.org/cases/rilr-v-johnson.

American College of Obstetricians and Gynecologists. "Oocyte Preservation. Committee Opinion No. 584." *Obstetrics and Gynecology* 123 (January 2014): 221–22.

American Society for Emergency Contraception. "Inching towards Progress: ASEC's 2015 Pharmacy Access Study." American Society for Emergency Contraception, December 2015. http://americansocietyforec.org/uploads/3/4/5/6/34568220/asec_2015_ec_access_report_1.pdf.

American Society for Reproductive Medicine. "Frequently Asked Questions about Infertility." American Society for Reproductive Medicine, 2016. www.asrm.org/awards/index.aspx?id=3012.

———. "Practice Committee Guidelines." 2011. www.asrm.org/Guidelines/.

Anderson, Benedict. *Imagined Communities: Reflections on the Origin and Spread of Nationalism*. London: Verso, 1983.

Andrejevic, Mark. "Interactive (In)Security: The Participatory Promise of Ready.Gov." *Cultural Studies* 20, nos. 4–5 (2006): 441–58.

———. "The Kinder, Gentler Gaze of Big Brother: Reality TV in the Era of Digital Capitalism." *New Media and Society* 4, no. 2 (2002): 251–70.

———. "'Securitainment' in the Post-9/11 Era." *Continuum: Journal of Media and Cultural Studies* 25, no. 2 (2011): 165–75.

Antecol, Heather. "The Opt-Out Revolution: Recent Trends in Female Labor Supply." *Research in Labor Economics* 33 (2011): 45–83.

Arab American Institute. "AAI Issue Brief: Hate Crimes." Arab American Institute, http://www.aaiusa.org/aai_issue_brief_hate_crimes. Accessed August 2, 2018.

Aradau, Claudia, and Rens Van Munster. "Taming the Future: The Dispositif of Risk in the War on Terror." In *Risk and the War on Terror*, edited by Louise Amoore and Marieke de Goede, 23–40. New York: Routledge, 2008.

Argyle, Catrin E., Joyce C. Harper, and Melanie C. Davies. "Oocyte Cryopreservation: Where Are We Now?" *Human Reproduction Update* 22, no. 4 (June 2016): 440–49. https://doi.org/10.1093/humupd/dmw007.

"Arkansas Woman Has 15th Child." *NBC News*, May 25, 2004. www.nbcnews.com/id/5060048/#.UZz2t5WRCos.

Arrillaga, Pauline. "Some 'Lost Birds' Fly Away Home." *Los Angeles Times*, July 15, 2001.

Aschwanden, Christie. "Fertility 101." *Marie Claire*, February 2009.

ASIS International and Institute of Finance and Management. "The United States Security Industry: Size and Scope, Insights, Trends, and Data." Alexandria, VA: ASIS International, 2013.

Aubrey, Jennifer Stevens, Elizabeth Behm-Morawitz, and Kyungbo Kim. "Understanding the Effects of MTV's *16 and Pregnant* on Adolescent Girls' Beliefs, Attitudes, and Behavioral Intentions toward Teen Pregnancy." *Journal of Health Communication* 19, no. 10 (October 3, 2014): 1145–60. https://doi.org/10.1080/10810730.2013.872721.

Bailey, Alison. "Reconceiving Surrogacy: Toward a Reproductive Justice Account of Indian Surrogacy." *Hypatia* 26, no. 4 (2011): 715–41.

Bancroft, Caitlin. "What I Learned Undercover at a Crisis Pregnancy Center." Blog, Huffington Post, August 15, 2013. www.huffingtonpost.com/caitlin-bancroft/crisis-pregnancy-center_b_3763196.html.

Basile, Monica R. "Reproductive Justice and Childbirth Reform: Doulas as Agents of Social Change." University of Iowa, 2012. http://ir.uiowa.edu/etd/2819.

Bates, Karen Grigsby. "Octuplets Make 14 for Mom, Stirring Debate." *All Things Considered*. NPR, January 30, 2009.

Baumgardner, Jennifer. "Would You Pledge Your Virginity to Your Father?" *Glamour*, January 1, 2007. www.glamour.com.

Bazelon, Emily. "Purvi Patel Could Be Just the Beginning." *New York Times Magazine*, April 1, 2015. www.nytimes.com.

Beck, Ulrich. "Living in the World Risk Society." *Economy and Society* 35, no. 3 (2006): 329–45.

———. *World at Risk*. Translated by Ciaran Cronin. Malden, MA: Polity, 2009.

Becker, Ron. "'Help Is on the Way!': *Supernanny*, *Nanny 911*, and the Neoliberal Politics of the Family." In *The Great American Makeover: Television, History, Nation*, edited by Dana Heller, 175–92. New York: Palgrave Macmillan, 2006.

"Being Angelina Not an Easy Role." *Chicago Tribune*, February 12, 2009.

Belkin, Lisa. "The Opt-Out Revolution." *New York Times Magazine*, October 26, 2003.

Bellafante, Ginia. "In Documentary, an Obsessed 'Octomom.'" *New York Times*, August 20, 2009.

———. "Real Life Is Like 'Juno,' Except Maybe the Dialogue." *New York Times*, June 11, 2009.

Bennett, Jeffrey A. *Banning Queer Blood: Rhetorics of Citizenship, Contagion, and Resistance*. Tuscaloosa: University of Alabama Press, 2009.

———. "Troubled Interventions: Public Policy, Vectors of Disease, and the Rhetoric of Diabetes Management." *Journal of Medical Humanities* 34, no. 1 (March 2013): 15–32. https://doi.org/10.1007/s10912-012-9198-0.

Bennett, Jeffrey A., and Charles E. Morris, eds. "Rhetorical Criticism's Multitudes." Special issue, *Review of Communication* 16, no. 1 (January 2, 2016): 1–107.

Beresford, Annette D. "Homeland Security as an American Ideology: Implications for U.S. Policy and Action." *Journal of Homeland Security and Emergency Management* 1, no. 3 (January 1, 2004). https://doi.org/10.2202/1547-7355.1042.

Biesecker, Barbara A. "Homeland Security [Special Section]." *Communication and Critical/Cultural Studies* 4, no. 2 (2007): 204–31.

Bjerklie, David, Alice Park, and Sora Song. "A to Z Guide." *Time*, January 19, 2004.

Bleyer, Jennifer. "Should You Freeze Your Eggs?" *Cosmopolitan*, January 2012.

Boodman, Sandra G. "The 'Morning-After' Kit; New Emergency Contraceptive Gives Women a Second Chance to Prevent Pregnancy." *Washington Post*, September 22, 1998, final edition, sec. Health.

Boonstra, Heather D. "Advocates Call for a New Approach after the Era of Abstinence-Only Sex Education." *Guttmacher Policy Review* 12, no. 1 (2009): 6–11.

———. "Meeting the Sexual and Reproductive Health Needs of Adolescents in School-Based Health Centers." *Guttmacher Policy Review* 18, no. 1 (2015): 21–26.

Boushey, Heather. *Are Women Opting Out? Debunking the Myth*. Washington, DC: Center for Economic and Policy Research, 2005. http://cepr.net/documents/publications/opt_out_2005_11_2.pdf.

Braithwaite, D. O., B. W. Bach, L. A. Baxter, R. DiVerniero, J. R. Hammonds, A. M. Hosek, E. K. Willer, and B. M. Wolf. "Constructing Family: A Typology of Voluntary Kin." *Journal of Social and Personal Relationships* 27, no. 3 (May 1, 2010): 388–407. https://doi.org/10.1177/0265407510361615.

Brandzel, Amy L. *Against Citizenship: The Violence of the Normative*. Urbana: University of Illinois Press, 2016.

Brice, Arthur. "Guatemalan Army Stole Children for Adoption, Report Says." International CNN, April 4, 2012. http://edition.cnn.com/2009/world/americas/09/12/guatemala.child.abduction/index.html.

Brief Amici Curiae Supporting Petitioners. *Whole Woman's Health v. Cole*, No. 15-274 (Supreme Court of the United States 2016).

Briggs, Laura. *Somebody's Children: The Politics of Transracial and Transnational Adoption*. Durham, NC: Duke University Press, 2012.

Brown, Joanna D., Sion Kim Harris, Elizabeth R. Woods, Matthew P. Buman, and Joanne E. Cox. "Longitudinal Study of Depressive Symptoms and Social Support in Adolescent Mothers." *Maternal and Child Health Journal* 16, no. 4 (May 2012): 894–901. https://doi.org/10.1007/s10995-011-0814-9.

Brown, Liz. "Octomom Nadya Suleman's 'The View' Appearance Evokes Criticism, Anger." *View Examiner*, February 25, 2009.

Bryant, Amy G., and Erika E. Levi. "Abortion Misinformation from Crisis Pregnancy Centers in North Carolina." *Contraception* 86, no. 6 (December 2012): 752–56. https://doi.org/10.1016/j.contraception.2012.06.001.

Buchanan, Lindal. *Rhetorics of Motherhood*. Studies in Rhetorics and Feminisms. Carbondale: Southern Illinois University Press, 2013.

Burke, Kenneth. *Permanence and Change: An Anatomy of Purpose*. 3rd ed. Berkeley: University of California Press, 1984.

Butler, Judith. *Precarious Life: The Powers of Mourning and Violence*. New York: Verso, 2006.

Cadena, Micaela, Raquel Z. Rivera, Tannia Esparza, and Denicia Cadena. *Dismantling*

Teen Pregnancy Prevention. Albuquerque, NM: Young Women United, 2016. www.youngwomenunited.org/wp-content/uploads/2016/05/ywu-dismantlingtpp-may2016-digital.pdf.

Calafell, Bernadette Marie. *Monstrosity, Performance, and Race in Contemporary Culture*. New York: Peter Lang, 2015.

"California Woman Gives Birth to Rare Octuplets." CBSNews, January 26, 2009. www.cbsnews.com/news/calif-woman-gives-birth-to-rare-octuplets/.

Caplan, Arthur. "Ethics and Octuplets: Society Is Responsible." *Philadelphia Inquirer*, February 6, 2009.

Carmon, Irin. "MTV's Abortion Special Didn't Disappoint." *Jezebel*, December 29, 2010. https://jezebel.com/5720450/mtvs-abortion-special-didnt-disappoint.

Casper, Monica J., and Laura M. Carpenter. "Sex, Drugs, and Politics: The HPV Vaccine for Cervical Cancer." *Sociology of Health and Illness* 30, no. 6 (September 2008): 886–99. https://doi.org/10.1111/j.1467-9566.2008.01100.x.

Celizic, Mike. "First Look: Octuplet Mom Shows Off Babies." Today, February 10, 2009. www.today.com/id/29086126/ns/today-parenting_and_family/t/first-look-octuplet-mom-shows-babies/.

Center for Reproductive Rights. "House Committee Rejects Bare Minimum Exceptions to Dangerous Bill Restricting Abortion Access for Teens." Center for Reproductive Rights, March 28, 2012. https://www.reproductiverights.org/press-room/house-committee-rejects-bare-minimum-exceptions-to-dangerous-bill-restricting-abortion-ac.

Centers for Disease Control and Prevention. "National Survey of Family Growth." Centers for Disease Control and Prevention, February 14, 2011.

Chavarro, Jorge E., Walter C. Willett, and Patrick J. Skerrett. "Fertility & Diet: How What You Eat Affects Your Odds of Getting Pregnant." *Newsweek*, December 10, 2007.

Chavarro, Jorge E., Walter C. Willett, and Patrick J. Skerrett. *The Fertility Diet: Groundbreaking Research Reveals Natural Ways to Boost Ovulation and Improve Your Chances of Getting Pregnant*. New York: McGraw-Hill, 2008.

Cheyney, Melissa, Marit Bovbjerg, Courtney Everson, Wendy Gordon, Darcy Hannibal, and Saraswathi Vedam. "Outcomes of Care for 16,924 Planned Home Births in the United States: The Midwives Alliance of North America Statistics Project, 2004 to 2009." *Journal of Midwifery and Women's Health* 59, no. 1 (January 2014): 17–27. https://doi.org/10.1111/jmwh.12172.

Cho, Connie. "Regulating Assisted Reproductive Technology." *Yale Journal of Medicine and Law* 7, no. 1 (2010): 40–41.

Choy, Catherine Ceniza. *Global Families: A History of Asian International Adoption in America*. New York: New York University Press, 2013.

Chung, Andrew. "Supreme Court Lifts Block on Wisconsin 'Cocaine Mom' Law during Appeal." Reuters, July 7, 2017. www.reuters.com.

Cinnamon, Lynn. "MTV's *16 and Pregnant*–Catelynn Lowell." Starcasm, July 17, 2009. http://starcasm.net/archives/8416.

Cisneros, Natalie. "'Alien' Sexuality: Race, Maternity, and Citizenship." *Hypatia* 28, no. 2 (2013): 290–306.

Cohany, Sharon R., and Emy Sok. "Trends in Labor Force Participation of Married Mothers of Infants." *Monthly Labor Review*, February 2007, 9–16.

Cohn, D'Vera. "Divorce and the Great Recession." *Pew Research Center's Social and Demographic Trends Project* (blog), May 2, 2012. www.pewsocialtrends.org/2012/05/02/divorce-and-the-great-recession/.

Colen, Shellee. "'With Respect and Feelings': Voices of West Indian Child Care Workers in New York City." In *All American Women: Lines That Divide, Ties That Bind*, edited by Johnnetta Cole, 46–70. New York: Free Press, 1986.

Colino, Stacey. "Are You Gambling with Your Fertility?" *Shape*, June 2012.

Collins, Patricia Hill. *Black Feminist Thought: Knowledge, Consciousness, and the Politics of Empowerment*. 2nd ed. New York: Routledge, 2000.

———. *Black Sexual Politics: African Americans, Gender, and the New Racism*. New York: Routledge, 2005.

Condit, Celeste. *Decoding Abortion Rhetoric: Communicating Social Change*. Urbana: University of Illinois Press, 1990.

Coontz, Stephanie. "The Myth of the Opt-Out Mom." *Christian Science Monitor*, March 30, 2006.

———. *The Way We Never Were: American Families and the Nostalgia Trap*. New York: Basic Books, 1992.

Cotter, David, Paula England, and Joan Hermsen. "Moms and Jobs: Trends in Mothers' Employment and Which Mothers Stay Home." Coral Gables, FL: Council on Contemporary Families, 2007. https://www.contemporaryfamilies.org/wp-content/uploads/2013/10/2007_Briefing_Cotter_Moms-and-jobs1.pdf.

Coutts, Sharona. "Anti-Choice Groups Use Smartphone Surveillance to Target 'Abortion-Minded Women' during Clinic Visits." Rewire, May 25, 2016. https://rewire.news/article/2016/05/25/anti-choice-groups-deploy-smartphone-surveillance-target-abortion-minded-women-clinic-visits/.

Cox, J. Robert. "Argument and Environmental Advocacy." *Controversia: An International Journal of Debate and Democratic Renewal* 1 (fall 2002): 82–85.

———. "Nature's 'Crisis Disciplines': Does Environmental Communication Have an Ethical Duty?" *Environmental Communication* 1, no. 1 (May 2007): 5–20. https://doi.org/10.1080/17524030701333948.

Culley, Lorraine, Nicky Hudson, and Floor van Rooij, eds. *Marginalized Reproduction: Ethnicity, Infertility, and Reproductive Technologies*. London: Earthscan, 2009.

Cunningham, Carolyn M. "Sixteen and Not Pregnant: Teen-Created YouTube Parody Videos and Sexual Risk-Taking in the United States." *Journal of Children and Media* 8, no. 1 (January 2, 2014): 53–68. https://doi.org/10.1080/17482798.2014.863479.

Currah, Paisley. "Expecting Bodies: The Pregnant Man and Transgender Exclusion from the Employment Non-Discrimination Act." *Women's Studies Quarterly* 36, nos. 3–4 (fall–winter 2008): 330–36.

Daar, Judith. "Federalizing Embryo Transfers: Taming the Wild West of Reproductive Medicine?" *Columbia Journal of Gender and Law* 23, no. 2 (2012): 257–325.

Daniel, Clare. "'Taming the Media Monster': Teen Pregnancy and the Neoliberal Safety (Inter)Net." *Signs: Journal of Women in Culture and Society* 39, no. 4 (2014): 973–98.

———. "Teen Sex, an Equal Opportunity Menace: Multicultural Politics in 16 and Pregnant." In Guglielmo, *MTV and Teen Pregnancy*, 79–92. Lanham, MA: Scarecrow, 2013.

Davey, Monica, and Pam Belluck. "Pharmacies Balk on After-Sex Pill and Widen Fight." *New York Times*, April 19, 2005.

Davidson, Camille M. "Octomom and Multi-Fetal Pregnancies: Why Federal Legislation Should Require Insurers to Cover In Vitro Fertilization." *William & Mary Journal of Women and the Law* 17 (2010): 135–86.

Davidson, Sandra, and Anita Rao. *She and Her: Thank You, More Please*. Aired May 7, 2016. https://www.acast.com/sheher/episode19-thankyou-moreplease.

Davis, Angela Y. *Women, Race, and Class*. New York: Vintage Books, 1983.

Davis, Dana-Ain. "The Politics of Reproduction: The Troubling Case of Nadya Suleman and Assisted Reproductive Technology." *Transforming Anthropology* 17, no. 2 (2009): 105–16.

De Genova, Nicholas. "Antiterrorism, Race, and the New Frontier: American Exceptionalism, Imperial Multiculturalism, and the Global Security State." *Identities* 17, no. 6 (December 15, 2010): 613–40. https://doi.org/10.1080/1070289X.2010.533523.

———. "The Production of Culprits: From Deportability to Detainability in the Aftermath of 'Homeland Security.'" *Citizenship Studies* 11, no. 5 (November 2007): 421–48. https://doi.org/10.1080/13621020701605735.

de Onís, Catalina (Kathleen) M. "Lost in Translation: Challenging (White, Monolingual Feminism's) with Justicia Reproductiva." *Women's Studies in Communication* 38, no. 1 (2015): 1–19.

———. "What's in an 'X'?: An Exchange about the Politics of 'Latinx.'" *Chiricú Journal: Latina/o Literatures, Arts, and Cultures* 1, no. 2 (2017): 78–91.

Demo, Anne Teresa. "The Guerrilla Girls' Comic Politics of Subversion." *Women's Studies in Communication* 23, no. 2 (2000): 133–56.

"Description of *Security Mom: An Unclassified Guide to Protecting Our Homeland and Your Home*." Amazon. Accessed May 17, 2016. www.amazon.com/Security-Mom-Unclassified-Protecting-Homeland/dp/1476733740.

DeSilver, Drew. "Chart of the Week: The Great Baby Recession." *Pew Research Center* (blog), July 25, 2014. www.pewresearch.org/fact-tank/2014/07/25/chart-of-the-week-the-great-baby-recession/.

Diaz, Daniella. "Kelly: DHS Is Considering Separating Undocumented Children from Their Parents at the Border." CNN, March 7, 2017. www.cnn.com/2017/03/06/politics/john-kelly-separating-children-from-parents-immigration-border/index.html.

Dillon, Raquel Maria. "Octuplets Born in California Doing 'Very Well.'" Associated Press, January 27, 2009.

Dinh, James. "MTV's '16 and Pregnant' Credited for Decline in Teen Pregnancy Rates." MTV News, December 12, 2010. www.mtv.com/news/1654818/mtvs-16-and-pregnant-credited-for-decline-in-teen-pregnancy-rates/.

Dolgen, Lauren. "Why I Created MTV's '16 and Pregnant,'" CNN, May 5, 2011. www.cnn.com/2011/SHOWBIZ/TV/05/04/teen.mom.dolgen/index.html.

Douglas, Susan J. *Enlightened Sexism: The Seductive Message That Feminism's Work Is Done*. New York: Times Books, 2010.

Douglas, Susan J., and Meredith W. Michaels. *The Mommy Myth: The Idealization of Motherhood and How It Has Undermined All Women*. New York: Free Press, 2004.

Dow, Bonnie J. "AIDS, Perspective by Incongruity, and Gay Identity in Larry Kramer's '1,112 and Counting.'" *Communication Studies* 45 (1994): 225–40.

———. "Criticism and Authority in the Artistic Mode." *Western Journal of Communication* 65, no. 3 (2001): 336–48.

———. "Michelle Obama, 'Mom-in-Chief': Gender, Race, and Familialism in Media Representations of the First Lady." In *The Rhetoric of Heroic Expectations: Establishing the Obama Presidency*, edited by Justin S. Vaughn and Jennifer R. Mercieca, 235–56. College Station: Texas A&M University Press, 2014.

———. *Prime-Time Feminism: Television, Media Culture, and the Women's Movement since 1970*. Philadelphia: University of Pennsylvania Press, 1996.

———. *Watching Women's Liberation: Feminism's Pivotal Years on the Network News*. Urbana: University of Illinois Press, 2014.

Doyle, Sady. *Trainwreck: The Women We Love to Hate, Mock, and Fear . . . and Why*. Brooklyn, NY: Melville House, 2016.

Dubriwny, Tasha N. "Consciousness-Raising as Collective Rhetoric: The Articulation of Experience in the Redstockings' Abortion Speak-Out of 1969." *Quarterly Journal of Speech* 91, no. 4 (11): 395–422.

———. "Mommy Blogs and the Disruptive Possibilities of Transgressive Drinking." In Hundley and Hayden, *Mediated Moms*, 203–20.

———. *The Vulnerable Empowered Woman: Feminism, Postfeminism, and Women's Health*. New Brunswick, NJ: Rutgers University Press, 2013.

Dubrofsky, Rachel E. "Surveillance on Reality Television and Facebook: From Authenticity to Flowing Data." *Communication Theory* 12 (2011): 111–29.

———. "Therapeutics of the Self: Surveillance in the Service of the Therapeutic." *Television and New Media* 8 (2007): 263–84.

Dunson, David B., Donna D. Baird, and Bernardo Colombo. "Increased Infertility with Age in Men and Women." *Obstetrics and Gynecology* 103, no. 1 (January 2004): 51–56. https://doi.org/10.1097/01.AOG.0000100153.24061.45.

Durham, M. Gigi. *The Lolita Effect: The Media Sexualization of Young Girls and What We Can Do about It*. Woodstock, NY: Overlook, 2008.

Eades, Claire E., Jill S. Ferguson, and Ronan E. O'Carroll. "Public Health in Community Pharmacy: A Systematic Review of Pharmacist and Consumer Views." *BMC Public Health* 11, no. 1 (2011): 582. https://doi.org/10.1186/1471-2458-11-582.

Eckholm, Erik. "Case Explores Rights of Fetus versus Mother." *New York Times*, October 23, 2013.

Edelman, Lee. *No Future: Queer Theory and the Death Drive*. Durham, NC: Duke University Press, 2004.

Edin, Kathryn, and Maria Kefalas. *Promises I Can Keep: Why Poor Women Put Motherhood before Marriage*. Berkeley: University of California Press, 2005.

Edwards, Janis L., and Amanda Leigh Brozana. "Gendering Anti-War Rhetoric: Cindy Sheehan's Symbolic Motherhood." *Journal of the Northwest Communication Association* 37 (2008): 78–102.

Ellison, Katherine, and Nina Martin. "Nearly Dying in Childbirth: Why Preventable Complications Are Growing in U.S." NPR, December 22, 2017. https://www.npr.org/2017/12/22/572298802/nearly-dying-in-childbirth-why-preventable-complications-are-growing-in-u-s.

Emily. "Interview: Farrah Abraham Talks Sophia, Misconceptions, Her New Restaurant and That Christian Parenting Book." Starcasm (blog), June 3, 2014. http://starcasm.net/archives/274344.

Enoch, Jessica. "Survival Stories: Feminist Historiographic Approaches to Chicana Rhetorics of Sterilization Abuse." *Rhetoric Society Quarterly* 35, no. 3 (2005): 5–30.

Essany, Michael. "*16 and Pregnant* Returns to MTV with Life after Labor Reunion and Dramatic Stories for Season 2." *Entertainment Examiner*, July 24, 2010.

Fabj, Valeria. "Motherhood as Political Voice: The Rhetoric of the Mothers of Plaza de Mayo." *Communication Studies* 44, no. 1 (March 1993): 1–18. https://doi.org/10.1080/10510979309368379.

Faderman, Lillian. *To Believe in Women: What Lesbians Have Done for America—A History*. Boston: Houghton Mifflin, 1999.

Fahs, Breanne. "Daddy's Little Girls: On the Perils of Chastity Clubs, Purity Balls, and Ritualized Abstinence." *Frontiers: A Journal of Women's Studies* 31, no. 3 (2010): 116–42.

Faludi, Susan. *Backlash: The Undeclared War against American Women*. 15th anniv. ed. New York: Three Rivers, 2006.

———. "Facebook Feminism, Like It or Not." *Baffler* 23 (August 2013). https://thebaffler.com/salvos/facebook-feminism-like-it-or-not.

———. *The Terror Dream: Myth and Misogyny in an Insecure America*. New York: Metropolitan Books, 2007.

Favara, Jeremiah. "A Maternal Heart: Angelina Jolie, Choices of Maternity, and Hegemonic Femininty in *People* Magazine." *Feminist Media Studies* 15, no. 4 (2015): 626–42.

Fay, Isabel. "The Home Front: Citizens behind the Camera." *Critical Studies in Media Communication* 33, no. 3 (May 26, 2016): 264–78. https://doi.org/10.1080/15295036.2016.1193210.

Feenberg, Andrew. *Critical Theory of Technology*. New York: Oxford University Press, 1991.

———. "Democratic Rationalization: Technology, Power, and Freedom." In *Philosophy of Technology: The Technological Condition*, edited by Robert C. Scharff and Val Dusek, 652–65. Malden, MA: Blackwell, 2003.

Ferguson, Michaele L. "Choice Feminism and the Fear of Politics." *Perspectives on Politics* 8, no. 1 (March 2010): 247–53.

Fernandez, Manny, and Erik Eckholm. "Pregnant, and Forced to Stay on Life Support." *New York Times*, January 7, 2014, sec. U.S. www.nytimes.com.

Fernández, Valeria. "Moms Go on a Hunger Strike to Get Themselves and Their Kids out of Immigration Detention." Public Radio International, August 25, 2016. https://www.pri.org/stories/2016-08-25/madres-berks-are-hunger-strike-get-their-kids-out-immigration-detention.

"Fertility Ethics." *Los Angeles Times*, February 3, 2009. http://articles.latimes.com/2009/feb/03/opinion/ed-octuplet3.

Fessler, Ann. *The Girls Who Went Away: The Hidden History of Women Who Surrendered Children for Adoption in the Decades before Roe v. Wade*. New York: Penguin, 2006.

Fiala, Christian, and Joyce H. Arthur. "'Dishonourable Disobedience'—Why Refusal to Treat in Reproductive Healthcare Is Not Conscientious Objection." *Woman—Psychosomatic Gynaecology and Obstetrics* 1 (December 2014): 12–23. https://doi.org/10.1016/j.woman.2014.03.001.

Fiegerman, Seth. "Actually, Sometimes It Sucks to Work at Apple—Here's Why." *Business Insider*, June 14, 2012. www.businessinsider.com/the-biggest-complaints-employees-have-about-working-at-apple-2012-6.

———. "Why Working at Apple Is a Dream Job." *Business Insider*, June 18, 2012. www.businessinsider.com/heres-what-employees-really-love-about-working-for-apple-2012-6.

Fieweger, Mary Ellen. "Stolen Children and International Adoptions." *Child Welfare* 70, no. 2 (1991): 285–91.

Finnigan, David. "First Peek at Octo-Cuties—Report Reveals Serial Mom Was Already on Food Stamps." *New York Post*, February 10, 2009.

"Fire Up Fertility." *Shape*, November 2011.

Fixmer-Oraiz, Natalie. "Contemplating Homeland Maternity." *Women's Studies in Communication* 38, no. 2 (2015): 129–34.

———. "(In)Conceivable: Risky Reproduction and the Rhetorical Labors of 'Octomom.'" *Communication and Critical/Cultural Studies* 11, no. 3 (2014): 231–49.

———. "No Exception Post-Prevention: 'Differential' Biopolitics on the Morning After." In *Contemplating Maternity in an Era of Choice: Explorations into Discourses of Reproduction*, edited by Sara Hayden and D. Lynn O'Brien Hallstein, 27–48. Lanham, MD: Lexington Books, 2010.

———. "Speaking of Solidarity: Surrogacy and the Rhetorics of Reproductive (in)Justice." *Frontiers: A Journal of Women's Studies* 34, no. 3 (2013): 126–64.

Flavin, Jeanne. *Our Bodies, Our Crimes: The Policing of Women's Reproduction in America*. New York: New York University Press, 2009.

Fontana, Roberta, and Sara Torre. "The Deep Correlation between Energy Metabolism and Reproduction: A View on the Effects of Nutrition for Women Fertility." *Nutrients* 8, no. 2 (February 11, 2016): 87. https://doi.org/10.3390/nu8020087.

Forman, Deborah L. "When 'Bad' Mothers Make Worse Law: A Critique of Legislative Limits on Embryo Transfer." *University of Pennsylvania Journal of Law and Social Change* 14 (2010): 273–312.

Forward Together (formerly Asian Communities for Reproductive Justice). "A New Vision for Advancing Our Movement for Reproductive Health, Reproductive Rights and Reproductive Justice." Forward Together, 2005. https://forwardtogether.org/tools/a-new-vision/.

———. "What Is Reproductive Justice?" Forward Together. Accessed August 14, 2018. https://forwardtogether.org/what-is-reproductive-justice/.

Foucault, Michel. *The History of Sexuality*. Vol. 1, *An Introduction*. Translated by Robert Hurley. New York: Vintage, 1990.

———. *Security, Territory, Population: Lectures at the Collège de France, 1977–78*. Translated by Graham Burchell. New York: Palgrave Macmillan, 2007.

Frey, Hillary. "How to Get Pregnant Exactly When You Want To." *Glamour*, June 2010.

Friedan, Betty. *The Feminine Mystique*. New York: Norton, 1963.

Friedman, May. "'100% Preventable': Teen Motherhood, Morality, and the Myth of Choice." In Guglielmo, *MTV and Teen Pregnancy*, 67–78.

Frost, Jennifer J. "Response to Inquiry Concerning Geographic Service Availability from Planned Parenthood Health Center." New York: Guttmacher Institute, August 14, 2015. www.guttmacher.org/pubs/guttmacher-cbo-memo-2015.pdf.

Fry, Richard, and D'Vera Cohn. "Women, Men and the New Economics of Marriage." *Pew Research Center's Social and Demographic Trends Project* (blog), January 19, 2010. www.pewsocialtrends.org/2010/01/19/women-men-and-the-new-economics-of-marriage/.

Gardner, Christine J. *Making Chastity Sexy: The Rhetoric of Evangelical Abstinence Campaigns*. Berkeley: University of California Press, 2001.

Gastelum, Amy. "Purvi Patel Faces 20 Years in Prison for Feticide and Child Neglect." Public Radio International, March 31, 2015. https://www.pri.org/stories/2015-03-30/purvi-patel-faces-20-years-prison-feticide-and-child-neglect.

Gates, Kelly. "The Globalization of Homeland Security." In *Routledge Handbook of Surveillance Studies*, edited by Kristie Ball, Kevin Haggerty, and David Lyon, 292–300. New York: Routledge, 2012.

Gentile, Katie. "What about the Baby? The New Cult of Domesticity and Media Images of Pregnancy." *Studies in Gender and Sexuality* 12 (2011): 38–58.

Gilbert, Kathryn E. "Commercial Speech in Crisis: Crisis Pregnancy Center Regulations and Definitions of Commercial Speech." *Michigan Law Review* 111, no. 4 (2013): 591–616.

Gill, Rosalind. "Postfeminist Media Culture: Elements of a Sensibility." *European Journal of Cultural Studies* 10, no. 2 (2007): 147–66.

———. "Post-Postfeminism? New Feminist Visibilities in Postfeminist Times." *Feminist Media Studies* 16, no. 4 (July 2016): 610–30. *CrossRef*, doi:10.1080/14680777.2016.1193293.

Gillan, Jennifer. "Extreme Makeover Homeland Security Edition." In *The Great American Makeover: Television, History, Nation*, edited by Dana Heller, 193–209. New York: Palgrave Macmillan, 2006.

Ginsburg, Faye D., and Rayna Rapp, eds. *Conceiving the New World Order: The Global Politics of Reproduction*. Berkeley: University of California Press, 1995.

Glasier, Anna. "Emergency Contraception: Clinical Outcomes." *Contraception* 87, no. 3 (March 2013): 309–13. https://doi.org/10.1016/j.contraception.2012.08.027.

Glennon, Theresa. "Choosing One: Resolving the Epidemic of Multiples in Assisted Reproduction." *Villanova Law Review* 55 (2010): 147–203.

Glenza, Jessica. "Purvi Patel Case: Legal Experts Warn on Reproductive Rights in Indiana." *Guardian*, April 2, 2015, sec. US news. www.theguardian.com/us-news/2015/apr/02/purvi-patel-case-alter-reproductive-rights-indiana.

Goede, Marieke de. "Beyond Risk: Premediation and the Post-9/11 Security Imagination." *Security Dialogue* 39, nos. 2–3 (April 2008): 155–76.

Gohmann, Johanna. "Chill Out." *Bust*, March 2013.

Goldberg, Stephanie. "The 'Teen Mom' Phenomenon." CNN, Entertainment, September 10, 2010. www.cnn.com/2010/SHOWBIZ/TV/09/10/teen.mom.mtv/index.html.

Goodman, Ellen. "A Workable Plan for Fewer Abortions." *Washington Post*, February 29, 2004, sec. Editorial, B07.

———. "Fertility Mistreatment." *New York Times*, February 6, 2009.

Goodnight, G. Thomas. "The Personal, Technical, and Public Spheres of Argument: A Speculative Inquiry into the Art of Public Deliberation." *Journal of the American Forensic Association* 18 (1982): 214–27.

Goodstein, Laurie. "Falwell: Blame Abortionists, Feminists and Gays." World News, *Guardian*, September 19, 2001, US ed. www.theguardian.com/world/2001/sep/19/september11.usa9.

Goodwin, Michele. "A Few Thoughts on Assisted Reproductive Technology." *Law and Inequality: A Journal of Theory and Practice* 27 (2009): 465–79.

Gordon, Linda. *The Moral Property of Women: A History of Birth Control Politics in America*. Chicago: University of Illinois Press, 2007.

———. *Pitied but Not Entitled: Single Mothers and the History of Welfare 1890–1935*. Cambridge: Harvard University Press, 1994.

Gottlieb, Jeff, and Sam Quinones. "The Eighth Baby Was a Surprise." *Los Angeles Times*, January 27, 2009.

Graff, E. J. "The Lie We Love." *Foreign Policy*, November–December 2008, 58–66.

Graham, Judith. "This Chicago Doctor Stumbled on a Hidden Epidemic of Fetal Brain Damage." *PBS NewsHour*, May 21, 2016. www.pbs.org/newshour/rundown/this-chicago-doctor-stumbled-on-a-hidden-epidemic-of-fetal-brain-damage/.

Greif, Mark. "Octomom, One Year Later." *N+1*, no. 9 (2010): 121–40.

Grewal, Inderpal. "'Security Moms' in the Early Twentieth-Century United States: The Gender of Security in Neoliberalism." *Women's Studies Quarterly* 34, nos. 1–2 (spring/summer 2006): 25–39.

Griffin, Rachel Alicia. "*Pushing* into *Precious*: Black Women, Media Representation, and the Glare of the White Supremacist Capitalist Patriarchal Gaze." *Critical Studies in Media Communication* 31, no. 3 (May 27, 2014): 182–97. https://doi.org/10.1080/15295036.2013.849354.

Grigoriadis, Vanessa. "Waking Up from the Pill." *New York Magazine*, December 6, 2010.

Grusin, Richard. "Premediation." *Criticism* 46, no. 1 (2004): 17–39.

Guglielmo, Letizia, ed. *MTV and Teen Pregnancy: Critical Essays on "16 and Pregnant" and "Teen Mom."* Lanham, MD: Scarecrow, 2013.

Guglielmo, Letizia, and Kimberly Wallace Stewart. "*16 and Pregnant* and the 'Unvarnished' Truth about Teen Pregnancy." In Guglielmo, *MTV and Teen Pregnancy*, 19–34.

Guillem, Susana Martínez, and Lisa A. Flores. "Maternal Transgressions, Racial Regressions: How Whiteness Mediates the (Worst) White Moms." In Hundley and Hayden, *Mediated Moms*, 77–101.

Gumbs, Alexis Pauline, China Martens, and Mai'a Williams, eds. *Revolutionary Mothering: Love on the Front Lines*. Oakland, CA: PM Press, 2016.

Guttmacher Institute. *Benefits of Contraceptive Use in the United States*. 2013. www.guttmacher.org.

———. "Fact Sheet: Induced Abortion in the United States." Guttmacher Institute, January 2017. https://www.guttmacher.org/fact-sheet/induced-abortion-united-states.

———. "Facts on Induced Abortion in the United States." New York: Guttmacher Institute, March 2016. Accessed March 23, 2016.

———. "Last Five Years Account for More than One-Quarter of All Abortion Restrictions Enacted since Roe." Guttmacher Institute, January 13, 2016. www.guttmacher.org/media/inthenews/2016/01/13/index.html.

———. "Minors' Rights as Parents." Guttmacher Institute, July 1, 2017. https://www.guttmacher.org/state-policy/explore/minors-rights-parents.

———. "The Number of States Considered Hostile to Abortion Skyrocketed between 2000 and 2014." Guttmacher Institute, November 12, 2015. https://www.guttmacher.org/infographic/2015/number-states-considered-hostile-abortion-skyrocketed-between-2000-and-2014.

———. "Parental Involvement in Minors' Abortions." Guttmacher Institute: State Laws and Policies, July 1, 2017. https://www.guttmacher.org/state-policy/explore/parental-involvement-minors-abortions.

———. "State Policies in Brief: Emergency Contraception." New York: Guttmacher Institute, March 2016.

———. "State Policies in Brief: Refusing to Provide Health Services." New York: Guttmacher Institute, March 2016.

Guzick, David S. "Age and Fertility: A Social-Biologic Balance." *Fertility and Sterility* 105, no. 6 (June 2016): 1461. https://doi.org/10.1016/j.fertnstert.2016.03.021.

Halkidis, Anna. "Bei Bei Shuai Case Exposes Pregnancy-Suicide Risk." Women's eNews, August 3, 2013. WomenseNews.org/2013/08/bei-bei-shuai-case-exposes-pregnancy-suicide-risk/.

Hall, Rachel. *The Transparent Traveler: The Performance and Culture of Airport Security*. Durham, NC: Duke University Press, 2015.

Hallstein, D. Lynn O'Brien. *Bikini-Ready Moms: Celebrity Profiles, Motherhood, and the Body*. Albany: State University of New York Press, 2015.

———. "Public Choices, Private Control: How Mediated Mom Labels Work Rhetorically to Dismantle the Politics of Choice and White Second Wave Feminist Successes." In *Contemplating Maternity in an Era of Choice: Explorations into Discourses of Reproduction*, edited by Sara Hayden and D. Lynn O'Brien Hallstein, 5–26. Lanham, MD: Lexington Books, 2010.

Halperin, Shirley. "The Business of *Glee*." *Hollywood Reporter*, February 2, 2011.

Happe, Kelly E. *The Material Gene: Gender, Race, and Heredity after the Human Genome Project*. New York: New York University Press, 2013.

Harris, Gardiner. "Official Quits on Pill Delay at the F.D.A." *New York Times*, September 1, 2005.

———. "U.S. Again Delays Decision on Sale of Next-Day Pill." *New York Times*, August 27, 2005.

Hartocollis, Anemona. "Mother Accuses Doctors of Forcing a C-Section and Files Suit." *New York Times*, May 16, 2014. www.nytimes.com.

Hartouni, Valerie. *Cultural Conceptions: On Reproductive Technologies and the Remaking of Life*. Minneapolis: University of Minnesota Press, 1997.

Hasinoff, Amy Adele. *Sexting Panic: Rethinking Criminalization, Privacy, and Consent*. Urbana: University of Illinois Press, 2015.

Hass, Nancy. "Time to Chill? Egg Freezing Technology Offers a Chance to Extend Fertility." *Vogue*, May 2011.

Hauser, Christine. "Florida Woman Whose 'Stand Your Ground' Defense Was Rejected Is Released." *New York Times*, February 7, 2017, sec. U.S. www.nytimes.com.

Hay, James. "Designing Homes to Be the First Line of Defense: Safe Households, Mobilization, and the New Mobile Privatization." *Cultural Studies* 20, nos. 4–5 (2006): 349–77.

Hay, James, and Mark Andrejevic, eds. "Homeland Insecurities." Special issue, *Cultural Studies* 20, nos. 4–5 (2006).

———. "Toward an Analytic of Governmental Experiments in These Times: Homeland Security as the New Social Security." *Cultural Studies* 20, nos. 4–5 (2006): 331–48.

Hayden, Sara. "Constituting Savvy Aunties: From Childless Women to Child-Focused Consumers." *Women's Studies in Communication* 34, no. 1 (May 5, 2011): 1–19. https://doi.org/10.1080/07491409.2011.566531.

———. "Family Metaphors and the Nation: Promoting a Politics of Care through the Million Mom March." *Quarterly Journal of Speech* 89, no. 3 (January 2003): 196–215. https://doi.org/10.1080/00335630320001253l3.

———. "Revitalizing the Debate between <Life> and <Choice>: The 2004 March for Women's Lives." *Communication and Critical/Cultural Studies* 6, no. 2 (2009): 111–31.

Henderson, J. Maureen. "Why We Should Be Alarmed that Apple and Facebook Are

Paying for Employee Egg Freezing." *Forbes*, October 15, 2014. www.forbes.com/sites/jmaureenhenderson/2014/10/15/dont-work-for-or-trust-a-company-that-pays-you-to-freeze-your-eggs/.

Hewlett, Sylvia Ann. *Creating a Life: Professional Women and the Quest for Children*. New York: Talk Miramax Books, 2002.

———. "Executive Women and the Myth of Having It All." *Harvard Business Review* 80, no. 4 (April 2002). https://hbr.org/2002/04/executive-women-and-the-myth-of-having-it-all.

Hoerl, Kristen, and Casey Ryan Kelly. "The Post-Nuclear Family and the Depoliticization of Unplanned Pregnancy in *Knocked Up*, *Juno*, and *Waitress*." *Communication and Critical/Cultural Studies* 7, no. 4 (2010): 360–80.

hooks, bell. "Dig Deep: Beyond 'Lean In.'" Feminist Wire, October 28, 2013. http://thefeministwire.com/2013/10/17973/.

———. *Yearning: Race, Gender, and Cultural Politics*. Boston: South End, 1990.

Hundley, Heather L., and Sara E. Hayden, eds. *Mediated Moms: Contemporary Challenges to the Motherhood Myth*. New York: Peter Lang, 2016.

Hymowitz, Kay. "Where in the World Is Octodad?" *Wall Street Journal*, February 20, 2009.

IMDb: The Internet Movie Database. "Awards for *Glee*." N.d. Accessed February 21, 2011.

———. "Awards for *Juno*." N.d. Accessed April 26, 2010.

Inbar, Michael. "First U.S. Octuplets Offer Advice to New Parents of Eight: Now Ten Years Old, Seven Surviving Chukwu Octuplets Are Healthy, 'Beautiful,'" Today, January 28, 2009, Parents. http://today.msnbc.msn.com/id/28891400/.

Inhorn, Marcia C. *Women, Consider Freezing Your Eggs*. CNN, updated April 9, 2013. www.cnn.com/2013/04/09/opinion/inhorn-egg-freezing.

Ivie, Robert L. "Productive Criticism." *Quarterly Journal of Speech* 81, no. 1 (1995): 2.

———. "Productive Criticism Then and Now." *American Communication Journal* 4, no. 3 (2001). http://ac-journal.org/journal/vol4/iss3/special/ivie.htm.

Jaffe, Sarah. "The Militarization of Everything." *Bitch* 17, no. 73 (2017): 36–42.

Jamal, Amaney A., and Nadine Christine Naber, ed. *Race and Arab Americans before and after 9/11: From Invisible Citizens to Visible Subjects*. Syracuse, NY: Syracuse University Press, 2008.

James, Susan Donaldson. "Octomom Lesson: More Couples Pressure Doctors." *ABC News*, October 25, 2010.

Jensen, Robin E. *Dirty Words: The Rhetoric of Public Sex Education, 1870–1924*. Urbana: University of Illinois Press, 2010.

———. "An Ecological Turn in Rhetoric of Health Scholarship: Attending to the Historical Flow and Percolation of Ideas, Assumptions, and Arguments." *Communication Quarterly* 63, no. 5 (October 20, 2015): 522–26. https://doi.org/10.1080/01463373.2015.1103600.

———. *Infertility: Tracing the History of a Transformative Term*. RSA Series in Transdisciplinary Rhetoric. University Park: Pennsylvania State University Press, 2016.

Johnson, Judith A., and Vanessa K. Burrows. *Emergency Contraception: Plan B*. CRS Report for Congress. Washington, DC: Congressional Research Service: Report for Congress, 2007. research.policyarchive.org/3017.pdf.

Jones, Bernie D. "Introduction: Women, Work, and Motherhood in American History." In *Women Who Opt Out: The Debate over Working Mothers and Work-Family Balance*, edited by Bernie D. Jones, 3–32. New York: New York University Press, 2012.

Jones, Rachel K., and Jenna Jerman. "Abortion Incidence and Service Availability In the United States, 2014." *Perspectives on Sexual and Reproductive Health* 49, no. 1 (March 1, 2017): 17–27. https://doi.org/10.1363/psrh.12015.

Jonsson, Patrik. "A Force behind the Lower Teen Birthrate: MTV's '16 and Pregnant.'" *Christian Science Monitor*, December 21, 2010. www.csmonitor.com/USA/Society/2010/1221/A-force-behind-the-lower-teen-birthrate-MTV-s-16-and-Pregnant.

Kalb, Claudia. "Fertility and the Freezer." *Newsweek*, 2004.

———. "Have Another 'Fertilitini.'" *Newsweek*, January 26, 2009.

Kaplan, Amy. "Homeland Insecurities: Some Reflections on Language and Space." *Radical History Review*, no. 85 (winter 2003): 82–93.

Kaproth-Joslin, Katherine, and Vikram Dogra. "Imaging of Female Infertility: A Pictorial Guide to the Hysterosalpingography, Ultrasonography, and Magnetic Resonance Imaging Findings of the Congenital and Acquired Causes of Female Infertility." *Radiologic Clinics of North America* 51, no. 6 (November 2013): 967–81. https://doi.org/10.1016/j.rcl.2013.07.002.

Kaufman, Marc. "Compromise May Restrict 'Morning-After' Pill." *Washington Post*, April 8, 2004, sec. A.

———. "FDA Delays Decision on Plan B Contraceptive." *Washington Post*, August 27, 2005.

———. "FDA Plan B Sales Rejected against Advice; Official Denies that Politics Blocked Contraceptive's Over-the-Counter Status." *Washington Post*, May 8, 2004, sec. A.

Kavanaugh, Megan L., Sanithia L. Williams, and E. Bimla Schwarz. "Emergency Contraception Use and Counseling after Changes in United States Prescription Status." *Fertility and Sterility* 95, no. 8 (June 2011): 2578–81. https://doi.org/10.1016/j.fertnstert.2011.03.011.

Kayyem, Juliette. "Juliette Kayyem on Homeland Security and Her Home: 'From Inside DHS It Was Logical. From My Kitchen? It Sucked.'" WGBH, April 11, 2016, News, https://news.wgbh.org/2016/04/11/news/juliette-kayyem-homeland-security-and-her-home-inside-dhs-it-was-logical-my-kitchen.

———. *Security Mom: An Unclassified Guide to Protecting Our Homeland and Your Home*. New York: Simon and Schuster, 2016.

Kelley, Raina. "Octomom Hypocrisy." *Newsweek*, March 3, 2009. www.newsweek.com/2009/03/02/octomom-hypocrisy.print.html.

Kelly, Casey Ryan. *Abstinence Cinema: Virginity and the Rhetoric of Sexual Purity in Contemporary Film*. New Brunswick, NJ: Rutgers University Press, 2016.

———. "'True' Love Waits: The Construction of Facts in Abstinence-until-Marriage

Discourse." In *Disturbing Argument: Selected Works from the 18th NCA/AFA Alta Conference on Argumentation*, edited by Catherine H. Palczewski, 376–81. New York: Routledge, 2015.

Kelly, Casey Ryan, and Kristen E. Hoerl. "Shaved or Saved? Disciplining Women's Bodies." *Women's Studies in Communication* 38, no. 2 (April 3, 2015): 141–45. https://doi.org/10.1080/07491409.2015.1027088.

Kelly, Kimberly. "In the Name of the Mother: Renegotiating Conservative Women's Authority in the Crisis Pregnancy Center Movement." *Signs* 38, no. 1 (September 2012): 203–30. https://doi.org/10.1086/665807.

Keranen, Lisa. "Concocting Viral Apocalypse: Catastrophic Risk and the Production of Bio(in)Security." *Western Journal of Communication* 75, no. 5 (2011): 451–72.

Kerber, Linda K. *Women of the Republic: Intellect and Ideology in Revolutionary America*. Chapel Hill: University of North Carolina Press, 1980.

King, Jamilah. "NYC Anti-Abortion Ad Is Coming Down—but the Real Battle's Just Begun." Text. Colorlines, February 24, 2011. www.colorlines.com/articles/nyc-anti-abortion-ad-coming-down-real-battles-just-begun.

Kingsbury, Kathleen. "Pregnancy Boom at Gloucester High." *Time*, June 18, 2008. http://content.time.com/time/magazine/article/0,9171,1816486,00.html.

Klein, Naomi. *The Shock Doctrine: The Rise of Disaster Capitalism*. New York: Metropolitan Books, 2007.

Knight, Nicole. "Report: Criminalizing Pregnancy a 'Noose around Your Neck.'" Rewire, May 23, 2017. https://rewire.news/article/2017/05/23/report-criminalizing-pregnancy-noose-around-neck/.

Knowles, Jon. *Issue Brief: Sex Education in the United States*. New York: Katharine Dexter McCormick Library and the Education Division of Planned Parenthood Federation of America, 2012. https://www.plannedparenthood.org/files/3713/9611/7930/Sex_Ed_in_the_US.pdf.

Knudson, Laura. "Cindy Sheehan and the Rhetoric of Motherhood: A Textual Analysis." *Peace and Change* 34, no. 2 (April 2009): 164–83. https://doi.org/10.1111/j.1468-0130.2009.00548.x.

Kochhar, Rakesh. "Employment in the Recession." *Pew Research Center's Social and Demographic Trends Project* (blog), July 6, 2011. www.pewsocialtrends.org/2011/07/06/iii-employment-in-the-recession/.

Kolata, Gina. "A Contraceptive Clears a Hurdle to Wider Access." *New York Times*, December 17, 2003.

———. "Debate on Selling Morning-After Pill over the Counter." *New York Times*, December 12, 2003.

Kost, Kathryn, Stanley Henshaw, and Liz Carlin. *U.S. Teenage Pregnancies, Births and Abortions: National and State Trends and Trends by Race and Ethnicity*. N.p.: Guttmacher Institute, January 2010.

Krawiec, Kimberly D. "Why We Should Ignore the 'Octomom.'" *Northwestern University Law Review* 104 (2009): 120–31.

Kristof, Nicholas. "TV Lowers Birthrate (Seriously)." *New York Times*, March 20, 2014, sec. A.

Kristof, Nicholas D., and Sheryl WuDunn. *Half the Sky: Turning Oppression into Opportunity for Women Worldwide*. New York: Vintage Books, 2009.

Lakoff, George. *Moral Politics: How Liberals and Conservatives Think*. 2nd ed. Chicago: University of Chicago Press, 2002.

Landau, Jamie. "Reproducing and Transgressing Masculinity: A Rhetorical Analysis of Women Interacting with Digital Photographs of Thomas Beatie." *Women's Studies in Communication* 35, no. 2 (2012): 178–203.

Last, Jonathan V. *What to Expect When No One's Expecting: America's Coming Demographic Disaster*. New York: Encounter Books, 2013.

Lawrence, Ryan E., Kenneth A. Rasinski, John D. Yoon, and Farr A. Curlin. "Obstetrician-Gynecologist Physicians' Beliefs about Emergency Contraception: A National Survey." *Contraception* 82, no. 4 (October 2010): 324–30.

Leadership Conference on Civil and Human Rights et al. Letter to Congress. "Stand Up for Women's Access to Healthcare Services: Oppose All Efforts to Defund Planned Parenthood." July 31, 2015. https://lulac.org/advocacy/PPFADefundingLetter7-31.pdf.

Letourneau, Nicole L., Miriam J. Stewart, and Alison K. Barnfather. "Adolescent Mothers: Support Needs, Resources, and Support-Education Interventions." *Journal of Adolescent Health* 35, no. 6 (December 2004): 509–25. https://doi.org/10.1016/j.jadohealth.2004.01.007.

Livingston, Gretchen. "Growing Number of Dads Home with the Kids." *Pew Research Center's Social and Demographic Trends Project* (blog), June 5, 2014. www.pewsocialtrends.org/2014/06/05/growing-number-of-dads-home-with-the-kids/.

Logsdon, M. Cynthia, John C. Birkimer, Amelia Ratterman, Krista Cahill, and Nancy Cahill. "Social Support in Pregnant and Parenting Adolescents: Research, Critique, and Recommendations." *Journal of Child and Adolescent Psychiatric Nursing* 15, no. 2 (2002): 75–83.

Lombardi, Lisa. "Protect Your Fertility." *Shape*, September 2003.

Lopez, Lori Kido. "The Radical Act of 'Mommy Blogging': Redefining Motherhood through the Blogosphere." *New Media and Society* 11, no. 5 (2009): 729–47.

Lorenzo, Rachel. "Young Women United Releases New Report, 'Dismantling Teen Pregnancy Prevention' for Immediate Release." June 1, 2016. Accessed August 8, 2016. www.youngwomenunited.org/press-advisories-and-releases/ (dead).

Lovell, Elyse D'nn. "College Students Who Are Parents Need Equitable Services for Retention." *Journal of College Student Retention: Research, Theory and Practice* 16, no. 2 (January 1, 2014): 187–202. https://doi.org/10.2190/CS.16.2.b.

Low, Setha, and Neil Smith, eds. *The Politics of Public Space*. New York: Routledge, 2006.

Lowrey, Annie. "MTV's '16 and Pregnant,' Derided by Some, May Resonate as a Cautionary Tale." *New York Times*, January 13, 2014.

Lozano-Reich, Nina M., and Dana L. Cloud. "The Uncivil Tongue: Invitational Rhetoric and the Problem of Inequality." *Western Journal of Communication* 73, no. 2 (2009): 220–26.

Ludden, Jennifer. "Egg Freezing Puts the Biological Clock on Hold." *Morning Edition*. NPR, aired May 31, 2011.

———. "States Fund Pregnancy Centers That Discourage Abortion." *All Things Considered*. NPR, March 9, 2015. www.npr.org/sections/health-shots/2015/03/09/391877614/states-fund-pregnancy-centers-that-discourage-abortion.

Luibhéid, Eithne. *Entry Denied: Controlling Sexuality at the Border*. Minneapolis: University of Minnesota Press, 2002.

———. *Pregnant on Arrival: Making the Illegal Immigrant*. Minneapolis: University of Minnesota Press, 2013.

Lyall, Sarah. "Britain Allows Over-the-Counter Sales of Morning-After Pill." *New York Times*, January 15, 2001, sec. A4.

Manning, Jimmie. "Exploring Family Discourses about Purity Pledges: Connecting Relationships and Popular Culture." *Qualitative Research Reports in Communication* 15, no. 1 (January 2014): 92–99. https://doi.org/10.1080/17459435.2014.955597.

———. "Paradoxes of (Im)Purity: Affirming Heteronormativity and Queering Heterosexuality in Family Discourses of Purity Pledges." *Women's Studies in Communication* 38, no. 1 (January 2, 2015): 99–117. https://doi.org/10.1080/07491409.2014.954687.

Marcos, Cristina. "Bill Would Ban Abortions across State Lines." Text. Hill, February 9, 2015. http://thehill.com/blogs/floor-action/house/232155-bill-would-ban-abortions-across-state-lines.

Marsh, Margaret, and Wanda Ronner. *The Empty Cradle: Infertility in America from Colonial Times to the Present*. Baltimore: Johns Hopkins University Press, 1996.

Martin, Nina, and Renee Montagne. "Black Mothers Keep Dying After Giving Birth." *All Things Considered*. NPR, December 7, 2017. https://www.npr.org/2017/12/07/568948782/black-mothers-keep-dying-after-giving-birth-shalon-irvings-story-explains-why.

———. "Focus on Infants during Childbirth Leaves U.S. Moms in Danger." *Morning Edition*. NPR, March 12, 2017. https://www.npr.org/2017/05/12/527806002/focus-on-infants-during-childbirth-leaves-u-s-moms-in-danger.

Marvin, Carolyn. *When Old Technologies Were New: Thinking about Communications in the Late Nineteenth Century*. New York: Oxford University Press, 1988.

Mask, Mia. "The Precarious Politics of *Precious*: A Close Reading of a Cinematic Text." *Black Camera* 4, no. 1 (winter 2012): 96–116.

Matson, Erin. "'Freeze Your Eggs, Free Your Career' Is Insulting to Women." RH Reality Check, April 22, 2014. http://rhrealitycheck.org/article/2014/04/22/freeze-eggs-free-career-insulting-women/.

May, Elaine Tyler. *Homeward Bound: American Families during the Cold War Era*. 20th ann. ed. New York: Basic Books, 2008.

Mayo Clinic Staff. "Female Infertility: Causes." Mayo Clinic. Accessed July 27, 2016. www.mayoclinic.org/diseases-conditions/female-infertility/basics/causes/con-20033618 (dead).

McGee, Summer Johnson. "Don't Blame Momma." *Bioethics.Net* (blog), February 6, 2009. http://www.bioethics.net/2009/02/dont-blame-momma.

McIntire, Lisa. *Crisis Pregnancy Centers Lie: The Insidious Threat to Reproductive Freedom*. NARAL Pro-Choice America, 2015. www.prochoiceamerica.org/assets/download-files/cpc-report-2015.pdf.

McKinnon, Sara L. "Essentialism, Intersectionality, and Recognition: A Feminist Rhetorical Approach to the Audience." In *Standing in the Intersection: Feminist Voices, Feminist Practices in Communication Studies*, edited by Karma R. Chávez and Cindy L. Griffin, 189–210. Albany: State University of New York Press, 2012.

McRobbie, Angela. *The Aftermath of Feminism: Gender, Culture and Social Change*. Thousand Oaks, CA: Sage, 2009.

Mead, Rebecca. "Cold Comfort: Tech Jobs and Egg Freezing." *New Yorker*, October 17, 2014. www.newyorker.com/news/daily-comment/facebook-apple-egg-freezing-benefits.

Meadows-Oliver, Mikki, Lois S. Sadler, Martha K. Swartz, and Patricia Ryan-Krause. "Sources of Stress and Support and Maternal Resources of Homeless Teenage Mothers." *Journal of Child and Adolescent Psychiatric Nursing* 20, no. 2 (2007): 116–25.

Meyer, Jennifer L., Melanie A. Gold, and Catherine L. Haggerty. "Advance Provision of Emergency Contraception among Adolescent and Young Adult Women: A Systematic Review of Literature." *Journal of Pediatric and Adolescent Gynecology* 24, no. 1 (February 2011): 2–9. https://doi.org/10.1016/j.jpag.2010.06.002.

Meyer, Michelle N. "States' Regulation of Assisted Reproductive Technologies: What Does the U.S. Constitution Allow?" Nelson A. Rockefeller Institute of Government, Harvard Public Law Working Paper, July 1, 2009.

Michaels, Meredith W. "Mothers 'Opting Out': Facts and Fiction." *Women's Studies Quarterly* 37, nos. 3–4 (2009): 317–22.

Midwives Alliance. "New Studies Confirm Safety of Home Birth with Midwives in the U.S." Midwives Alliance of North America, January 30, 2014. http://mana.org/blog/home-birth-safety-outcomes.

Miller, Carolyn R. "The Presumptions of Expertise: The Role of Ethos in Risk Analysis." *Configurations* 11 (2004): 163–202.

———. "Risk, Controversy, and Rhetoric: Response to Goodnight." *Argumentation and Advocacy* 42 (2005): 34–37.

Miller, Lisa. "The Retro Wife: Feminists Who Say They're Having It All—by Choosing to Stay Home." *New York Magazine*, March 17, 2013.

Mink, Gwendolyn. *Welfare's End*. Ithaca, NY: Cornell University Press, 1998.

Mitchell, Don. *The Right to the City: Social Justice and the Fight for Public Space*. New York: Guilford, 2003.

Modarressy-Tehrani, Caroline. "'Cocaine Mom Law' That Locks up Pregnant Women Might Be Done in Wisconsin." Vice News, May 28, 2017. https://news.vice.com/story/cocaine-mom-law-that-locks-up-pregnant-women-might-be-done-in-wisconsin.

Mollborn, Stefanie. "Making the Best of a Bad Situation: Material Resources and Teenage Parenthood." *Journal of Marriage and Family* 69 (2007): 92–104.

"MomsRising." MomsRising.org. Accessed June 3, 2016. www.momsrising.org/.

Moore, Tina. "Octuplet Grandma's Shame: Daughter Has 14 Kids, No Husband." *New York Daily News*, January 31, 2009.

Morgan, Lynn M., and Meredith W. Michaels, eds. *Fetal Subjects, Feminist Positions*. Philadelphia: University of Pennsylvania Press, 1999.

"Mothers Gone Wild." *Maclean's*, February 23, 2009.

Motluk, Alison. "When Eight Is Seven Too Many." *New Scientist* 201, no. 2695 (2009): 24.

Mshaka, Thembisa S. "Commentary: Why ThatsAbortion.Com Billboard Is an Ad *Fail*." *Thembisa S. Mshaka* (blog), February 24, 2011. https://thembisamshaka.com/2011/02/24/commentary-why-thatsabortion-com-billboard-is-an-ad-fail/.

"MTV's Premiere of 'Teen Mom' Marks the Highest-Rated New Series Launch in Over a Year." *TV by the Numbers* (blog), December 9, 2009. http://tvbythenumbers.zap2it.com/network-press-releases/mtvs-premiere-of-teen-mom-marks-the-highest-rated-new-series-launch-in-over-a-year/.

Mutsaerts, Meike A. Q., Anne M. van Oers, Henk Groen, Jan M. Burggraaff, Walter K. H. Kuchenbecker, Denise A. M. Perquin, Carolien A. M. Koks, et al. "Randomized Trial of a Lifestyle Program in Obese Infertile Women." *New England Journal of Medicine* 374, no. 20 (May 19, 2016): 1942–53. https://doi.org/10.1056/NEJMoa1505297.

Naaman, Lara. "Now that Everyone's Freezing Their Eggs, Should You?" *Glamour*, April 2013.

Naber, Nadine Christine. "Introduction: Arab Americans and US Racial Formations." In *Race and Arab Americans before and after 9/11: From Invisible Citizens to Visible Subjects*, edited by Amaney A. Jamal and Nadine Christine Naber, 1–45. Syracuse, NY: Syracuse University Press, 2008.

Nadasen, Premilla. *Welfare Warriors: The Welfare Rights Movement in the United States*. New York: Routledge, 2005.

Nash, Elizabeth, Rachel Benson Gold, Gwendolyn Rathbun, and Yana Vierboom. "Laws Affecting Reproductive Health and Rights: 2014 State Policy Review." Guttmacher Institute, January 5, 2015. www.guttmacher.org/statecenter/updates/2014/statetrends42014.html.

National Abortion Federation. "NAF Violence and Disruption Statistics." 2015. http://prochoice.org/education-and-advocacy/violence/violence-statistics-and-history/.

National Advocates for Pregnant Women. "Federal Court Declares Wisconsin 'Unborn Child Protection' Law Unconstitutional: Law Permitting Forced Treatment and

Detention of Pregnant Women Is Struck Down, Effective Immediately." *National Advocates for Pregnant Women* (blog), May 1, 2017. http://advocatesforpregnantwomen.org/blog/2017/05/federal_court_declares_wiscons.php.

National Campaign to Prevent Teen and Unplanned Pregnancy. "National Data." 2015. Accessed August 14, 2018. https://powertodecide.org/what-we-do/information/national-state-data/national.

National Women's Law Center. *Emergency Contraception Coverage under Family Planning §1115 Waivers*. Washington, DC: National Women's Law Center, December 2007.

———. "Pharmacy Refusals 101." *National Women's Law Center: Expanding the Possibilities* (blog), August 4, 2015. http://nwlc.org/resources/pharmacy-refusals-101/.

National Women's Law Center, and Law Students for Reproductive Justice. *Fact Sheet: If You Really Care about Criminal Justice, You Should Care about Reproductive Justice!* National Women's Law Center, October 3, 2014. https://nwlc.org/resources/if-you-really-care-about-criminal-justice-you-should-care-about-reproductive-justice/.

Native American Community Board. "Indian Health Service and Tribal Health Center Plan B Accessibility Survey." 2017. www.nativeshop.org/images/pdf/2017-05-Plan-B-IHS-and-Tribal-Health-Center-final-report-2.pdf.

Native American Women's Health Education Resource Center. "Lack of Access to Emergency Contraception Continues." 2014. www.nativeshop.org/m/news-110/783-the-lack-of-access-to-emergency-contraception-continues.html.

Naylor, Brian. "Senate Limits Interstate Abortions for Minors." *Morning Edition*. NPR, July 26, 2006. https://www.npr.org/templates/story/story.php?storyId=5582615.

Nebbe, Charity. "Talk of Iowa on Iowa Public Radio." *Childless by Choice*, March 4, 2016. http://iowapublicradio.org/post/childless-choice#stream/0.

Negra, Diane. "Structural Integrity, Historical Reversion, and the Post-9/11 Chick Flick." *Feminist Media Studies* 8, no. 1 (2008): 51–68.

Newman, Amie. "Iowa 'Feticide' Law Could Be Used to Target Mothers." Huffington Post (blog), April 18, 2010. www.huffingtonpost.com/amie-newman/iowa-feticide-law-could-b_b_463153.html.

Nixon, Laura. "The Right to (Trans) Parent: A Reproductive Justice Approach to Reproductive Rights, Fertility, and Family-Building Issues Facing Transgender People." *William & Mary Journal of Women and the Law* 20 (2013): 73–103.

NYU School of Law Global Justice Clinic, and the Fordham Law School Center for International Law and Justice. "Suppressing Protest: Human Rights Violations in the U.S. Response to Occupy Wall Street." Protest and Assembly Rights Project. New York, 2012. http://chrgj.org/wp-content/uploads/2012/10/suppressingprotest.pdf.

O'Brien Cherry, C., N. Chumbler, J. Bute, and A. Huff. "Building a 'Better Life': The Transformative Effects of Adolescent Pregnancy and Parenting." *Sage Open* 5, no. 1 (February 11, 2015). https://doi.org/10.1177/2158244015571638.

O'Connell, Michael. "TV Ratings: 'Glee' Exits Stage Left." Hollywood Reporter, March 21, 2015. www.hollywoodreporter.com/live-feed/tv-ratings-glee-exits-stage-783509.

"Octomom vs. Illegal Aliens." *Topix: Immigration Reform Form*, February 16, 2009. www.topix.com.

"Octuplets' Family Filed for Bankruptcy." CBSNews, January 30, 2009. https://www.cbsnews.com/news/octuplets-family-filed-for-bankruptcy/.

"Octuplets' Mom: 'All I Ever Wanted.'" CNN, February 6, 2009. http://articles.cnn.com/2009-02-06/us/octuplets.mom_1_octuplets-birth-nadya-suleman-octuplets-mom?_s=PM:US.

Office of Population Research at Princeton University. "Get Emergency Contraception Now." Emergency Contraception Website, August 14, 2017. http://ec.princeton.edu/locator/concerned-about-cost.html#Medicaid.

O'Reilly, Andrea, ed. *Feminist Mothering*. Albany: State University of New York Press, 2008.

———. *Maternal Theory: Essential Readings*. Toronto: Demeter, 2007.

Orman, Suz. "Suz Orman's Intervention with 'Octomom' Nadya Suleman." *Oprah Show*, January 14, 2011.

Ouellette, Laurie. *Lifestyle TV*. New York: Routledge, 2016.

Ouellette, Laurie, and James Hay. *Better Living through Reality TV: Television and Post-Welfare Citizenship*. Malden, MA: Blackwell, 2008.

Palmer, Gareth. "On Our Best Behaviour." *FlowTV* 5, December 15, 2006. http://flowtv.org/2006/12/on-our-best-behaviour/.

Palmer-Mehta, Valerie. "Subversive Maternities: Staceyann Chin's Contemplative Voice." *QED: A Journal in GLBTQ Worldmaking* 3, no. 1 (2016): 34–60.

Palmer-Mehta, Valerie, and Sherianne Shuler. "'Devil Mamas' of Social Media: Resistant Maternal Discourses in Sanctimommy." In Hundley and Hayden, *Mediated Moms*, 221–46.

Paltrow, Lynn, and Jeanne Flavin. "Arrests of and Forced Interventions on Pregnant Women in the United States (1973–2005): The Implications for Women's Legal Status and Public Health." *Journal of Health Politics, Policy and Law* 38, no. 2 (2013): 299–343.

Parker, Willie. *Life's Work: A Moral Argument for Choice*. New York: Atria Books, 2017.

Parsons, Sabrina. "Female Tech CEO: Egg-Freezing 'Benefit' Sends the Wrong Message to Women." *Business Insider*, October 20, 2014. www.businessinsider.com/apple-facebook-egg-freezing-benefit-is-bad-for-women-2014-10.

Pearson, Catherine. "Montana County Has Plan for Moms-to-Be Who Drink or Do Drugs: Jail 'Em." AOL.com, January 27, 2018. https://www.aol.com/article/news/2018/01/27/montana-county-has-plan-for-moms-to-be-who-drink-or-do-drugs-jail-em/23345328/.

Peeples, Jennifer A., and Kevin M. DeLuca. "The Truth of the Matter: Motherhood, Community and Environmental Justice." *Women's Studies in Communication* 29, no. 1 (April 2006): 59–87. https://doi.org/10.1080/07491409.2006.10757628.

Percheski, Christine. "Opting Out? Cohort Differences in Professional Women's Employment Rates from 1960 to 2005." *American Sociological Review* 73, no. 3 (June 2008): 497–517.

Perry, David. "Anti-Choice Legislators Try to Force Wedge between Reproductive, Disability Rights Activists." Rewire, January 16, 2015. https://rewire.news/article/2015/01/16/anti-choice-legislators-try-force-wedge-reproductive-disability-rights-activists/.

Petchesky, Rosalind Pollack. "Fetal Images: The Power of Visual Culture in the Politics of Reproduction." *Feminist Studies* 13, no. 2 (1987): 263–92.

Peters, Mark, and David Wessel. "Idled Americans: More Men in Their Prime Are Out of Work and at Home." *Wall Street Journal*, February 6, 2014, sec. J.

Peterson, James D. *Tamara M. Loertscher v. Eloise Anderson, Brad D. Schimel, and Taylor County*, no. 14–cv–870–jdp (United States District Court for the Western District of Wisconsin, April 28, 2017).

Pew Research Center. "Black-White Conflict Isn't Society's Largest." *Pew Research Center's Social and Demographic Trends Project* (blog), September 24, 2009. www.pewsocialtrends.org/2009/09/24/black-white-conflict-isnt-societys-largest/.

———. *Few Say Police Forces Nationally Do Well in Treating Races Equally*. Pew Research Center/*USA Today*, August 25, 2014. www.people-press.org/2014/08/25/few-say-police-forces-nationally-do-well-in-treating-races-equally/.

———. "Psychology of Bad Times Fueling Consumer Cutbacks: Job Worries Mount, 73% Spending Less on Holidays." Pew Research Center for the People and the Press (press release). December 12, 2008. http://assets.pewresearch.org/wp-content/uploads/sites/5/legacy-pdf/475.pdf.

———. "Public Attitudes toward the War in Iraq: 2003–2008." *Pew Research Center* (blog), March 19, 2008. www.pewresearch.org/2008/03/19/public-attitudes-toward-the-war-in-iraq-20032008/.

Pezzullo, Phaedra C. *Toxic Tourism: Rhetorics of Pollution, Travel, and Environmental Justice*. Tuscaloosa: University of Alabama Press, 2007.

Phillips, Kyra. "DNA on Ice: The Next Step in Women's Equality." CNN, April 20, 2015. www.cnn.com/2015/04/20/opinions/phillips-egg-freezing/.

Pieklo, Jessica Mason. "Pregnant Wisconsin Woman Jailed under State's 'Personhood'-Like Law." Rewire, December 12, 2014. https://rewire.news/article/2014/12/12/pregnant-wisconsin-woman-jailed-states-personhood-like-law/.

Piepmeier, Alison. "The Inadequacy of 'Choice': Disability and What's Wrong with Feminist Framings of Reproduction." *Feminist Studies* 39, no. 1 (2013): 159–86.

Planned Parenthood Action Fund. "The Cost of Defunding Planned Parenthood." September 9, 2015. https://istandwithpp.org/facts/cost-defunding-planned-parenthood/.

Pollitt, Katha. "Protect Pregnant Women: Free Bei Bei Shuai." *Nation*, March 7, 2012. www.thenation.com/article/protect-pregnant-women-free-bei-bei-shuai/.

Practice Committee of the American Society for Reproductive Medicine, and Society for Assisted Reproductive Technology. "Mature Oocyte Cryopreservation: A Guideline." *Fertility and Sterility* 99, no. 1 (2013): 37–43.

Prescott, Heather Munro. *The Morning After: A History of Emergency Contraception in the*

United States. Critical Issues in Health and Medicine. New Brunswick, NJ: Rutgers University Press, 2011.

Prison Birth Project. "About." Prison Birth Project. Accessed July 19, 2016. http://theprisonbirthproject.org/about/.

Projansky, Sarah. "Mass Magazine Cover Girls: Some Reflections on Postfeminist Girls and Postfeminism's Daughters." In *Interrogating Postfeminism: Gender and the Politics of Popular Culture*, edited by Yvonne Tasker and Diane Negra, 40–72. Durham, NC: Duke University Press, 2007.

"A Public Health Victory." Opinion, *New York Times*, December 18, 2003, sec. A42.

Quraishi, Jen. "New Act Prohibits Minors Traveling for Abortions." *Mother Jones* (blog), June 22, 2011. https://www.motherjones.com/politics/2011/06/new-act-prohibits-minors-traveling-abortions/.

Rabin, Nina, and Roxana Bacon. "Women on the Run." *Ms.* 27, no. 2 (summer 2017): 18–23.

Rafie, Sally, Grace Kim, Lily Lau, Connie Tang, Colette Brown, and Nicole Maderas. "Assessment of Family Planning Services at Community Pharmacies in San Diego, California." *Pharmacy* 1, no. 2 (October 11, 2013): 153–59. https://doi.org/10.3390/pharmacy1020153.

Rankin, Kenrya. "Black Lives Matter Partners with Reproductive Justice Groups to Fight for Black Women." Text. Colorlines, February 9, 2016. https://www.colorlines.com/articles/black-lives-matter-partners-reproductive-justice-groups-fight-black-women.

Rao, Radhika. "How (Not) to Regulate ARTs: Lessons from Octomom." *Albany Law Journal of Science and Technology* 21, no. 2 (2011): 313–21.

Raymond, Elizabeth G., and David A. Grimes. "The Comparative Safety of Legal Induced Abortion and Childbirth in the United States:" *Obstetrics and Gynecology* 119, no. 2, part 1 (February 2012): 215–19. https://doi.org/10.1097/AOG.0b013e31823fe923.

Redfearn, Suz. "Preparing for a Mistake: For Emergency Birth Control, Plan Ahead." *Washington Post*, May 21, 2002, sec. Health.

Reeves, Joshua. "If You See Something, Say Something: Lateral Surveillance and the Uses of Responsibility." *Surveillance and Society* 10, nos. 3–4 (2012): 235–48.

Rein, Lisa, and Craig Timberg. "Emergency Birth Control Approved; Bill Calls for Access without Prescription." *Washington Post*, February 21, 2001, sec. A.

Reitman, Janet. "Abortion Rights at Risk: The GOP's War on Women Rages On." *Rolling Stone*, April 22, 2015. www.rollingstone.com/politics/news/abortion-rights-at-risk-the-gop-opens-a-new-front-in-the-war-on-women-20150422.

Reitman, Jason, dir. *Juno*. Fox Searchlight Pictures, 2007.

RESOLVE: The National Infertility Association. "Insurance Coverage in Your State." RESOLVE: The National Infertility Association, 2013.

Rettner, Rachael. "US Infertility Rates Drop Over Last 3 Decades." *Live Science*, August 14, 2013. https://www.livescience.com/38877-infertility-rates-drop-united-states.html.

Richards, Sarah Elizabeth. "Do You Know Where Your Eggs Are?" *Cosmopolitan*, June 2013.

———. "The Freedom of Freezing." *Marie Claire*, May 2013.

———. "Freezing Your Eggs—Is This What We're All Doing Now?" *Cosmopolitan*, June 13, 2013. www.cosmopolitan.com/lifestyle/advice/a4477/fertility-fears/.

———. *Motherhood, Rescheduled: The New Frontier of Egg Freezing and the Women Who Tried It*. New York: Simon and Schuster, 2013.

———. "Should You Freeze Your Eggs?" *Marie Claire*, May 2007.

———. "Why I Froze My Eggs (and You Should, Too)." *Wall Street Journal*, May 3, 2013.

Riggs, Damien W. "What Makes a Man? Thomas Beatie, Embodiment, and 'Mundane Transphobia.'" *Feminism and Psychology* 24, no. 2 (2014): 157–71.

Roberts, Dorothy. *Killing the Black Body: Race, Reproduction, and the Meaning of Liberty*. New York: Pantheon Books, 1997.

———. "Race, Gender, and Genetic Technologies: A New Reproductive Dystopia?" *Signs: Journal of Women in Culture and Society* 34, no. 4 (summer 2009): 783–804.

———. *Shattered Bonds: The Color of Child Welfare*. New York: Basic Civitas Books, 2003.

Robinson, Jessica. "Idaho Woman Arrested for Abortion Is Uneasy Case for Both Sides." NPR, April 9, 2012. www.npr.org/templates/story/story.php?storyId=150312812.

Rochman, Bonnie. "Octuplets Fallout: Should Fertility Doctors Set Limits?" *Time*, February 2, 2009.

Rodriguez, Maria I., Kathryn M. Curtis, Mary Lyn Gaffield, Emily Jackson, and Nathalie Kapp. "Advance Supply of Emergency Contraception: A Systematic Review." *Contraception* 87, no. 5 (May 2013): 590–601. https://doi.org/10.1016/j.contraception.2012.09.011.

Rogers, Adam. "Options beyond the Pill." *Newsweek*, Spring/Summer Special Edition 1999.

Romesburg, Don. "Where She Comes From: Locating Queer Transracial Adoption." *QED: A Journal in GLBTQ Worldmaking* 1, no. 3 (2014): 1–29.

Rose, Melody, and Mark O. Hatfield. "Republican Motherhood Redux?: Women as Contingent Citizens in 21st Century America." *Journal of Women, Politics, and Policy* 29, no. 1 (2008): 5–30.

Rose, Nikolas S. *The Politics of Life Itself: Biomedicine, Power, and Subjectivity in the Twenty-First Century*. Princeton, NJ: Princeton University Press, 2007.

Rose, Nikolas, and Peter Miller. *Governing the Present: Administering Economic, Social and Personal Life*. Cambridge, UK: Polity, 2008.

Rosen, Joanne D. "The Public Health Risks of Crisis Pregnancy Centers." *Perspectives on Sexual and Reproductive Health* 44, no. 3 (2012): 201–5.

Rosenblum, Emma. "Freeze Your Eggs, Free Your Career." *Bloomberg Business Week*, April 17, 2014.

Ross, Loretta J. "The Color of Choice: White Supremacy and Reproductive Justice." In *The Color of Violence: The Incite! Anthology*, edited by Incite! Women of Color Against Violence, 53–65. Cambridge, MA: South End, 2006.

———. "The Movement for Reproductive Justice: Six Years Old and Growing." *Collective Voices* 4, no. 10 (2009): 8–9.

———. "Understanding Reproductive Justice." Trust Black Women, March 2011. www.trustblackwomen.org/our-work/what-is-reproductive-justice/9-what-is-reproductive-justice.

Ross, Loretta J., and Rickie Solinger. *Reproductive Justice: An Introduction*. Oakland: University of California Press, 2017.

Rubin, Rita. "A Singular Approach to IVF." *USA Today*, March 4, 2009.

Salazar, Layldua. "Activist's Detainment Reminds Us Immigration Is a Reproductive Justice Issue." Rewire, March 12, 2108. https://rewire.news/article/2018/03/12/activists-detainment-reminds-us-immigration-reproductive-justice-issue/.

Salter, Mark B. "Conclusion: Risk and Imagination in the War on Terror." In *Risk and the War on Terror*, edited by Louise Amoore and Marieke de Goede, 233–46. New York: Routledge, 2008.

Samerski, Silja. "Genetic Counseling and the Fiction of Choice: Taught Self-Determination as a New Technique of Social Engineering." *Signs: Journal of Women in Culture and Society* 34, no. 4 (summer 2009): 735–61.

Sampson, Olivia, Sandy K. Navarro, Amna Khan, Norman Hearst, Tina R. Raine, Marji Gold, Suellen Miller, and Heike Thiel de Bocanegra. "Barriers to Adolescents' Getting Emergency Contraception through Pharmacy Access in California: Differences by Language and Region." *Perspectives on Sexual and Reproductive Health* 41, no. 2 (June 2009): 110–18. https://doi.org/10.1363/4111009.

Sandberg, Sheryl. *Lean In: Women, Work, and the Will to Lead*. New York: Knopf, 2013.

Sandler, Lauren, and Kate Witteman. "None Is Enough." *Time* 182, no. 7 (August 12, 2013): 38.

Saul, Stephanie. "Birth of Octuplets Puts Focus on Fertility Clinics." *New York Times*, February 11, 2009.

Schein, Margot, and NARAL Pro-Choice North Carolina. Letter to Natalie Fixmer-Oraiz. "The Truth about CPCs: Targeting Vulnerable Communities." July 18, 2017.

Schmidt, Mitchell. "Organization Marks 25 Years of Teen Parent Program." *Cedar Rapids Gazette*, September 20, 2015. www.thegazette.com/subject/news/business/organization-marks-45-years-of-teen-parent-program-20150920.

Schoen, Johanna. *Abortion after Roe*. Chapel Hill: University of North Carolina Press, 2015.

———. *Choice and Coercion: Birth Control, Sterilization, and Abortion in Public Health and Welfare*. Chapel Hill: University of North Carolina Press, 2005.

Schuster Institute for Investigative Journalism. "Adoption: Cambodia." February 22, 2011. www.brandeis.edu/investigate/gender/adoption/cambodia.html.

———. "The Baby Business: Policy Proposals for Fairer Practice." *Fraud and Corruption in International Adoptions*. Waltham, MA: Schuster Institute for Investigative Journalism, April 5, 2012.

Scott, J. Blake. *Risky Rhetoric: AIDS and the Cultural Practices of HIV Testing*. Carbondale: Southern Illinois University Press, 2003.

"Season Finale for MTV's 'Teen Mom' Scores Series High 3.6 Million Viewers." *TV by the Numbers* (blog), January 27, 2010. http://tvbythenumbers.zap2it.com/ratings/season-finale-for-mtvs-teen-mom-scores-series-high-3-6-million-viewers/.

Seery, John. "The Juno Effect." Blog, Huffington Post, January 22, 2008. www.huffingtonpost.com/john-seery/the-juno-effect_b_82582.html.

Sellers, Patricia. "Power: Do Women Really Want It?" *Fortune*, October 13, 2003. http://archive.fortune.com/magazines/fortune/fortune_archive/2003/10/13/350932/index.htm.

Sexuality Information and Education Council of the U.S. (SIECUS). "President's FY 2017 Budget Applauded by the Sexuality Information and Education Council of the U.S. (SIECUS)." February 9, 2016. www.siecus.org/index.cfm?fuseaction=Feature.showFeature&featureid=2437&pageid=611.

Shales, Tom. "*16 & Pregnant* Deftly Plumbs the Parent Trap." *Washington Post*, June 11, 2009.

Sheffield, Rob. "*Glee*'s Unstoppable Roll." *Rolling Stone*, November 25, 2010.

Shome, Raka. *Diana and Beyond: White Femininity, National Identity, and Contemporary Media Culture*. Urbana: University of Illinois Press, 2014.

Shorto, Russell. "Contra-Contraception." *New York Times Magazine*, May 7, 2006.

SIECUS: Sexuality Information and Education Council of the United States. "A History of Federal Funding for Abstinence-Only-Until-Marriage Programs." SIECUS: Sexuality Information and Education Council of the United States. Accessed April 13, 2016. www.siecus.org/index.cfm?fuseaction=page.viewpage&pageid=1340&nodeid=1.

Silliman, Jael, et al. *Undivided Rights: Women of Color Organize for Reproductive Justice*. Cambridge, MA: South End, 2004.

Sistas on the Rise. "Sistas on the Rise Herstory." Accessed October 20, 2011. http://sistasontherise.com/About%20Us.shtml.

Sivinski, Stephanie N. "Putting Too Many (Fertilized) Eggs in One Basket: Methods of Reducing Multifetal Pregnancies in the United States." *Texas Law Review* 88, no. 4 (March 2010): 897–916.

Slaughter, Anne-Marie. "Why Women Still Can't Have It All." *Atlantic*, August 2012. www.theatlantic.com/magazine/archive/2012/07/why-women-still-cant-have-it-all/309020/.

Sloop, John M. "Disciplining the Transgendered: Brandon Teena, Public Representation, and Normativity." *Western Journal of Communication* 64, no. 2 (2000): 165–89.

Smith, Andrea. *Conquest: Sexual Violence and American Indian Genocide*. Cambridge, MA: South End, 2005.

———. "Not-Seeing: State Surveillance, Settler Colonialism, and Gender Violence." In *Feminist Surveillance Studies*, edited by Rachel E. Dubrofsky and Shoshana Amielle Magnet, 21–38. Durham, NC: Duke University Press, 2015.

Smith, Hortense. "Abstinence, the 'Sexy' Way." *Jezebel*, August 9, 2009. http://jezebel.com/5333434/abstinence-the-sexy-way.

SmithBattle, L. "'I Wanna Have a Good Future': Teen Mothers' Rise in Educational

Aspirations, Competing Demands, and Limited School Support." *Youth and Society* 38, no. 3 (March 1, 2007): 348–71. https://doi.org/10.1177/0044118X06287962.
Smolin, David M. "Child Laundering: How the Intercountry Adoption System Legitimizes and Incentivizes the Practices of Buying, Trafficking, Kidnapping, and Stealing Children." *Wayne Law Review* 52, no. 1 (2006): 113–200.
Smolowe, Jill, Johnny Dodd, Howard Breuer, and Lorenzo Benet. "A Mom's Controversial Choice." *People*, February 16, 2009.
Smolowe, Jill, Johnny Dodd, Howard Breuer, and Lorenzo Benet. "The Challenge of Her Life." *People*, February 23, 2009.
Solinger, Rickie. *Beggars and Choosers: How the Politics of Choice Shapes Adoption, Abortion, and Welfare in the United States*. New York: Hill and Wang, 2001.
———. *Pregnancy and Power: A Short History of Reproductive Politics in America*. New York: New York University Press, 2005.
Solomon, Akiba. "9 Reasons to Hate Anti-Abortion Billboards That Target Black Women." Text. Colorlines, February 25, 2011. www.colorlines.com/articles/9-reasons-hate-anti-abortion-billboards-target-black-women.
———. "The Missionary Movement to 'Save' Black Babies." Colorlines, May 2, 2013. www.colorlines.com/articles/missionary-movement-save-black-babies.
SPARK Reproductive Justice Now. "Guiding Principles and Central Voices." Accessed October 28, 2011. http://sparkrj.org/content/about/guidingprinciplesandcentralvoices.
Spector-Bagdady, Kayte K. "Artificial Parentage: Screening Parents for Assisted Reproductive Technologies." *Michigan State University Journal of Medicine and Law* 14 (2010): 457–76.
Spigel, Lynn. *Welcome to the Dreamhouse: Popular Media and Postwar Suburbs*. Durham, NC: Duke University Press, 2001.
Spivak, Gayatri. *The Spivak Reader: Selected Works of Gayatri Spivak*. Edited by Donna Landry and MacLean. New York: Routledge, 1996.
Squier, Susan Merrill. *Liminal Lives: Imagining the Human at the Frontiers of Biomedicine*. Durham, NC: Duke University Press, 2004.
Stabile, Carol A. "'Sweetheart, This Ain't Gender Studies': Sexism and Superheroes." *Communication and Critical/Cultural Studies* 6, no. 1 (2009): 86–92.
Stabile, Carol A., and Carrie Rentschler. "States of Insecurity and the Gendered Politics of Fear." *NWSA Journal* 17, no. 3 (2005): vii–xxv.
Stacey, Michelle. "How to Keep Your Body Baby-Ready." *Cosmopolitan*, January 2009.
Stahl, Lesley. "Staying at Home." *60 Minutes*, October 10, 2004.
Stateman, Alison. "The Octuplets' Mom Speaks, and the Questions Grow." *Time*, February 7, 2009.
Steiner, Anne Z., and Anne Marie Z. Jukic. "Impact of Female Age and Nulligravidity on Fecundity in an Older Reproductive Age Cohort." *Fertility and Sterility* 105, no. 6 (June 2016): 1584–1588.e1. https://doi.org/10.1016/j.fertnstert.2016.02.028.
Steiner, Linda, and Carolyn Bronstein. "When Tiger Mothers Transgress: Amy Chua,

Dara-Lynn Weiss and the Cultural Imperative of Intensive Mothering." In Hundley and Hayden, *Mediated Moms*, 247–74.
Stepp, Laura Sessions. "With Birth Control, Plan B Is Topic A." *Washington Post*, February 10, 2004, sec. Style C01.
Stewart, Susan. "Big Brood Spawns Big Ratings." *New York Times*, February 15, 2009.
Stone, Pamela. *Opting Out? Why Women Really Quit Careers and Head Home*. Berkeley: University of California Press, 2008.
Stone, Pamela, and Lisa Ackerly Hernandez. "The Rhetoric and Reality of 'Opting Out.'" In *Women Who Opt Out: The Debate over Working Mothers and Work-Family Balance*, edited by Bernie D. Jones, 33–56. New York: New York University Press, 2012.
Stoop, D., E. Maes, N. P. Polyzos, G. Verheyen, H. Tournaye, and J. Nekkebroeck. "Does Oocyte Banking for Anticipated Gamete Exhaustion Influence Future Relational and Reproductive Choices? A Follow-Up of Bankers and Non-Bankers." *Human Reproduction* (Oxford, UK) 30, no. 2 (February 2015): 338–44. https://doi.org/10.1093/humrep/deu317.
Stopczynski, Kelli. "Lawyer Wants Woman's Feticide Charge Dropped, Some Evidence Excluded." WSBT, November 20, 2014. wsbt.com/news/local/lawyer-wants-womans-feticide-charge-dropped-some-evidence-excluded.
Stormer, Nathan. "Embodying Normal Miracles." *Quarterly Journal of Speech* 83, no. 2 (5): 172.
Story, Louise. "Many Women at Elite Colleges Set Career Path to Motherhood." *New York Times*, September 20, 2005.
Suddath, Claire. "Labor Crisis: Maternity Leave Isn't Working for Working Women." *Bloomberg Businessweek*, January 19, 2015.
Suleman, Nadya. "A Conversation with Nadya Suleman." Interview by Oprah Winfrey. *Oprah Show*, April 20, 2010.
———. "Her Side of the Story." Interview by Ann Curry, *Dateline News*, NBC, February 10, 2009.
———. "Octuplets' Mom Talks with Dr. Phil." Interview by Phil McGraw, *Dr. Phil*, February 25, 2009.
Surdin, Ashley. "Octuplet Mother Also Gives Birth to Ethical Debate." *Washington Post*, February 4, 2009.
Szabo, Liz, and Laura Ungar. "Family Planning Budgets in Crisis before Planned Parenthood Controversy." *USA Today*, July 31, 2015. www.usatoday.com/story/news/2015/07/30/family-planning-budgets-crisis-before-planned-parenthood-controversy/30861853/.
Tapia, Ruby C. "Impregnating Images: Visions of Race, Sex, and Citizenship in California's Teen Pregnancy Prevention Campaigns." *Feminist Media Studies* 5, no. 1 (2005): 7–22.
Tasker, Yvonne, and Diane Negra. *Interrogating Postfeminism: Gender and the Politics of Popular Culture*. Durham, NC: Duke University Press, 2007.
Taylor, Bruce, Geoffrey Alpert, Bruce Kubu, Daniel Woods, and Roger G. Dunham.

"Changes in Officer Use of Force over Time: A Descriptive Analysis of a National Survey." *Policing: An International Journal of Police Strategies and Management* 34, no. 2 (May 31, 2011): 211–32. https://doi.org/10.1108/13639511111131058.

Thoma, Pamela. "Buying Up Baby: Modern Feminine Subjectivity, Assertions of 'Choice,' and the Repudiation of Reproductive Justice in Postfeminist Unwanted Pregnancy Films." *Feminist Media Studies* 9, no. 4 (2009): 409–25.

Thomas, Christopher Scott. "The Mothers of East Los Angeles: (Other)Mothering for Environmental Justice." *Southern Communication Journal* (2018): 1–17.

Thomson, Katherine. "Does Nadya Suleman Think She's Angelina Jolie?" *HuffPost Entertainment*, February 10, 2009.

Thornton, Davi Johnson. "Race, Risk, and Pathology in Psychiatric Culture: Disease Awareness Campaigns as Governmental Rhetoric." *Critical Studies in Media Communication* 27, no. 4 (2010): 311–35.

Tinneberg, Hans-Rudolf, and Antonio Gasbarrini. "Infertility Today: The Management of Female Medical Causes." *International Journal of Gynaecology and Obstetrics: The Official Organ of the International Federation of Gynaecology and Obstetrics* 123, suppl. 2 (December 2013): S25–30. https://doi.org/10.1016/j.ijgo.2013.09.004.

Tischler, Linda. "Where Are the Women?" *Fast Company*, no. 79 (February 2004): 52–60.

Tonn, Mari Boor. "Militant Motherhood: Labor's Mary Harris 'Mother' Jones." *Quarterly Journal of Speech* 82 (1996): 1–21.

Trafford, Abigail. "Second Opinion." *Washington Post*, May 15, 2001.

Trenka, Jane Jeong, Sun Yung Shin, Julia Chinyere Oparah, Jae Ran Kim, and Shannon Gibney. "Transnational and Transracial Adoption: The Right of Poor Women of Color to Keep and Raise Their Children." In *Reproductive Justice Briefing Book: A Primer on Reproductive Justice and Social Change*, edited by SisterSong Women of Color Reproductive Health Collective, 56. N.p.: N.p., 2007.

Trudeau, Jennifer. "The Role of New Media on Teen Sexual Behaviors and Fertility Outcomes—the Case of *16 and Pregnant*." *Southern Economic Journal*, March 17, 2015. https://doi.org/10.1002/soej.12034.

Trust Black Women Partnership. "Our Story." Trust Black Women. Accessed July 19, 2017. www.trustblackwomen.org/about-trust-black-women/our-story.

Twenge, Jean. "How Long Can You Wait to Have a Baby?" *Atlantic*, August 2013. www.theatlantic.com/magazine/archive/2013/07/how-long-can-you-wait-to-have-a-baby/309374/.

Tyagi, Amelia Warren. "Why Women Have to Work." *Time* 163, no. 12 (March 22, 2004): 56.

Tyre, Peg. "Daddy's Home, and a Bit Lost." *New York Times*, January 11, 2009.

Unborn Child Protection Act, Wis. Stat. (1997).

United Health Foundation. "America's Health Rankings: Maternal Mortality." America's Health Rankings, 2018. https://www.americashealthrankings.org/explore/2018-health-of-women-and-children-report/measure/maternal_mortality/state/ALL.

United Nations. "Senior UN Officials Spotlight Women's Health Rights to Accelerate Global Development." *UN News Centre*, May 30, 2013.

U.S. Centers for Disease Control and Prevention. "More than 3 Million US Women at Risk for Alcohol-Exposed Pregnancy." CDC Newsroom, February 2, 2016. www.cdc.gov/media/releases/2016/p0202-alcohol-exposed-pregnancy.html.

———. "Pregnancy Mortality Surveillance System." Centers for Disease Control and Prevention, November 9, 2017. https://www.cdc.gov/reproductivehealth/maternalinfanthealth/pmss.html.

U.S. Department of Health and Human Services. "Voluntary Relinquishment for Adoption." Washington, DC, 2005.

U.S. Department of Justice, Civil Rights Division. "Investigation of the Albuquerque Police Department." April 10, 2014. https://www.justice.gov/sites/default/files/crt/legacy/2014/04/10/apd_findings_4-10-14.pdf.

———. "Investigation of the Ferguson Police Department." March 4, 2015. http://apps.washingtonpost.com/g/documents/national/department-of-justice-report-on-the-ferguson-mo-police-department/1435/.

U.S. Department of State. "Intercountry Adoption: FY 2016 Annual Report on Intercountry Adoption." Washington, DC: Bureau of Consular Affairs, 2017.

U.S. Food and Drug Administration. "Postmarket Drug Safety Information for Patients and Providers—Plan B: Questions and Answers—August 24, 2006; Updated December 14, 2006." WebContent, August 24, 2006. https://www.fda.gov/Drugs/DrugSafety/PostmarketDrugSafetyInformationforPatientsandProviders/ucm109783.htm.

Valenti, Jessica. *The Purity Myth: How America's Obsession with Virginity Is Hurting Young Women*. Berkeley, CA: Seal, 2009.

———. *Why Have Kids?: A New Mom Explores the Truth about Parenting and Happiness*. Boston: New Harvest, 2012.

———. "Why No Abortions on MTV's '16 and Pregnant'?" February 10, 2010. Accessed July 24, 2015.

Vasquez, Emily, and Kate Hammer. "Easier Access to Plan B Pill Evokes Praise, and Concern." *New York Times*, August 2006.

Vasquez, Tina. "'Anti-Choice Fanaticism' in the U.S. Immigration System: The Real Reason Jane Doe's Abortion Request Is Being Denied." Rewire, October 16, 2017. https://rewire.news/article/2017/10/16/anti-choice-fanaticism-u-s-immigration-system-real-reason-jane-abortion-request-denied/.

———. "Immigrant Minor Held 'Hostage' in Texas Because She Wants Abortion Care." Rewire, October 11, 2017. https://rewire.news/article/2017/10/11/immigrant-minor-held-hostage-texas-wants-abortion-care/.

———. "Teenage Immigrant Forced by Government to Remain Pregnant." Rewire, October 20, 2017. https://rewire.news/article/2017/10/20/teenage-immigrant-forced-remain-pregnant/.

Vavrus, Mary Douglas. "Opting Out Moms in the News: Selling New Traditionalism in the New Millennium." *Feminist Media Studies* 7, no. 1 (2007): 47–63.

Velez-Mitchell, Jane. "Issues with Jane Velez-Mitchell." HLN, November 24, 2009.

Ventura, Stephanie J., Brady E. Hamilton, and T. J. Mathews. "National and State Patterns of Teen Births in the United States, 1940–2013." *National Vital Statistics Reports* 63, no. 4 (2014): 1–34.

Wade, Lisa. "Sexing Up Abstinence—Sociological Images." August 8, 2009. http://thesocietypages.org/socimages/2009/08/08/sexing-up-abstinence/.

Waggoner, Miranda R. "Motherhood Preconceived: The Emergence of the Preconception Health and Health Care Initiative." *Journal of Health Politics, Policy and Law* 38, no. 2 (January 1, 2013): 345–71. https://doi.org/10.1215/03616878-1966333.

———. *The Zero Trimester: Pre-Pregnancy Care and the Politics of Reproductive Risk.* Oakland: University of California Press, 2017.

Wahlberg, David. "Judge Who Blocked 'Cocaine Mom' Law Partially Lifts Ruling as State Appeals." *Wisconsin State Journal*, May 5, 2017. http://host.madison.com/news/local/health-med-fit/judge-who-blocked-cocaine-mom-law-partially-lifts-ruling-as/article_68f095a9-ebff-5222-98f4-a90f42f4b420.html.

Wallis, Claudia. "The Case for Staying Home." *Time* 163, no. 12 (March 22, 2004): 50–59.

Wang, Wendy, Kim Parker, and Paul Taylor. "Breadwinner Moms." *Pew Research Center's Social and Demographic Trends Project* (blog), May 29, 2013. www.pewsocialtrends.org/2013/05/29/breadwinner-moms/.

Warner, Judith. *Perfect Madness: Motherhood in the Age of Anxiety*. New York: Riverhead Books, 2005.

———. "The Opt-Out Generation Wants Back In." *New York Times Magazine*, August 7, 2013.

Waxman, Henry. "False and Misleading Health Information Provided by Federally Funded Pregnancy Resource Centers." Washington, DC: U.S. House of Representatives Committee on Government Reform—Minority Staff Special Investigations Division, 2006.

———. "The Content of Federally Funded Abstinence-Only Education Programs." Washington, DC: U.S. House of Representatives Committee on Government Reform—Minority Staff Special Investigations Division, 2004.

Welter, Barbara. "The Cult of True Womanhood: 1820–1860." *American Quarterly* 18, no. 2 (1966): 151–74.

West, Isaac. "Performing Resistance in/from the Kitchen: The Practice of Maternal Pacifist Politics and la WISP's Cookbooks." *Women's Studies in Communication* 30, no. 3 (fall 2007): 358–383.

———. *Transforming Citizenships: Transgender Articulations of the Law*. New York: New York University Press, 2014.

"What He Thinks about Your, Um, Eggs." *Glamour*, January 2014.

Wheaton, Sarah, and Ben Schreckinger. "Police Union Accuses White House of Politicizing Cop Safety." Politico, May 18, 2015. www.politico.com/story/2015/05/white-house-limiting-military-equipment-for-police-118041.

White House, Office of the Press Secretary. "Fact Sheet: The White House Summit on Working Families." WhiteHouse.gov, June 23, 2014. https://obamawhitehouse.archives.gov/the-press-office/2014/06/23/fact-sheet-white-house-summit-working-families.

Wihbey, John, and Leighton Walter Kille. "Excessive or Reasonable Force by Police? Research on Law Enforcement and Racial Conflict." *Journalist's Resource* (blog), July 28, 2016. https://journalistsresource.org/studies/government/criminal-justice/police-reasonable-force-brutality-race-research-review-statistics.

Wilkinson, Tracey A., Nisha Fahey, Christine Shields, Emily Suther, Howard J. Cabral, and Michael Silverstein. "Pharmacy Communication to Adolescents and Their Physicians Regarding Access to Emergency Contraception." *Pediatrics* 129, no. 4 (April 1, 2012): 624–29. https://doi.org/10.1542/peds.2011-3760.

Wilkinson, Tracey A., Nisha Fahey, Emily Suther, Howard J. Cabral, and Michael Silverstein. "Access to Emergency Contraception for Adolescents." *JAMA* 307, no. 4 (January 25, 2012). https://doi.org/10.1001/jama.2011.1949.

Wilkinson, Tracey A., Sally Rafie, Porsche D. Clark, Aaron E. Carroll, and Elizabeth Miller. "Evaluating Community Pharmacy Responses about Levonorgestrel Emergency Contraception by Mystery Caller Characteristics." *Journal of Adolescent Health*, February 2018. https://doi.org/10.1016/j.jadohealth.2017.11.303.

Wilkinson, Tracey A., Gabriela Vargas, Nisha Fahey, Emily Suther, and Michael Silverstein. "'I'll See What I Can Do': What Adolescents Experience When Requesting Emergency Contraception." *Journal of Adolescent Health* 54, no. 1 (January 2014): 14–19. https://doi.org/10.1016/j.jadohealth.2013.10.002.

Williams, Joan. "The Opt-Out Revolution Revisited." *American Prospect*, February 19, 2007.

Williams, Raymond. *The Long Revolution*. London: Chatto and Windus, 1961.

Wilson, Jacque. "Study: '16 and Pregnant,' 'Teen Mom' Led to Fewer Teen Births." CNN, January 13, 2014. www.cnn.com/2014/01/13/health/16-pregnant-teens-childbirth/index.html.

Wilson, Julie A., and Emily Chivers Yochim. *Mothering through Precarity: Women's Work and Digital Media*. Durham, NC: Duke University Press, 2017.

Wilson, Teddy. "Mississippi Woman Criminally Charged for Pregnancy Outcome After Home Birth." Rewire, February 6, 2018. https://rewire.news/article/2018/02/06/mississippi-woman-criminally-charged-pregnancy-outcome-home-birth.

Winter, Meaghan. "'Save the Mother, Save the Baby': An Inside Look at a Pregnancy Center Conference." *Cosmopolitan*, April 6, 2015. www.cosmopolitan.com/politics/a38642/heartbeat-international-conference-crisis-pregnancy-centers-abortion/.

Wolf, Joan. *Is Breast Best? Taking on the Breastfeeding Experts and the New High Stakes of Motherhood*. New York: New York University Press, 2011.

Wood, Susan F. "Inappropriate Obstructions to Access: The FDA's Handling of Plan B." *American Medical Association Journal of Ethics* 16, no. 4 (April 2014): 295–301.

Wright, Paul J., Ashley K. Randall, and Analisa Arroyo. "Father–Daughter Communication about Sex Moderates the Association between Exposure to MTV's *16 and Pregnant/Teen Mom* and Female Students' Pregnancy-Risk Behavior." *Sexuality and Culture* 17, no. 1 (March 2013): 50–66. https://doi.org/10.1007/s12119-012-9137-2.

Wynn, Lisa L. "United States: Activism, Sexual Archetypes, and the Politicization of Science." In *Emergency Contraception: The Story of a Global Reproductive Health Technology*, edited by Angelina Marguerite Foster and Lisa L. Wynn, 39–55. New York: Palgrave Macmillan, 2012.

Yandoli, Krystie Lee. "Why 'Obvious Child' Is the Abortion Movie We All Need." Bustle, December 26, 3013. www.bustle.com/articles/11370-why-obvious-child-is-the-abortion-movie-we-all-need.

Yao, David F., and Jesse N. Mills. "Male Infertility: Lifestyle Factors and Holistic, Complementary, and Alternative Therapies." *Asian Journal of Andrology* 18, no. 3 (June 2016): 410–18. https://doi.org/10.4103/1008-682X.175779.

Young Women United. "Why We Do YWU: Young Women United's Vision of Purpose." Accessed October 20, 2011. www.youngwomenunited.org/whoweare/whywedoywu.html (dead).

Zernike, Kate. "Use of Morning-After Pill Rising and It May Go over the Counter." *New York Times*, May 19, 2003, sec. A1.

Zimmerman, Toni Schindler, Jennifer T. Aberle, Jennifer L. Krafchick, and Ashley M. Harvey. "Deconstructing the 'Mommy Wars': The Battle over the Best Mom." *Journal of Feminist Family Therapy* 20, no. 3 (2008): 203–19.

Index

NATALIE FIXMER-ORAIZ is an assistant professor of communication studies and gender, women's, and sexuality studies at the University of Iowa.

FEMINIST MEDIA STUDIES

Queer Migration Politics: Activist Rhetoric and Coalitional Possibilities Karma R. Chávez
Sexting Panic: Rethinking Criminalization, Privacy, and Consent Amy Adele Hasinoff
Cupcakes, Pinterest, and Ladyporn: Feminized Popular Culture in the Early Twenty-First Century Edited by Elana Levine
Gendered Asylum: Race and Violence in U.S. Law and Politics Sara L. McKinnon
Football and Manliness: An Unauthorized Feminist Account of the NFL Thomas P. Oates
Alice in Pornoland: Hardcore Encounters with the Victorian Gothic Laura Helen Marks
Homeland Maternity: US Security Culture and the New Reproductive Regime Natalie Fixmer-Oraiz